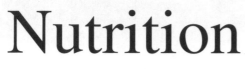

A·N·N·U·A·L E·D·I·T·I·O·N·S

Nutrition

Seventeenth Edition

05/06

D0792438

EDITOR

Dorothy Klimis-Zacas

University of Maine-Orono

Dorothy Klimis-Zacas is a Professor of Clinical Nutrition at the University of Maine and cooperating professor of nutrition and dietetics at Harokopio University, Athens, Greece. She teaches undergraduate and graduate classes in nutrition and its relation to health and disease for students of dietetics, nurses, and physicians.

Her current research interests relate to basic investigations in the area of trace mineral nutrition and its role in the development of atherosclerosis and to applied investigations that utilize nutritional interventions to reduce cardiovascular disease risk in adolescents both in the United States and in the Mediterranean region.

A Ph.D. and Fullbright Fellow, Dr. Klimis-Zacas is the author of numerous research articles and the editor of two books, *Manganese in Health and Disease* and the recently published second edition of *Nutritional Concerns for Women*. She is a member of Sigma Delta Epsilon, The American Society of Nutritional Sciences, The International Atherosclerosis Society, the American Dietetic Association, The Society for Nutrition Education, and The American Heart Association.

McGraw-Hill/Dushkin

2460 Kerper Blvd., Dubuque, Iowa 52001

Visit us on the Internet
http://www.dushkin.com

Credits

1. **Nutrition Trends**
   Unit photo—© Getty Images/PhotoLink/C. Sherburne.
2. **Nutrients**
   Unit photo—© PhotoDisc, Inc.
3. **Diet and Disease: Through the Life Span**
   Unit photo—© Getty Images/PhotoLink/S. Pearce.
4. **Obesity and Weight Control**
   Unit photo—© PhotoDisc, Inc.
5. **Health Claims**
   Unit photo—© The McGraw-Hill Companies, Inc./Jill Braaten.
6. **Food Safety/Technology**
   Unit photo—© CORBIS/Royalty Free.
7. **World Hunger and Malnutrition**
   Unit photo—Photograph courtesy of USAID.

Copyright

Cataloging in Publication Data
Main entry under title: Annual Editions: Nutrition. 2005/2006.
1. Nutrition—Periodicals. I. Klimis-Zacas, Dorothy, *comp.* II. Title: Nutrition.
ISBN 0–07–311220–8   658'.05   ISSN 1055–6990

Seventeenth Edition

Cover image © Photos.com/C. Sherburne/PhotoLink/Getty Images
Printed in the United States of America   1234567890QPDQPD98765   Printed on Recycled Paper

Preface

In publishing ANNUAL EDITIONS we recognize the enormous role played by the magazines, newspapers, and journals of the public press in providing current, first-rate educational information in a broad spectrum of interest areas. Many of these articles are appropriate for students, researchers, and professionals seeking accurate, current material to help bridge the gap between principles and theories and the real world. These articles, however, become more useful for study when those of lasting value are carefully collected, organized, indexed, and reproduced in a low-cost format, which provides easy and permanent access when the material is needed. That is the role played by ANNUAL EDITIONS.

Since nutrition is an evolving science, it necessitates updating *Annual Editions: Nutrition* annually to keep up with the plethora of topics and controversies raised in the field. The main goal of this anthology is to provide the reader with up-to-date information by presenting current topics of information based on scientific evidence. *Annual Editions: Nutrition* also presents controversial topics in a balanced and unbiased manner. Where appropriate, international perspectives are presented. We hope that the reader will develop critical thinking and be empowered to ask questions and to seek answers.

We are presently experiencing an obesity and diabetes epidemic with detrimental effects on the health of not only adults but also of children and teens. Globalization and the role a few mega food companies play in providing consumers with products loaded with fat and sugars along with the increased caloric intake from large portion sizes and a reduction of activity have all contributed to the onset of these degenerative diseases. Also, lately obesity has been observed in third world countries where it coexists with hunger and malnutrition. Actually, the World Health Organization in its recent report on "Diet, Nutrition and the prevention of Chronic Diseases" questions the role and contribution of global companies in the increasing incidence of obesity in developing countries.

The decoding of the genome has heralded the area of Nutrigenomics, which has enabled us to appreciate the interactions between genotype and nutrition and the effect of nutrients on gene expression. Thus the era of custom-made diets rather than "one diet fits all" was ushered to the forefront. This revolution will affect the way we diagnose and treat disease, design dietary interventions to reduce risk, and set nutrient requirements among many others.

"Nutrition experts" and "health advisors" seem to appear everywhere. We are at the parapet of a revolution in information technology and of nutritional research. Information is distributed at a very fast pace, across continents, and without consideration of country borders. Thus, informing the consumer regularly with reliable and current nutrition information is the duty of the professional.

Annual Editions: Nutrition 05/06 is to be used as a companion to a standard nutrition text so that it may update, expand, or emphasize certain topics that are covered in the text or present a totally new topic not covered in a standard text.

To accomplish this, *Annual Editions: Nutrition 05/06* is composed of seven units that review current knowledge and controversies in the area of nutrition. The first unit describes current trends in the field of nutrition in the United States and the rest of the world, including the new dietary guidelines for the United States and the "New Food Guide Pyramid"—an alternative to the U.S.D.A.'s Food Guide Pyramid. Units two, three, and four include topics that focus on nutrients and their relationship to health and disease, recent research finding on the role nutrients play in degenerative disease, and the worldwide obesity epidemic. Units five and six cover topics on health claims and focus on food safety, including subjects about which consumers are misinformed and are thus vulnerable to quackery. Finally, unit seven focuses on world hunger and malnutrition, including environmental sustainability and biotechnology. A *topic guide* will assist the reader in finding other articles on a given subject and the *World Wide Web* sites will help in further exploring a particular topic.

Your input is most valuable to improving this anthology, which we update yearly. We would appreciate your comments and suggestions as you review the current edition.

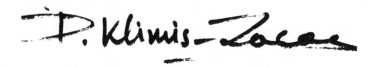

Dorothy Klimis-Zacas
Editor

Contents

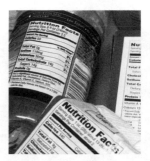

UNIT 1
Nutrition Trends

The concepts in bold italics are developed in the article. For further expansion, please refer to the Topic Guide and the Index.

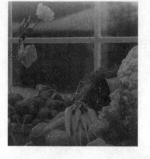

UNIT 2
Nutrients

The concepts in bold italics are developed in the article. For further expansion, please refer to the Topic Guide and the Index.

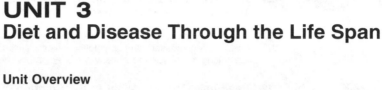

UNIT 3
Diet and Disease Through the Life Span

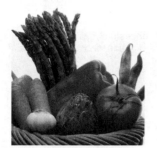

The concepts in bold italics are developed in the article. For further expansion, please refer to the Topic Guide and the Index.

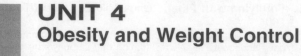

UNIT 4
Obesity and Weight Control

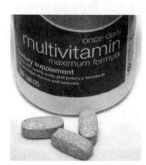

UNIT 5
Health Claims

The concepts in bold italics are developed in the article. For further expansion, please refer to the Topic Guide and the Index.

UNIT 6
Food Safety/Technology

The concepts in bold italics are developed in the article. For further expansion, please refer to the Topic Guide and the Index.

UNIT 7
World Hunger and Malnutrition

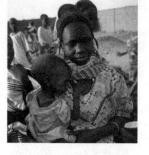

The concepts in bold italics are developed in the article. For further expansion, please refer to the Topic Guide and the Index.

The concepts in bold italics are developed in the article. For further expansion, please refer to the Topic Guide and the Index.

Topic Guide

This topic guide suggests how the selections in this book relate to the subjects covered in your course. You may want to use the topics listed on these pages to search the Web more easily.

On the following pages a number of Web sites have been gathered specifically for this book. They are arranged to reflect the units of this *Annual Edition.* You can link to these sites by going to the DUSHKIN ONLINE support site at *http://www.dushkin.com/online/.*

ALL THE ARTICLES THAT RELATE TO EACH TOPIC ARE LISTED BELOW THE BOLD-FACED TERM.

Adolescents

1. The Changing American Diet: A Report Card

Age related eye disorders

13. Eye Wise: Seeing Into the Future
14. Feast For Your Eyes: Nutrients That May Help Save Your Sight

Attitudes and knowledge

1. The Changing American Diet: A Report Card
3. Rebuilding the Food Pyramid
5. Getting Personal with Nutrition
6. Food, Spirituality, Mindful Eating
7. Who's Filling Your Grocery Bag?
8. Moving Towards Healthful Sustainable Diets
32. Are Your Supplements Safe?

Biotechnology

15. Fortifying with Fiber
46. Assessment of Allergenic Potential of Genetically Modified Foods: An Agenda for Future Research

Cancer

17. Prostate Cancer: More Questions than Answers

Carbohydrates

3. Rebuilding the Food Pyramid
4. The Low-Carb Frenzy: The Force That is Reshaping the Food Industry and Our Bodies
11. Going Beyond Atkins
12. Good Carbs, Bad Carbs

Children

19. Meeting Children's Nutritional Needs
23. A Call to Action: Seeking Answers to Childhood Weight Issues

Controversies

4. The Low-Carb Frenzy: The Force That is Reshaping the Food Industry and Our Bodies
11. Going Beyond Atkins
27. Herbal Lottery
29. How Low Can You Go?: Cutting Calories to Extend Life?

Coronary heart disease

9. Omega-3 Choices: Fish or Flax?
18. Coffee, Spices, Wine: New Dietary Ammo Against Diabetes?
28. The Latest Scoop on Soy
30. Multiple Choices: The Right Vitamins For You

Diabetes

11. Going Beyond Atkins
12. Good Carbs, Bad Carbs
18. Coffee, Spices, Wine: New Dietary Ammo Against Diabetes?
30. Multiple Choices: The Right Vitamins For You

Diet

14. Feast For Your Eyes: Nutrients That May Help Save Your Sight
28. The Latest Scoop on Soy

Diet and disease

12. Good Carbs, Bad Carbs
13. Eye Wise: Seeing Into the Future
16. Diet and Genes
17. Prostate Cancer: More Questions than Answers
18. Coffee, Spices, Wine: New Dietary Ammo Against Diabetes?
19. Meeting Children's Nutritional Needs
21. How We Grew So Big

Diet and genes

5. Getting Personal with Nutrition
16. Diet and Genes

Disease

14. Feast For Your Eyes: Nutrients That May Help Save Your Sight
28. The Latest Scoop on Soy

Fats and substitutes

9. Omega-3 Choices: Fish or Flax?
10. Revealing Trans Fats
36. Hooked on Fish? There Might Be Some Catches

Fiber

15. Fortifying with Fiber

Food

1. The Changing American Diet: A Report Card
6. Food, Spirituality, Mindful Eating
15. Fortifying with Fiber
31. Food-Friendly Bugs Do The Body Good
32. Are Your Supplements Safe?
33. Tainted Food
34. Certified Organic
35. Send in the Clones
36. Hooked on Fish? There Might Be Some Catches

Food allergies

46. Assessment of Allergenic Potential of Genetically Modified Foods: An Agenda for Future Research

Food labeling

35. Send in the Clones

Food safety and technology

33. Tainted Food
34. Certified Organic
35. Send in the Clones
36. Hooked on Fish? There Might Be Some Catches
37. Ensuring the Safety of Dietary Supplements

Food supply

38. Hunger and Mortality
39. The Scourge of "Hidden Hunger": Global Dimensions of Micronutrient Deficiencies
40. Undernurishment, Poverty and Development
42. Food Security, Overweight, and Agricultural Research—A View From 2003

World Wide Web Sites

The following World Wide Web sites have been carefully researched and selected to support the articles found in this reader. The easiest way to access these selected sites is to go to our DUSHKIN ONLINE support site at *http://www.dushkin.com/online/*.

AE: Nutrition 05/06

The following sites were available at the time of publication. Visit our Web site—we update DUSHKIN ONLINE regularly to reflect any changes.

General Sources

American Dietetic Association
http://www.eatright.org

This consumer link to nutrition and health includes resources, news, marketplace, search for a dietician, government information, and a gateway to related sites. The site includes a tip of the day and special features.

The Blonz Guide to Nutrition
http://www.blonz.com

The categories in this valuable site report news in the fields of nutrition, food science, foods, fitness, and health. There is also a selection of search engines and links.

CSPI: Center for Science in the Public Interest
http://www.cspinet.org

CSPI is a nonprofit education and advocacy organization that is committed to improving the safety and nutritional quality of our food supply. CSPI publishes the *Nutrition Action Healthletter,* which has monthly information about food.

Institute of Food Technologists
http://www.ift.org

This site of the Society for Food Science and Technology is full of important information and news about every aspect of the food products that come to market.

International Food Information Council Foundation (IFIC)
http://ific.org

IFIC's purpose is to be the link between science and communications by offering the latest scientific information on food safety, nutrition, and health in a form that is understandable and useful for opinion leaders and consumers to access.

U.S. National Institutes of Health (NIH)
http://www.nih.gov

Consult this site for links to extensive health information and scientific resources. Comprised of 24 separate institutes, centers, and divisions, the NIH is one of eight health agencies of the Public Health Service, which, in turn, is part of the U.S. Department of Health and Human Services.

UNIT 1: Nutrition Trends

Food Science and Human Nutrition Extension
http://www.fshn.uiuc.edu/

This extensive Iowa State University site links to latest news and reports, consumer publications, food safety information, and many other useful nutrition-related sites.

Food Surveys Research Group
http://www.barc.usda.gov/bhnrc/foodsurvey/home.htm

Visit this site of the Beltsville Human Nutrition Research Center Food Surveys research group first, and then click on USDA to keep up with nutritional news and information.

UNIT 2: Nutrients

Dole 5 A Day: Nutrition, Fruits & Vegetables
http://www.dole5aday.com

The Dole Food Company, a founding member of the "National 5 A Day for Better Health Program," offers this site to entice children into taking an interest in proper nutrition.

Food and Nutrition Information Center
http://www.nal.usda.gov/fnic/

Use this site to find dietary and nutrition information provided by various USDA agencies and to find links to food and nutrition resources on the Internet.

Nutrient Data Laboratory
http://www.nal.usda.gov/fnic/foodcomp/

Information about the USDA Nutrient Database can be found on this site. Search here for answers to FAQs, a glossary of terms, facts about food composition, and useful links.

NutritionalSupplements.com
http://www.nutritionalsupplements.com

This source provides unbiased information about nutritional supplements and prescription drugs, submitted by consumers with no vested interest in the products.

U.S. National Library of Medicine
http://www.nlm.nih.gov

This site permits you to search databases and electronic information sources such as MEDLINE, learn about research projects, and keep up on nutrition-related news.

Fish Contamination Resource
www.epa.gov/waterscience/fishadvice/advice.html

This Environmental Protection Agency website gives the latest information on fish contamination issues.

UNIT 3: Diet and Disease Through the Life Span

American Cancer Society
http://www.cancer.org

Open this site and its various links to learn the concerns and lifestyle advice of the American Cancer Society. It provides information on alternative therapies, tobacco, other Web resources, and more.

American Heart Association (AHA)
http://www.americanheart.org

The AHA offers this site to provide the most comprehensive information on heart disease and stroke as well as late-breaking news. The site presents facts on warning signs, a reference guide, and explanations of diseases and treatments.

The Food Allergy and Anaphylaxis Network
http://www.foodallergy.org

The Food Allergy Network site, which welcomes consumers, health professionals, and reporters, includes product alerts and updates, information about food allergies, daily tips, and links to other sites.

Heinz Infant & Toddler Nutrition

http://www.heinzbaby.com

An educational section full of nutritional information and meal-planning guides for parents and caregivers as well as articles and reviews by leading pediatricians and nutritionists can be found on this page.

LaLeche League International

http://www.lalecheleague.org

Important information to mothers who are contemplating breast feeding can be accessed at this Web site. Links to other sites are also possible.

UNIT 4: Obesity and Weight Control

American Anorexia Bulimia Association/National Eating Disorders Association (AABA)

http://www.nationaleatingdisorders.org/

The AABA is a nonprofit organization of concerned people dedicated to the prevention and treatment of eating disorders. It offers many services, including help lines, referral networks, school outreach, support groups, and prevention programs.

American Society of Exercise Physiologists (ASEP)

http://www.asep.org/

The goal of the ASEP is to promote health and physical fitness. This extensive site provides links to publications related to exercise and career opportunities in exercise physiology.

Calorie Control Council

http://www.caloriecontrol.org

The Calorie Control Council's Web site offers information on cutting calories, achieving and maintaining healthy weight, and low-calorie, reduced-fat foods and beverages.

Eating Disorders: Body Image Betrayal

http://www.bibri.com/home/index.htm

This extensive collection of links leads to information on compulsive eating, bulimia, anorexia, and other disorders.

Shape Up America!

http://www.shapeup.org

At the Shape Up America! Web site you will find the latest information about safe weight management, healthy eating, and physical fitness. Links include Support Center, Cyberkitchen, Media Center, Fitness Center, and BMI Center.

UNIT 5: Health Claims

Federal Trade Commission (FTC): Diet, Health & Fitness

http://www.ftc.gov/bcp/menu-health.htm

This site of the FTC on the Web offers consumer education rules and acts that include a wide range of subjects, from buying exercise equipment to virtual health "treatments."

Food and Drug Administration (FDA)

http://www.fda.gov/default.htm

The FDA presents this site that addresses products they regulate, current news and hot topics, safety alerts, product approvals, reference data, and general information and directions.

National Council Against Health Fraud (NCAHF)

http://www.ncahf.org

The NCAHF does business as the National Council for Reliable Health Information. At its Web page it offers links to other related sites, including Dr. Terry Polevoy's "Healthwatcher Net."

QuackWatch

http://www.quackwatch.com

Quackwatch Inc., a nonprofit corporation, provides this guide to examine health fraud. Data for intelligent decision making on health topics are also presented.

UNIT 6: Food Safety/Technology

American Council on Science and Health (ACSH)

http://www.acsh.org/food/

The ACSH addresses issues that are related to food safety here. In addition, issues on nutrition and fitness, alcohol, diseases, environmental health, medical care, lifestyle, and tobacco may be accessed on this site.

Centers for Disease Control and Prevention (CDC)

http://www.cdc.gov

The CDC offers this home page, from which you can obtain information about travelers' health, data related to disease control and prevention, and general nutritional and health information, publications, and more.

FDA Center for Food Safety and Applied Nutrition

http://vm.cfsan.fda.gov

It is possible to access everything from this Web site that you might want to know about food safety and what government agencies are doing to ensure it.

Food Safety Project (FSP)

http://www.extension.iastate.edu/foodsafety/

This site from the Cooperative Extension Service at North Carolina State University has a database designed to promote food safety education via the Internet.

National Food Safety Programs

http://vm.cfsan.fda.gov/~dms/fs-toc.html

Data from the Food and Drug Administration, U.S. Department of Agriculture, Environmental Protection Agency, and Centers for Disease Control and Prevention expanding on the government policies and initiatives regarding food safety are presented on this site.

USDA Food Safety and Inspection Service (FSIS)

http://www.fsis.usda.gov

The FSIS, part of the U.S. Department of Agriculture, is the government agency "responsible for ensuring that the nation's commercial supply of meat, poultry, and egg products is safe, wholesome, and correctly labeled and packaged."

UNIT 7: World Hunger and Malnutrition

Population Reference Bureau

http://www.prb.org

A key source for global population information, this is a good place to pursue data on nutrition problems worldwide.

World Health Organization (WHO)

http://www.who.int/en/

This home page of the World Health Organization will provide you with links to a wealth of statistical and analytical information about health and nutrition around the world.

WWW Virtual Library: Demography & Population Studies

http://demography.anu.edu.au/VirtualLibrary/

A multitude of important links to information about global poverty and hunger can be found here.

We highly recommend that you review our Web site for expanded information and our other product lines. We are continually updating and adding links to our Web site in order to offer you the most usable and useful information that will support and expand the value of your Annual Editions. You can reach us at: *http://www.dushkin.com/annualeditions/*.

UNIT 1
Nutrition Trends

Unit Selections

1. **The Changing American Diet: A Report Card**, Bonnie Liebman
2. **Dietary Guidelines for Americans 2005: Executive Summary**, U.S. Department of Health and Human Services, U.S. Department
3. **Rebuilding the Food Pyramid**, Walter C. Willett and Meir J. Stampfer
4. **The Low-Carb Frenzy: The Force That is Reshaping the Food Industry and Our Bodies**, Daniel Kadlec
5. **Getting Personal with Nutrition**, Food Insight
6. **Food, Spirituality, Mindful Eating**, Mary Kaye Sawyer-Morse
7. **Who's Filling Your Grocery Bag?**, James E. Tillotson
8. **Moving Towards Healthful Sustainable Diets**, Barbara Storper

Key Points to Consider

• Based on new scientific evidence, how should the Food Guide Pyramid be modified?

• Name some changes that have occurred in the American diet since the 1970s

• How is the individual going to ensure that he/she is eating a healthful and sustainable diet?

• Which are the factors that lead us to overeat?

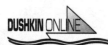 **Links: www.dushkin.com/online/**
These sites are annotated in the World Wide Web pages.

Food Science and Human Nutrition Extension
http://www.fshn.uiuc.edu/
Food Surveys Research Group
http://www.barc.usda.gov/bhnrc/foodsurvey/home.htm

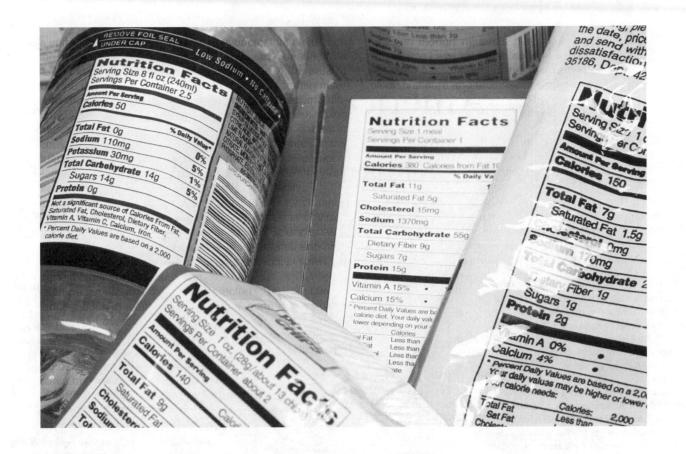

Consumers worldwide are bombarded with daily messages about nutrients and health. The first unit describes current trends and developments in the field of nutrition and explores the role the food industry, agribusiness, and other special interest groups and institutions play in the increasing incidence of obesity. It also presents the "new" dietary guidelines and describes a new "type" of pyramid as an alternate to the U.S.D.A's food guide pyramid.

The first article describes how Americans are doing with their eating. Compared to the decade of the 70's, Americans are now eating more cheeses, breads, chicken, and vegetables—but have also increased their soda consumption dramatically. The good news is that they have decreased beef and whole-milk consumption. This unit addresses the challenges nutritionists face in educating consumers toward healthful sustainable diets that will improve quality of life and benefit the environment and support local agriculture.

Americans can refer to the newly announced 2005 U.S. Dietary Guidelines for guidance to construct a healthy diet. Physical activity and weight management, increasing consumption of fruits and vegetables to ensure adequate levels of antioxidant vitamins, minerals, and fiber are the main focal points of the new Dietary Guidelines. The traditional U.S.D.A. Food Guide Pyramid focuses on meat and dairy, does not give advice on cholesterol and saturated fat, and does not distinguish among types of carbohydrates. Drs. Willet and Stampfer offer an alternative to the traditional U.S.D.A. Food Guide Pyramid. Their "New Food Guide Pyramid" encourages the consumption of healthy fats, whole-grain foods, distinguishes among types of carbohydrates, and encourages exercise.

Most Americans think that eating certain types of food while avoiding others is more critical to weight management than reducing their portion sizes and thus caloric intake. However, the role of packaging, size and shape of containers, influences consumers' buying decisions, and their impression that they eat less than they actually do.

The monopoly large food companies have on the kind of food we eat and on our wallet is tremendous. Most snack foods are loaded with salt, sugar, and fat and a big percentage of Americans' food dollar goes there. So not only personal behavior but also mega snack companies contribute to the obesity epidemic.

Recently Americans are becoming alarmed by the high incidence of obesity and have started to demand low-carbohydrate items and are going on low-carbohydrate diets. The food industry has been ready once again to meet this demand by producing a myriad of "low carb" food items.

The importance and immediacy of nutritionists educating consumers toward a healthful diet that will benefit the environment, support local economy and agriculture, and prevent disease is discussed in the last article of this unit by Barbara Storper.

The Changing American Diet

A Report Card

BY BONNIE LIEBMAN

What are Americans eating? Are we turning towards vegetarian diets or indulging in more steak? Are we getting fat on fat-free ice cream, cake, and cookies or rewarding ourselves with fat-laden cheesecake, ice cream, and pastries? Are we eating more fruits and vegetables or more french fries?

Since the early 1900s, the U.S. Department of Agriculture has been tracking the amount of food available for Americans to eat. (The numbers over-estimate what we actually swallow, since some food never gets sold, some spoils, and some gets left on our plate. But they're valid for year-to-year comparisons.)

Every few years, we use that data to size up the American diet. The "grades" look not just at what we're eating, but whether we're moving in the right direction. Here's our latest report card.

Beverages: D

In 1977, soda became the most popular American beverage, and it never looked back. We now drink roughly 50 gallons of soda per person per year. And that doesn't include the eight gallons of uncarbonated soda that masquerades as "fruit" drinks. Of the healthier beverages—milk, fruit *juice*, and bottled water—only water is clearly climbing. The bottom line: The soft-drink industry keeps filling our ever-larger cups with its high-calorie sugar water, and we keep drinking as though there were no (bathroom scale to get on) tomorrow.

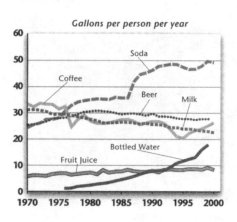

Gallons per person per year

Dairy Products: D

We're eating only slightly less ice cream than we did in 1970. And most of it is as fatty as it was 30 years ago (except for Ben & Jerry's and Häagen-Dazs, which are even fattier).

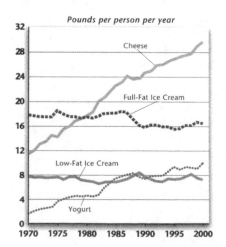

Pounds per person per year

As for cheese: The sky's the limit. We eat more than twice as much as we did in 1970. Cheese has now passed beef as our number-one source of saturated fat. Pizza and cheeseburgers started the trend back in the 1960s. But now cheese is everywhere: in your tacos and nachos, your soups and salads, your rice and potatoes, your chicken and fish… and your arteries.

Flour & Cereal: B

We're eating more flour than we did in the 1970s (in the U.S., flour means wheat). Some goes into breads, bagels, pasta, and pancakes; some ends up in cakes, cookies, Cinnabons, doughnuts, and other sweets.

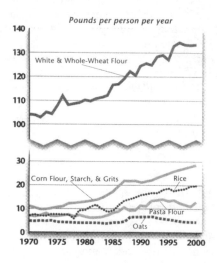

Pounds per person per year

Are all those carbs making us fat? You bet they are … along with all the fat, protein, and alcohol we scarf down. And only a tiny fraction of the wheat flour is whole-grain, the kind that may help lower the risk of heart disease and diabetes.

Added Fats & Oils: B

The big trends in fats and oils are clear: Since 1970, we've been eating slightly less butter and margarine, more shortening, and (much) more oil.

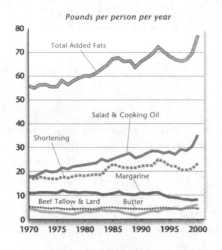

Pounds per person per year

Shortening, butter, and some margarines have saturated or trans fat, which clogs arteries. Oils don't. But all fats have calories…and that's one thing we don't need more of. Some people blame America's obesity epidemic on a low-fat diet (see "Big Fat Lies," November 2002). Can you find the low-fat diet on this graph?

Sweeteners: F

We now produce 152 pounds of added sugars each year for every man, woman, and child in America. That's 25 percent more than in 1970. Soft drinks account for a third of our intake. So-called "fruit" drinks supply another ten percent, while cookies, cakes, and other sweet baked goods contribute 14 percent (thank you, Mrs. Fields and Cinnabon). Candy, breakfast cereals, and ice cream each chip in about five percent. Does the tiny dip in 2000 signal the end of our runaway sweet tooth? Stay tuned.

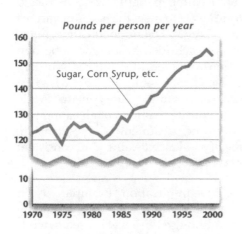

Pounds per person per year

Meat, Poultry, & Seafood: B

Beef and pork were neck-and-neck for the first half of the 20th century. But in the 1950s, beef started a steep climb that finally peaked in the mid-1970s. Chicken's growth keeps clucking along. But we still eat far more red meat (111 pounds per person) than poultry and seafood (83 pounds) each year.

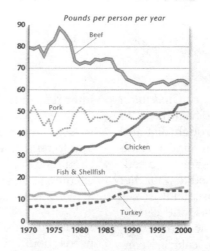

Pounds per person per year

Fruits & Vegetables: A

We're eating more fruits and vegetables than we did 30 years ago. On the upswing are bell peppers, broccoli, carrots, cucumbers, mushrooms, onions, spinach, squash, and tomatoes (but not brussels sprouts, cabbage, celery, or sweet potatoes). Also rising are bananas, grapes, mangos, melons, papayas, pears, pineapples and strawberries (but not apples, apricots, cherries, grapefruit, oranges, peaches, or plums). We still don't eat enough fruits and vegetables, but at least we're moving in the right direction.

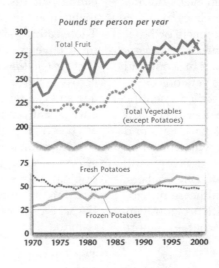

Pounds per person per year

Milk: C

Whole milk is down (that's good). So is reduced-fat (2 percent) milk (also good). But low-fat (1 percent) and skim (fat-free) aren't replacing the fattier milks. And we still drink more than twice as much of the two fattier milks than their two low-fat cousins.

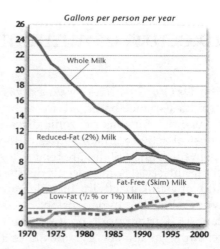

Gallons per person per year

Heather Jones DeMino helped compile the information for this article. Source: Economic Research Service, U.S. Department of Agriculture. (To access the U.S.D.A.'s per capita food consumption database on-line, go to www.ers.usda.gov/data/foodconsumption.)

Dietary Guidelines for Americans 2005

Executive Summary

The *Dietary Guidelines for Americans [Dietary Guidelines]* provides science-based advice to promote health and to reduce risk for major chronic diseases through diet and physical activity. Major causes of morbidity and mortality in the United States are related to poor diet and a sedentary lifestyle. Some specific diseases linked to poor diet and physical inactivity include cardiovascular disease, type 2 diabetes, hypertension, osteoporosis, and certain cancers. Furthermore, poor diet and physical inactivity, resulting in an energy imbalance (more calories consumed than expended), are the most important factors contributing to the increase in overweight and obesity in this country. Combined with physical activity, following a diet that does not provide excess calories according to the recommendations in this document should enhance the health of most individuals.

An important component of each 5-year revision of the *Dietary Guidelines* is the analysis of new scientific information by the Dietary Guidelines Advisory Committee (DGAC) appointed by the Secretaries of the U.S. Department of Health and Human Services (HHS) and the U.S. Department of Agriculture (USDA). This analysis, published in the DGAC Report (http://www.health.gov/dietary guidelines/dga2005 /report/), is the primary resource for development of the report on the Guidelines by the Departments. The *Dietary Guidelines* and the report of the DGAC differ in scope and purpose compared to reports for previous versions of the *Guidelines*. The 2005 DGAC report is a detailed scientific analysis. The scientific report was used to develop the *Dietary Guidelines* jointly between the two Departments and forms the basis of recommendations that will be used by USDA and HHS for program and policy development. Thus it is a publication oriented toward policymakers, nutrition educators, nutritionists, and healthcare providers rather than to the general public, as with previous versions of the *Dietary Guidelines*, and contains more technical information.

The intent of the *Dietary Guidelines* is to summarize and synthesize knowledge regarding individual nutrients and food components into recommendations for a pattern of eating that can be adopted by the public. In this publication, Key Recommendations are grouped under nine inter-related focus areas. The recommendations are based on the preponderance of scientific evidence for lowering risk of chronic disease and promoting health. It is important to remember that these are integrated messages that should be implemented as a whole. Taken together, they encourage most Americans to eat fewer calories, be more active, and make wiser food choices.

A basic premise of the *Dietary Guidelines* is that nutrient needs should be met primarily through consuming foods. Foods provide an array of nutrients and other compounds that may have beneficial effects on health. In certain cases, fortified foods and dietary supplements may be useful sources of one or more nutrients that otherwise might be consumed in less than recommended amounts. However, dietary supplements, while recommended in some cases, cannot replace a healthful diet.

Two examples of eating patterns that exemplify the *Dietary Guidelines* are the USDA Food Guide (http://www.usda. gov/cnpp/pyramid.html) and the DASH (Dietary Approaches to Stop Hypertension) Eating Plan.[1] Both of these eating patterns are designed to integrate dietary recommendations into a healthy way to eat for most individuals. These eating patterns are not weight loss diets, but rather illustrative examples of how to eat in accordance with the *Dietary Guidelines*. Both eating patterns are constructed across a range of calorie levels to meet the needs of various age and gender groups. For the USDA Food Guide, nutrient content estimates for each food group and subgroup are based on population-weighted food intakes. Nutrient content estimates for the DASH Eating Plan are based on selected foods chosen for a sample 7-day menu. While originally developed to study the effects of an eating pattern on the prevention and treatment of hypertension, DASH is one example of a balanced eating plan consistent with the 2005 *Dietary Guidelines*.

Throughout most of this publication, examples use a 2,000-calorie level as a reference for consistency with the Nutrition Facts Panel. Although this level is used as a reference, recommended calorie intake will differ for individuals based on age, gender, and activity level. At each calorie level, individuals who eat nutrient-dense foods may be able to meet their recommended nutrient intake without consuming their full calorie allotment. The remaining calories—the *discretionary calorie allowance*—allow individuals flexibility to consume some foods and beverages that may contain added fats, added sugars, and alcohol.

The recommendations in the *Dietary Guidelines* are for Americans over 2 years of age. It is important to incorporate the food preferences of different racial/ethnic groups, vegetarians, and other groups when planning diets and developing educational programs and materials. The USDA Food Guide and the DASH Eating Plan are flexible enough to accommodate a range of food preferences and cuisines.

Taken together, [the *Dietary Guidelines*] encourage most Americans to eat fewer calories, be more active, and make wiser food choices.

The *Dietary Guidelines* is intended primarily for use by policymakers, healthcare providers, nutritionists, and nutrition educators. The information in the *Dietary Guidelines* is useful for the development of educational materials and aids policymakers in designing and implementing nutrition-related programs, including federal food, nutrition education, and information programs. In addition, this publication has the potential to provide authoritative statements as provided for in the Food and Drug Administration Modernization Act (FDAMA). Because the *Dietary Guidelines* contains discussions where the science is emerging, only statements included in the Executive Summary and the sections titled "Key Recommendations," which reflect the preponderance of scientific evidence, can be used for identification of authoritative statements. The recommendations are interrelated and mutually dependent; thus the statements in this document should be used together in the context of planning an overall healthful diet. However, even following just some of the recommendations can have health benefits.

The following is a listing of the *Dietary Guidelines* by chapter.

ADEQUATE NUTRIENTS WITHIN CALORIE NEEDS

Key Recommendations

- Consume a variety of nutrient-dense foods and beverages within and among the basic food groups while choosing foods that limit the in-

take of saturated and *trans* fats, cholesterol, added sugars, salt, and alcohol.
- Meet recommended intakes within energy needs by adopting a balanced eating pattern, such as the USDA Food Guide or the DASH Eating Plan.

Key Recommendations for Specific Population Groups

- *People over age 50.* Consume vitamin B12 in its crystalline form (i.e., fortified foods or supplements).
- *Women of childbearing age who may become pregnant.* Eat foods high in heme-iron and/or consume iron-rich plant foods or iron-fortified foods with an enhancer of iron absorption, such as vitamin C-rich foods.
- *Women of childbearing age who may become pregnant and those in the first trimester of pregnancy.* Consume adequate synthetic folic acid daily (from fortified foods or supplements) in addition to food forms of folate from a varied diet.
- *Older adults, people with dark skin, and people exposed to insufficient ultraviolet band radiation (i.e., sunlight).* Consume extra vitamin D from vitamin D-fortified foods and/or supplements.

WEIGHT MANAGEMENT

Key Recommendations

- To maintain body weight in a healthy range, balance calories from foods and beverages with calories expended.
- To prevent gradual weight gain over time, make small decreases in food and beverage calories and increase physical activity.

Key Recommendations for Specific Population Groups

- *Those who need to lose weight.* Aim for a slow, steady weight loss by decreasing calorie intake while maintaining an adequate nutrient intake and increasing physical activity.
- *Overweight children.* Reduce the rate of body weight gain while allowing growth and development. Consult a healthcare provider before placing a child on a weight-reduction diet.
- *Pregnant women.* Ensure appropriate weight gain as specified by a healthcare provider.
- *Breastfeeding women.* Moderate weight reduction is safe and does not compromise weight gain of the nursing infant.
- *Overweight adults and overweight children with chronic diseases and/or on medication.* Consult a healthcare provider about weight loss strategies prior to starting a weight-reduction program to ensure appropriate management of other health conditions.

PHYSICAL ACTIVITY

Key Recommendations

- Engage in regular physical activity and reduce sedentary activities to promote health, psychological well-being, and a healthy body weight.
  - To reduce the risk of chronic disease in adulthood: Engage in at least 30 minutes of moderate-intensity physical activity, above usual activity, at work or home on most days of the week.
  - For most people, greater health benefits can be obtained by engaging in physical activity of more vigorous intensity or longer duration.
  - To help manage body weight and prevent gradual, unhealthy body weight gain in adulthood: Engage in approximately 60 minutes of moderate- to vigorous-intensity activity on most days of the week while not exceeding caloric intake requirements.
  - To sustain weight loss in adulthood: Participate in at least 60 to 90 minutes of daily moderate-intensity physical activity while not exceeding caloric intake requirements. Some people may need to consult with a healthcare provider before participating in this level of activity.
- Achieve physical fitness by including cardiovascular conditioning, stretching exercises for flexibility, and resistance exercises or calisthenics for muscle strength and endurance.

Key Recommendations for Specific Population Groups

- *Children and adolescents.* Engage in at least 60 minutes of physical activity on most, preferably all, days of the week.
- *Pregnant women.* In the absence of medical or obstetric complications, incorporate 30 minutes or more of moderate-intensity physical activity on most, if not all, days of the week. Avoid activities with a high risk of falling or abdominal trauma.
- *Breastfeeding women.* Be aware that neither acute nor regular exercise adversely affects the mother's ability to successfully breastfeed.
- *Older adults.* Participate in regular physical activity to reduce functional declines associated with aging and to achieve the other benefits of physical activity identified for all adults.

FOOD GROUPS TO ENCOURAGE

Key Recommendations

- Consume a sufficient amount of fruits and vegetables while staying within energy needs. Two cups of fruit and 2 ½ cups of vegetables per day are recommended for a reference 2,000-calorie intake, with higher or lower amounts depending on the calorie level.
- Choose a variety of fruits and vegetables each day. In particular, select from all five vegetable subgroups (dark green, orange, legumes, starchy vegetables, and other vegetables) several times a week.
- Consume 3 or more ounce-equivalents of whole-grain products per day, with the rest of the recommended grains coming from enriched or whole-grain products. In general, at least half the grains should come from whole grains.
- Consume 3 cups per day of fat-free or low-fat milk or equivalent milk products.

Key Recommendations for Specific Population Groups

- *Children and adolescents.* Consume whole-grain products often; at least half the grains should be whole grains. Children 2 to 8 years should consume 2 cups per day of fat-free or low-fat milk or equivalent milk products. Children 9 years of age and older should consume 3 cups per day of fat-free or low-fat milk or equivalent milk products.

FATS

Key Recommendations

- Consume less than 10 percent of calories from saturated fatty acids and less than 300 mg/day of cholesterol, and keep *trans* fatty acid consumption as low as possible.
- Keep total fat intake between 20 to 35 percent of calories, with most fats coming from sources of polyunsaturated and monounsaturated fatty acids, such as fish, nuts, and vegetable oils.
- When selecting and preparing meat, poultry, dry beans, and milk or milk products, make choices that are lean, low-fat, or fat-free.
- Limit intake of fats and oils high in saturated and/or *trans* fatty acids, and choose products low in such fats and oils.

Key Recommendations for Specific Population Groups

- *Children and adolescents.* Keep total fat intake between 30 to 35 percent of calories for children 2 to 3 years of age and between 25 to 35 percent of calories for children and adolescents 4 to 18 years of age, with most fats coming from sources of polyunsaturated and monounsaturated fatty acids, such as fish, nuts, and vegetable oils.

6

CARBOHYDRATES

Key Recommendations
- Choose fiber-rich fruits, vegetables, and whole grains often.
- Choose and prepare foods and beverages with little added sugars or caloric sweeteners, such as amounts suggested by the USDA Food Guide and the DASH Eating Plan.
- Reduce the incidence of dental caries by practicing good oral hygiene and consuming sugar- and starch-containing foods and beverages less frequently.

SODIUM AND POTASSIUM

Key Recommendations
- Consume less than 2,300 mg (approximately 1 tsp of salt) of sodium per day.
- Choose and prepare foods with little salt. At the same time, consume potassium-rich foods, such as fruits and vegetables.

Key Recommendations for Specific Population Groups
- *Individuals with hypertension, blacks, and middle-aged and older adults.* Aim to consume no more than 1,500 mg of sodium per day, and meet the potassium recommendation (4,700 mg/day) with food.

ALCOHOLIC BEVERAGES

Key Recommendations
- Those who choose to drink alcoholic beverages should do so sensibly and in moderation—defined as the consumption of up to one drink per day for women and up to two drinks per day for men.
- Alcoholic beverages should not be consumed by some individuals, including those who cannot restrict their alcohol intake, women of childbearing age who may become pregnant, pregnant and lactating women, children and adolescents, individuals taking medications that can interact with alcohol, and those with specific medical conditions.

- Alcoholic beverages should be avoided by individuals engaging in activities that require attention, skill, or coordination, such as driving or operating machinery.

FOOD SAFETY

Key Recommendations
- To avoid microbial food borne illness:
  - Clean hands, food contact surfaces, and fruits and vegetables. Meat and poultry should *not* be washed or rinsed.
  - Separate raw, cooked, and ready-to-eat foods while shopping, preparing, or storing foods.
  - Cook foods to a safe temperature to kill microorganisms.
  - Chill (refrigerate) perishable food promptly and defrost foods properly.
  - Avoid raw (unpasteurized) milk or any products made from unpasteurized milk, raw or partially cooked eggs or foods containing raw eggs, raw or undercooked meat and poultry, unpasteurized juices, and raw sprouts.

Key Recommendations for Specific Population Groups
- *Infants and young children, pregnant women, older adults, and those who are immunocompromised.* Do not eat or drink raw (unpasteurized) milk or any products made from unpasteurized milk, raw or partially cooked eggs or foods containing raw eggs, raw or undercooked meat and poultry, raw or undercooked fish or shellfish, unpasteurized juices, and raw sprouts.
- *Pregnant women, older adults, and those who are immunocompromised:* Only eat certain deli meats and frankfurters that have been reheated to steaming hot.

Note
1. N/H Publication No. 03-4082, Facts about the DASH Eating Plan, United States Department of Health and Human Services, National Institutes of Health, National Heart, Lung, and Blood Institute, Karanja NM et al. *Journal of the American Dietetic Association (JADA)* 8:S19-27, 1999. http://www.nhlbi.nih.gov/health/public/heart/hbp/dash/.

United States Department of Health and Human Services, 2005.

REBUILDING

the

Food Pyramid

The dietary guide introduced a decade ago has led people astray. Some fats are healthy for the heart, and many carbohydrates clearly are not.

By Walter C. Willett and Meir J. Stampfer

In 1992 the U.S. Department of Agriculture officially released the Food Guide Pyramid, which was intended to help the American public make dietary choices that would maintain good health and reduce the risk of chronic disease. The recommendations embodied in the pyramid soon became well known: people should minimize their consumption of fats and oils but should eat six to 11 servings a day of foods rich in complex carbohydrates—bread, cereal, rice, pasta and so on. The food pyramid also recommended generous amounts of vegetables (including potatoes, another plentiful source of complex carbohydrates), fruit and dairy products, and at least two servings a day from the meat and beans group, which lumped together red meat with poultry, fish, nuts, legumes and eggs.

Even when the pyramid was being developed, though, nutritionists had long known that some types of fat are essential to health and can reduce the risk of cardiovascular disease. Furthermore, scientists had found little evidence that a high intake of carbohydrates is beneficial.

Since 1992 more and more research has shown that the USDA pyramid is grossly flawed. By promoting the consumption of all complex carbohydrates and eschewing all fats and oils, the pyramid provides misleading guidance. In short, not all fats are bad for you, and by no means are all complex carbohydrates good for you. The USDA's Center for Nutrition Policy and Promotion is now reassessing the pyramid, but this effort is not expected to be completed until 2004. In the meantime, we have drawn up a new pyramid that better reflects the current understanding of the relation between diet and health. Studies indicate that adherence to the recommendations in the revised pyramid can significantly reduce the risk of cardiovascular disease for both men and women.

How did the original USDA pyramid go so wrong? In part, nutritionists fell victim to a desire to simplify their dietary recommendations. Researchers had known for decades that saturated fat—found in abundance in red meat and dairy products—raises cholesterol levels in the blood. High cholesterol levels, in turn, are associated with a high risk of coronary heart disease (heart attacks and other ailments caused by the blockage of the arteries to the heart). In the 1960s controlled feeding studies, in which the participants eat carefully prescribed diets for several weeks, substantiated that saturated fat increases cholesterol levels. But the studies also showed that polyunsaturated fat—found in vegetable oils and fish—reduces cholesterol. Thus, dietary advice during the 1960s and 1970s emphasized the replacement of saturated fat with polyunsaturated fat, not total fat reduction. (The subsequent doubling of polyunsaturated fat consumption among Americans probably contributed greatly to the halving of coronary heart disease rates in the U.S. during the 1970s and 1980s.)

The notion that fat in general is to be avoided stems mainly from observations that affluent Western countries have both high intakes of fat and high rates of coronary heart disease. This correlation, however, is limited to saturated fat. Societies in which people eat relatively large portions of monounsaturated and polyunsaturated

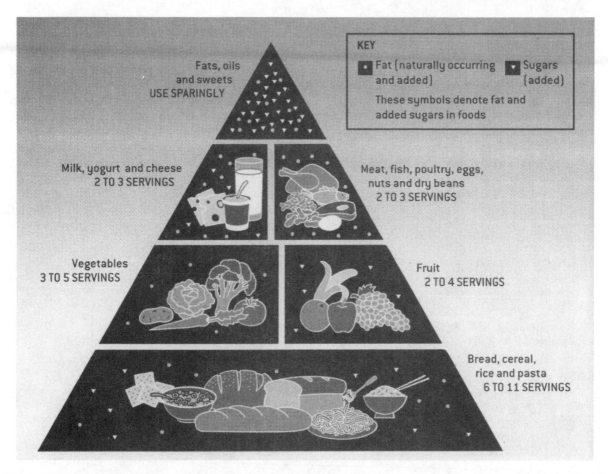

Old Food Pyramid conceived by the U.S. Department of Agriculture was intended to convey the message "Fat is bad" and its corollary "Carbs are good." These sweeping statements are now being questioned.

For information on the amount of food that counts as one serving, visit www.nal.usda.gov: 8001/py/pmap.htm

fat tend to have lower rates of heart disease [*see illustration on next page*]. On the Greek island of Crete, for example, the traditional diet contained much olive oil (a rich source of monounsaturated fat) and fish (a source of polyunsaturated fat). Although fat constituted 40 percent of the calories in this diet, the rate of heart disease for those who followed it was lower than the rate for those who followed the traditional diets of Japan, in which fat made up only 8 to 10 percent of the calories. Furthermore, international comparisons can be misleading: many negative influences on health, such as smoking, physical inactivity and high amounts of body fat, are also correlated with Western affluence.

Unfortunately, many nutritionists decided it would be too difficult to educate the public about these subtleties. Instead they put out a clear, simple message: "Fat is bad." Because saturated fat represents about

40 percent of all fat consumed in the U.S., the rationale of the USDA was that advocating a low-fat diet would naturally reduce the intake of saturated fat. This recommendation was soon reinforced by the food industry, which began selling cookies, chips and other products that were low in fat but often high in sweeteners such as high-fructose corn syrup.

When the food pyramid was being developed, the typical American got about 40 percent of his or her calories from fat, about 15 percent from protein and about 45 percent from carbohydrates. Nutritionists did not want to suggest eating more protein, because many sources of protein (red meat, for example) are also heavy in saturated fat. So the "Fat is bad" mantra led to the corollary "Carbs are good." Dietary guidelines from the American Heart Association and other groups recommended that people get at least half their calories from carbohydrates and

no more than 30 percent from fat. This 30 percent limit has become so entrenched among nutritionists that even the sophisticated observer could be forgiven for thinking that many studies must show that individuals with that level of fat intake enjoyed better health than those with higher levels. But no study has demonstrated long-term health benefits that can be directly attributed to a low-fat diet. The 30 percent limit on fat was essentially drawn from thin air.

The wisdom of this direction became even more questionable after researchers found that the two main cholesterol-carrying chemicals—low-density lipoprotein (LDL), popularly known as "bad cholesterol," and high-density lipoprotein (HDL), known as "good cholesterol"—have very different effects on the risk of coronary heart disease. Increasing the ratio of LDL to HDL in the blood raises the risk, whereas decreasing

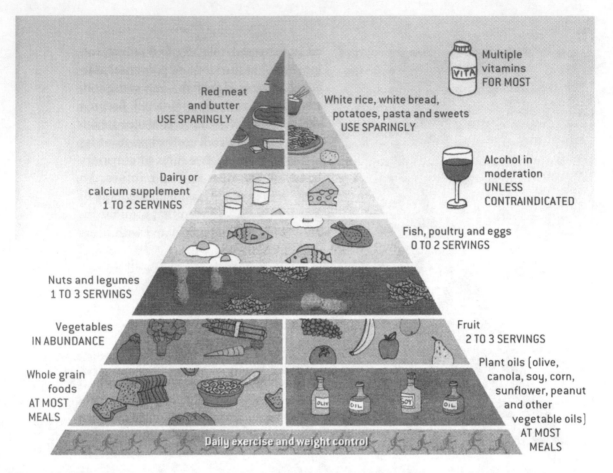

New Food Pyramid outlined by the authors distinguishes between healthy and unhealthy types of fat and carbohydrates. Fruits and vegetables are still recommended, but the consumption of dairy products should be limited.

the ratio lowers it. By the early 1990s controlled feeding studies had shown that when a person replaces calories from saturated fat with an equal amount of calories from carbohydrates the levels of LDL and total cholesterol fall, but the level of HDL also falls. Because the ratio of LDL to HDL does not change, there is only a small reduction in the person's risk of heart disease. Moreover, the switch to carbohydrates boosts the blood levels of triglycerides, the component molecules of fat, probably because of effects on the body's endocrine system. High triglyceride levels are also associated with a high risk of heart disease.

The effects are more grievous when a person switches from either monounsaturated or polyunsaturated fat to carbohydrates. LDL levels rise and HDL levels drop, making the cholesterol ratio worse. In contrast, replacing saturated fat with ei-ther monounsaturated or polyunsaturated fat improves this ratio and would be expected to reduce heart disease. The only fats that are significantly more deleterious than carbohydrates are the trans-unsaturated fatty acids; these are produced by the partial hydrogenation of liquid vegetable oil, which causes it to solidify. Found in many margarines, baked goods and fried foods, trans fats are uniquely bad for you because they raise LDL and triglycerides while reducing HDL.

THE BIG PICTURE

TO EVALUATE FULLY the health effects of diet, though, one must look beyond cholesterol ratios and triglyceride levels. The foods we eat can cause heart disease through many other pathways, including raising blood pressure or boosting the tendency of blood to clot. And other foods can prevent heart disease in surprising ways; for instance, omega-3 fatty acids (found in fish and some plant oils) can reduce the likelihood of ventricular fibrillation, a heart rhythm disturbance that causes sudden death.

The ideal method for assessing all these adverse and beneficial effects would be to conduct large-scale trials in which individuals are randomly assigned to one diet or another and followed for many years. Because of practical constraints and cost, few such studies have been conducted, and most of these have focused on patients who already suffer from heart disease. Though limited, these studies have supported the benefits of replacing saturated fat with polyunsaturated fat, but not with carbohydrates.

The best alternative is to conduct large epidemiological studies in which the diets of many people are periodically assessed and the participants are monitored for the development of heart disease and other conditions. One of the best-known examples of this research is the Nurses' Health Study, which was begun in 1976 to evaluate the effects of oral contraceptives but was soon extended to nutrition as well. Our group at Harvard University has followed nearly 90,000 women in this study who first completed detailed questionnaires on diet in 1980, as well as more than 50,000 men who were enrolled in the Health Professionals Follow-Up Study in 1986.

After adjusting the analysis to account for smoking, physical activity and other recognized risk factors, we found that a participant's risk of heart disease was strongly influenced by the type of dietary fat consumed. Eating trans fat increased the risk substantially, and eating saturated fat increased it slightly. In contrast, eating monounsaturated and polyunsaturated fats decreased the risk—just as the controlled feeding studies predicted. Because these two effects counterbalanced each other, higher overall consumption of fat did not lead to higher rates of coronary heart disease. This finding reinforced a 1989 report by the National Academy of Sciences that concluded that total fat intake alone was not associated with heart disease risk.

But what about illnesses besides coronary heart disease? High rates of breast, colon and prostate cancers in affluent Western countries have led to the belief that the consumption of fat, particularly animal fat, may be a risk factor. But large epidemiological studies have shown little evidence that total fat consumption or intakes of specific types of fat during midlife affect the risks of breast or colon cancer. Some studies have indicated that prostate cancer and the consumption of animal fat may be associated, but reassuringly there is no suggestion that vegetable oils increase any cancer risk. Indeed, some studies have suggested that vegetable oils may slightly reduce such risks. Thus, it is reasonable to

make decisions about dietary fat on the basis of its effects on cardiovascular disease, not cancer.

Finally, one must consider the impact of fat consumption on obesity, the most serious nutritional problem in the U.S. Obesity is a major risk factor for several diseases, including type 2 diabetes (also called adult-onset diabetes), coronary heart disease, and cancers of the breast, colon, kidney and esophagus. Many nutritionists believe that eating fat can contribute to weight gain because fat contains more calories per gram than protein or carbohydrates. Also, the process of storing dietary fat in the body may be more efficient than the conversion of carbohydrates to body fat. But recent controlled feeding studies have shown that these considerations are not practically important. The best way to avoid obesity is to limit your total calories, not just the fat calories. So the critical issue is whether the fat composition of a diet can influence one's ability to control caloric intake. In other words, does eating fat leave you more or less hungry than eating protein or carbohydrates? There are various theories about why one diet should be better than another, but few long-term studies have been done. In randomized trials, individuals assigned to low-fat diets tend to lose a few pounds during the first months but then regain the weight. In studies lasting a year or longer, low-fat diets have consistently not led to greater weight loss.

CARBO-LOADING

NOW LET'S LOOK at the health effects of carbohydrates. Complex carbohydrates consist of long chains of sugar units such as glucose and fructose; sugars contain only one or two units. Because of concerns that sugars offer nothing but "empty calories"—that is, no vitamins, minerals or other nutrients—complex carbohydrates form the base of the USDA food pyramid. But refined carbohydrates, such as white bread and white rice, can be very quickly bro-

ken down to glucose, the primary fuel for the body. The refining process produces an easily absorbed form of starch—which is defined as glucose molecules bound together—and also removes many vitamins and minerals and fiber. Thus, these carbohydrates increase glucose levels in the blood more than whole grains do. (Whole grains have not been milled into fine flour.)

Or consider potatoes. Eating a boiled potato raises blood sugar levels higher than eating the same amount of calories from table sugar. Because potatoes are mostly starch, they can be rapidly metabolized to glucose. In contrast, table sugar (sucrose) is a disaccharide consisting of one molecule of glucose and one molecule of fructose. Fructose takes longer to convert to glucose, hence the slower rise in blood glucose levels.

A rapid increase in blood sugar stimulates a large release of insulin, the hormone that directs glucose to the muscles and liver. As a result, blood sugar plummets, sometimes even going below the baseline. High levels of glucose and insulin can have negative effects on cardiovascular health, raising triglycerides and lowering HDL (the good cholesterol). The precipitous decline in glucose can also lead to more hunger after a carbohydrate-rich meal and thus contribute to overeating and obesity.

In our epidemiological studies, we have found that a high intake of starch from refined grains and potatoes is associated with a high risk of type 2 diabetes and coronary heart disease. Conversely, a greater intake of fiber is related to a lower risk of these illnesses. Interestingly, though, the consumption of fiber did not lower the risk of colon cancer, as had been hypothesized earlier.

The best way to avoid obesity is to LIMIT YOUR TOTAL CALORIES, not just the fat calories.

Overweight, inactive people can become resistant to insulin's effects and therefore require more of the hormone to regulate their blood sugar. Recent evidence indicates that the adverse metabolic response to carbohydrates is substantially worse among people who already have insulin resistance. This finding may account for the ability of peasant farmers in Asia and elsewhere, who are extremely lean and active, to consume large amounts of refined carbohydrates without experiencing diabetes or heart disease, whereas the same diet in a more sedentary population can have devastating effects.

EAT YOUR VEGGIES

HIGH INTAKE OF FRUITS and vegetables is perhaps the least controversial aspect of the food pyramid. A reduction in cancer risk has been a widely promoted benefit. But most of the evidence for this benefit has come from case-control studies, in which patients with cancer and selected control subjects are asked about their earlier diets. These retrospective studies are susceptible to numerous biases, and recent findings from large prospective studies (including our own) have tended to show little relation between overall fruit and vegetable consumption and cancer incidence. (Specific nutrients in fruits and vegetables may offer benefits, though; for instance, the folic acid in green leafy vegetables may reduce the risk of colon cancer, and the lycopene found in tomatoes may lower the risk of prostate cancer.)

The real value of eating fruits and vegetables may be in reducing the risk of cardiovascular disease. Folic acid and potassium appear to contribute to this effect, which has been seen in several epidemiological studies. Inadequate consumption of folic acid is responsible for higher risks of serious birth defects as well, and low intake of lutein, a pigment in green leafy vegetables, has been associated with greater risks of cataracts and degeneration of the retina. Fruits and vegetables are also the primary source of many vitamins needed for good health. Thus, there are good reasons to consume the recommended five servings a day, even if doing so has little impact on cancer risk. The inclusion of potatoes as a vegetable in the USDA pyramid has little justification, however; being mainly starch, potatoes do not confer the benefits seen for other vegetables.

Another flaw in the USDA pyramid is its failure to recognize the important health differences between red meat (beef, pork and lamb) and the other foods in the meat and beans group (poultry, fish, legumes, nuts and eggs). High consumption of red meat has been associated with an increased risk of coronary heart disease, probably because of its high content of saturated fat and cholesterol. Red meat also raises the risk of type 2 diabetes and colon cancer. The elevated risk of colon cancer may be related in part to the carcinogens produced during cooking and the chemicals found in processed meats such as salami and bologna.

Poultry and fish, in contrast, contain less saturated fat and more unsaturated fat than red meat does. Fish is a rich source of the essential omega-3 fatty acids as well. Not surprisingly, studies have shown that people who replace red meat with chicken and fish have a lower risk of coronary heart disease and colon cancer. Eggs are high in cholesterol, but consumption of up to one a day does not appear to have adverse effects on heart disease risk (except among diabetics), probably because the effects of a slightly higher cholesterol level are counterbalanced by other nutritional benefits. Many people have avoided nuts because of their high fat content, but the fat in nuts, including peanuts, is mainly unsaturated, and walnuts in particular are a good source of omega-3 fatty acids. Controlled feeding studies show that nuts improve blood cholesterol ratios, and epidemiological studies indicate that they lower the risk of heart disease and diabetes. Also, people who eat nuts are actually less likely to be obese; perhaps because nuts are more satisfying to the appetite, eating them seems to have the effect of significantly reducing the intake of other foods.

Yet another concern regarding the USDA pyramid is that it promotes over-consumption of dairy products, recommending the equivalent of two or three glasses of milk a day. This advice is usually justified by dairy's calcium content, which is believed to prevent osteoporosis and bone fractures. But the highest rates of fractures are found in countries with high dairy consumption, and large prospective studies have not shown a lower risk of fractures among those who eat plenty of dairy products. Calcium is an essential nutrient, but the requirements for bone health have probably been overstated. What is more, we cannot assume that high dairy consumption is safe: in several studies, men who consumed large amounts of dairy products experienced an increased risk of prostate cancer, and in some studies, women with high intakes had elevated rates of ovarian cancer. Although fat was initially assumed to be the responsible factor, this has not been supported in more detailed analyses. High calcium intake itself seemed most clearly related to the risk of prostate cancer.

More research is needed to determine the health effects of dairy products, but at the moment it seems imprudent to recommend high consumption. Most adults who are following a good overall diet can get the necessary amount of calcium by consuming the equivalent of one glass of milk a day. Under certain circumstances, such as after menopause, people may need more calcium than usual, but it can be obtained at lower cost and without saturated fat or calories by taking a supplement.

A HEALTHIER PYRAMID

ALTHOUGH THE USDA'S food pyramid has become an icon of nutrition over the past decade, until recently no studies had evaluated the health of individuals who followed its guidelines. It very likely has some benefits, especially from a high intake of fruits and vegetables. And a decrease in total fat intake would tend to reduce the consumption of harmful saturated and trans fats. But the pyramid could also lead people to eat fewer of the healthy unsaturated fats and more refined starches, so the benefits might be negated by the harm.

To evaluate the overall impact, we used the Healthy Eating Index (HEI), a score developed by the USDA to measure adherence to the pyramid and its accompanying dietary guidelines in federal nutrition programs. From the data collected in our large epidemiological studies, we calculated each participant's HEI score and then examined the relation of these scores to subsequent risk of major chronic disease (defined as heart attack, stroke, cancer or nontraumatic death from any cause). When we compared people in the same age groups, women and men with the highest HEI scores did have a lower risk of major chronic disease. But these individuals also smoked less, exercised more and had generally healthier lifestyles than the other participants. After adjusting for these variables, we found that participants with the highest HEI scores did not experience significantly better overall health outcomes. As predicted, the pyramid's harms counterbalanced its benefits.

Because the goal of the pyramid was a worthy one—to encourage healthy dietary choices—we have tried to develop an alternative derived from the best available knowledge. Our revised pyramid emphasizes weight control through exercising daily and avoiding an excessive total intake of calories. This pyramid recommends that the bulk of one's diet should consist of healthy fats (liquid vegetable oils such as olive, canola, soy, corn, sunflower and peanut) and healthy carbohydrates (whole grain foods such as whole wheat bread, oatmeal and brown rice). If both the fats and carbohydrates in your diet are healthy, you probably do not have to worry too much about the percentages of total calories coming from each. Vegetables and fruits should also be eaten in abundance. Moderate amounts of healthy sources of protein (nuts, legumes, fish, poultry and eggs) are encouraged, but dairy consumption should be limited to one to two servings a day. The revised pyramid recommends minimizing the consumption of red meat, butter, refined grains (including white bread, white rice and white pasta), potatoes and sugar.

Trans fat does not appear at all in the pyramid, because it has no place in a healthy diet. A multiple vitamin is suggested for most people, and moderate alcohol consumption can be a worthwhile option (if not contraindicated by specific health conditions or medications). This last recommendation comes with a caveat: drinking no alcohol is clearly better than drinking too much. But more and more studies are showing the benefits of moderate alcohol consumption (in any form: wine, beer or spirits) to the cardiovascular system.

Men and women eating in accordance with THE NEW PYRAMID had a lower risk of major chonic disease.

Can we show that our pyramid is healthier than the USDA's? We created a new Healthy Eating Index that measured how closely a person's diet followed our recommendations. Applying this revised index to our epidemiological studies, we found that men and women who were eating in accordance with the new pyramid had a lower risk of major chronic disease [*see illustration on opposite page*]. This benefit resulted almost entirely from significant reductions in the risk of cardiovascular disease—up to 30 percent for women and 40 percent for men. Following the new pyramid's guidelines did not, however, lower the risk of cancer. Weight control and physical activity, rather than specific food choices, are associated with a reduced risk of many cancers.

Of course, uncertainties still cloud our understanding of the relation between diet and health. More research is needed to examine the role of dairy products, the health effects of specific fruits and vegetables, the risks and benefits of vitamin supplements, and the long-term effects of diet during childhood and early adult life. The interaction of dietary factors with genetic predisposition should also be investigated, although its importance remains to be determined.

Another challenge will be to ensure that the information about nutrition given to the public is based strictly on scientific evidence. The USDA may not be the best government agency to develop objective nutritional guidelines, because it may be too closely linked to the agricultural industry. The food pyramid should be rebuilt in a setting that is well insulated from political and economic interests.

WALTER C. WILLETT and *MEIR J. STAMPFER* are professors of epidemiology and nutrition at the Harvard School of Public Health. Willett chairs the school's department of nutrition, and Stampfer heads the department of epidemiology. Willett and Stampfer are also professors of medicine at Harvard Medical School. Both of them practice what they preach by eating well and exercising regularly.

The Low-Carb Frenzy

THE FORCE THAT IS RESHAPING THE FOOD INDUSTRY—AND OUR BODIES

By DANIEL KADLEC

LET GO FROM HIS JOB AS A HOTEL MANAGER LAST SUMMER, BRAD SALTZMAN had begun to panic by fall. Sure, his bank account was evaporating. But equally upsetting, he says, was that he was seeking too much comfort in the kitchen and was busting out of his belt. Physically and fiscally, Saltzman, 36, was a mess. Then he hit upon a cure-all: low carbs. Saltzman went on the Atkins diet at about the same time he helped launch Pure Foods, a specialty retailer based in Beverly Hills, Calif., that sells only products with comparatively few carbohydrates. Today Saltzman is 25 lbs. lighter, and his wallet is weighty. He has 24 employees, up from just four when he started, and will have 40 full-timers by June. "It was a eureka moment for me," Saltzman says of his carb-counting catharsis in October. "I needed to lose weight, and I needed a job in the next 30 days or—all kidding aside—I'd have had to move in with my grandmother." Instead, he's college-trim and planning a chain of stores and low-carb cafes and vending machines that he believes will ring up $100 million in sales annually within five years.

Critics of the carb counters' revolution may scoff at Saltzman's enthusiasm, believing that Atkins, South Beach, Zone and other protein-packed eating regimens are part of a fad that will soon run its course, like low-fat diets in the 1980s. But they can't deny his weight loss or that of countless others who have dropped 20 or 50 or 100 lbs. after cutting carbs from their meals. Exactly why all those pounds melt away when we give up potatoes and bread remains something of a mystery to the dieting public. Is it mostly the temporary loss of water weight? Do low-carb fanatics lose weight while consuming more calories, as a Harvard study suggests, or do they end up eating less because they simply get bored with the high-protein life? Or is there some sort of metabolic magic when steak, eggs and cheese replace the starches in our diet? The late Dr. Robert Atkins, who got the ball rolling in 1972, controversially ascribed the weight loss to ketosis, the fat-burning state a body reaches when deprived of carbs. His critics have bordered on fanatic, their stridency growing in proportion to the diet's increase in popularity.

Many Americans figure they will let the nutritionists hash all this out—and take all the time you please, thank you. In the meantime, as Saltzman discovered, there are pounds to drop and profits to crop. It seems as if everyone is giving the low-carb culture a whirl. Whoopi Goldberg does it. So do Jennifer Aniston and Bill Clinton. What's good enough for the stars is, of course, appealing to the rest of us. Some 26 million Americans are on a hard-core low-carb diet right now. And 70 million more limit their carb intake without formally dieting, according to a new poll by Opinion Dynamics Corp.

Counting carbs has become as powerful a fixture in the economy as

> ## $30 BILLION
>
> Expected sales of low-carb products this year. That's more than Coca-Cola generates in revenue from soft-drink sales worldwide

it has in society. Some 586 distinct new low-carb foods and beverages hit the grocery shelves last quarter, up from 633 in all of last year and 339 in 2002, bringing the total over just two years to 1,558 new entries. The average carb-conscious shopper spends $85 a month on specialty foods. Low-carb-related sales from such consumables as Michelob Ultra beer and books like *Dr. Atkins' New Diet Revolution* are expected to hit $30 billion this year, reports *LowCarbiz*, a trade publication that owes its existence to carbophobia.

Carb awareness is building by the day—to the consternation of companies even loosely in the business of selling the dreaded carbs. They are fighting back any way they can. Anheuser-Busch, which has launched Michelob Ultra and helped publicize that all light beers (including Bud Light) are relatively low in carbs, spent nearly $1 million for full-page ads that ran in 31 major newspapers last Friday. The ads pointedly attack the claim in Dr. Arthur Agatston's *South Beach Diet* that beer is laden with the carb maltose, a sugar. "The South Beach diet is enormously popular," says Francine Katz, a spokeswoman for Anheuser. "But there is information in there about beer that is incorrect, and a call to any brewer would have cleared it up." She says that all maltose turns to alcohol and carbonation in the brewing process and that Anheuser won't rule out legal action if Agatston fails to set the record straight.

Those with less at stake are embracing the trend. When baseball opened for business this spring, many ballparks were promoting low-carb concessions, from bison burgers on low-carb buns at Cleveland's Jacobs Field to braised pork "wings" at St. Louis Busch Stadium. This month burger chain Hardee's signed baseball great Mark McGwire, known as Big Mac, to flog its bunless Thickburger, playing catch-up with the other Big Mac, McDonald's, which is phasing out supersize portions and offering adult Happy Meals that are carb conscious. Burger King is launching an Angus steakburger that can come wrapped in lettuce and slathered with low-carb steak sauce. Krispy Kreme says it will have a low-sugar—and therefore lower-carb—doughnut by year's end.

Even before the food chains caught on, local eateries were offering Atkins-friendly menus. "We'll never take French fries and onion rings off the menu," says Miles Angelo, a chef at the upscale Caribou Club in Aspen, Colo. "But I was forced to read the Atkins book and immerse myself in the whole diet. Now 50% of our menu can be prepared Atkins-approved."

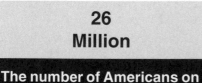

26 Million

The number of Americans on a hard-core low-carb diet right now

In grocery stores, niche firms like Atkins Nutritionals, founded by Atkins (the bulk of it was recently sold for more than $500 million), and Ketogenics have so far been responsible for most of the low-carb breakfast bars and other packaged foods to hit the grocery aisles. But now the big boys are crowding into the act.

Frito-Lay has unveiled Tostitos and Doritos Edge, in which soy protein is used in place of starch to lower the chips' carb count. Unilever has a Carb Options line of 32 products that include reformulated Ragú sauce, Wish-Bone salad dressing and Lipton tea with fewer carbs. Coors has begun marketing its new low-carb Aspen Edge to compete with Michelob Ultra. "The mainstream food and beverage manufacturers have finally made low carb a priority," says Suzanna Prong Eygabroat, an analyst at market-research firm Productscan Online.

What has shaken the food giants to act is surveys like the one from research firm Mintel International showing that 3 of every 5 low-carb dieters say they plan to limit carb intake for life. Half the people who tried a low-carb diet in the past 12 months and 1 in 3 who tried a low-carb diet more than a year ago are still limiting their carb intake, according to a Morgan Stanley study. Says Morgan analyst Bill Pecoriello: "Carb watching should hold pretty steady long after low-carb diets lose their popularity."

Americans are the most overweight population on the planet, and obesity is fast becoming a national health crisis. The Centers for Disease Control and Prevention reported that poor diet and lack of exercise, which killed 400,000 Americans in 2000, may soon overtake tobacco, which killed 435,000 people that year, as the leading preventable cause of death in the U.S.

You would think that any development—fad or not—that takes an inch or two off our collective girth would be well received. "Other countries are laughing at us," says Harry Balzer, vice president at NPD Group, a market-research firm that studies eating patterns in the U.S. Those slim, wine-drinking, chain-smoking Europeans chuckle at our diet and health obsessiveness, since we continue to overeat. Yet there are signs that carb counting may be working. In its latest annual report, NPD found that after six consecutive years of weight gain, the number of overweight adult Americans fell 1 percentage point, to 55%. Was it carb counting? No one really knows. But at fast-food restaurants, salad orders (low in carbs) rose 12%, while French-fries consumption (carb mountain) fell 10%.

The more carb counting becomes ingrained in our lives, the more worried many nutritionists grow. They argue that low-carb weight loss, while real, will not last for many folks, who once they stop dieting will obey their taste buds and return to the junk foods they love. "I work with a lot of people who have obsessive-compulsive food issues," says Darlene Kvist, a nutritionist in St. Paul, Minn. "Once they get that taste back in their mouth, then it's really hard for them not to want more and more."

What if they stay off carbs indefinitely? This is where the jury is out. A growing body of medical evidence supports the notion that in the short term, low-carbing can work for weight loss and that getting slimmer is beneficial in fighting heart disease and diabetes. The study of long-term effects is only now getting under way, and one worry is the higher cholesterol counts that can accompany a diet rich in fatty meats. Unequivocally, high cholesterol levels contribute to heart disease.

How does carb counting work? In simple terms, carbs are digested or broken down into sugars, which then circulate in the bloodstream. As sugar levels in the blood rise, so does insulin. Peaks of insulin push the body to store excess sugar as fat. By cutting carbs, you effectively cut sugar surges and not only store less fat but also start to burn off more of the fat you have. If this were the whole story, of course, there would be little controversy and none of the colossal food frenzy being waged among companies desperate to get on the right side of the carb culture.

But there is a second front in carb wars—good carbs vs. bad carbs. The good ones are found in whole-grain breads, beans, fruits and vegetables. They contain fiber and break down slowly when digested, avoiding those damaging sugar and insulin spikes. The bad ones are found in white rice, potatoes, most commercial breads and all manner of processed crackers, cookies, chips, soda and candy bars. Bad carbs break down more quickly and result in sugar overload.

As you might imagine, those in the carb business are trying to claim that their carbs are the benevolent ones. The most extensive push has come from pasta manufacturers, which in February footed most of the bill for a global summit in Rome, gathering scientists, physicians, nutritionists and chefs to address the carb issue. Their somewhat predictable finding: pasta is wonderful; the cereal grains used to make some types contain critical nutrients that break down slowly.

If science is unavailing, there is always marketing. The U.S. Potato Board and Idaho Potato Commission, alarmed at a 5% drop in potato consumption, have launched separate ad campaigns playing up the vitamin C and potassium in spuds and the energy value of carbs for active people. Orange-juice manufacturers are bitter over a similar decline in consumption that they attribute to Agatston's South Beach diet, which holds that o.j. carries an excessive sugar load. "Obesity? Diabetes? These are not a by-product of people drinking too much orange juice," says Eric Boomhower of the Florida department of citrus. At one point, citrus growers looked into whether they could use an obscure state law against disparaging agriculture to sue Agatston. "There is a shift in consumer demand," Agatston responds. "People should get on the bandwagon and stop complaining." The growers have done both. They launched a $7 million ad campaign last week playing up their product's nutritional value, and they have started offering lower-carb juice.

ALL THIS SPIN CAN MAKE THE LOW-CARB universe difficult to navigate.

But there are a few simple things to keep in mind. First, any bald-faced low-carb claims can get foodmakers into trouble—call it carbage. That's because the Food and Drug Administration has yet to define what constitutes a low-or light-or reduced-carb anything. Hence the proliferation of fuzzier labeling terms like carb smart, carb conscious, carb aware and carb fit. Russell Stover, for example, received a warning letter from the agency about the name of its Low Carb line of chocolates. The company has offered to change the name but hopes it won't have to since the FDA announced in March that the agency will come up with a definition for *low carb*.

Second, there is the confusing notion of net carbs. Some manufacturers subtract the good carbs from the bad ones and advertise the difference. This is a slippery slope because the FDA insists that a carb is a carb is a carb. So net carbs are not the same as fewer carbs.

Third, some low-carb products are so loaded with extra calories that they pose an unnecessary hurdle to weight loss. Take Subway's traditional 280-calorie 6-in. sandwich, the one that helped Jared slim down and find a gig as Subway's pitchman. That's about half the calories of the Atkins-friendly Subway chicken bacon ranch wrap. Want real results? Order the traditional sandwich on the tortilla wrap for fewer carbs *and* fewer calories.

Finally, some low-carb products never had many carbs to begin with. Wish-Bone Carb Options ranch dressing has zero carbs, but the regular version has just 1 g per 2tbsp. serving. Unless you're knocking the stuff back like beer at a frat party, the difference is a joke. And speaking of beer, Miller Lite now markets itself as a low-carb brew though it never changed the recipe. It just happened to be low carb all along (3.2 g per 12 oz., vs. 12 g for the typical beer).

No matter where you stand on the carb issue, what should be clear by now is the staying power of a trend that is sending tremors through the

economic food chain. Not even December's mad-cow scare has put a dent in beef consumption. Pork bellies, which give us bacon, are trading at record high prices. Egg prices have hit a 20-year high. The stock price of Cal-Maine Foods, a leading fresh-egg producer, has soared nearly sevenfold in 12 months. Some economists go so far as to credit the low-carb culture as a chief force in revitalizing our farm-belt economy.

Here is how a diet revolution is rippling through the economy:

■ THE FOOD GIANTS WEIGH IN

THE LOW-CARB CRAZE IS ALSO ROILING THE world's biggest food-manufacturing companies. H.J. Heinz Co., whose frozen entrees have been hammered by the low-carb lifestyle, is taking carbs out of its Smart Ones lineup; Nestlé is doing the same with Lean Cuisine. Heinz pulled 75% of the carbs out of its flagship ketchup for a One Carb version that hit stores last week. Hershey has introduced 1 gram Sugar Carb chocolate bars.

Meanwhile, General Mills has acknowledged that higher egg demand suggests that many consumers are eating omelets instead of cereal. The company, which partly attributed poor financial results last quarter to carb counting, is responding with a higher-protein/lower-carb version of Total cereal. It will unveil 40 new products in May, including low-carb Hamburger Helper. Kraft is working on a CarbWell line of salad dressings and barbecue sauces, and is recasting its marketing to feature the meager carb content of sugar-free Jell-O. Breyers is rolling out CarbSmart Klondike bars.

On it goes. Launching a new food line is no small undertaking. Consumer research and continual tinkering with the formula can cost millions of dollars and require two years from concept to shelf. Diet foods are trickiest because a company must determine the trade-off between taste and calorie count that will please the most people. Sara Lee, recognizing that its carbcentric baked-goods line is vulnerable, has begun marketing Delightful breads with fewer carbs. The company sees a secondary market for low-carb products: the world's 171 million diabetics, for whom carbs can be a deadly sin. The number of diabetics will grow to 366 million by 2030, according to World Health Organization estimates released this week. "Low-carb products will make it easier for diabetics to control their diets while giving them access to foods that were formerly strictly limited," says Edward O'Neill, associate director of the food-processing center at the University of Nebraska in Lincoln. The diabetic market alone can sustain many of the low-carb products coming to life, he notes.

1,558

Number of new low-carb products that have hit stores since 2002

Unilever is investing more aggressively than most in carb counting. It rushed the Carb Options line—the company's largest brand launch in two years—to market in a blistering 12 months, half the usual time for new products. Mike Polk, chief operating officer of Unilever Bestfoods North America, predicts that sales of low-carb packaged foods will almost double, to $700 million, this year and will rise to $1 billion in 2005. "We want to be a big share of that market," he says. One reason that Unilever is embracing low carbs is that its Slim-Fast line of meal-replacement shakes (low calorie but not so low carb), whose sales peaked at $1 billion in 2002, has dropped off the radar; sales fell 21% last year. Kraft's SnackWells and other diet products have ridden the same roller coaster. Slim-Fast's recovery plan is to tailor 40% of its products to low-carb dieters.

■ THE LOW-CARB AISLE

YOU MAY HAVE NOTICED THE ADDITIONAL shelf space that low-carb goods are getting in your supermar-

ket. The Albertson's chain now offers more than 100 low-carb products, compared with just 10 less than a year ago. "We found it's having a profound effect," says Andrew Kramer, Albertson's director of ethnic marketing and specialty foods. Sales in his category more than doubled last year, led by growth in low-carb lines. Meanwhile, the central action alley at Wal-Mart SuperCenters crammed some 200 low-carb products into a 16-ft. run during prime dieting season after New Year's. The company is considering launching its own line of low-carb foods, which would surely narrow the price premium that many of these items carry.

■ THE LOW-CARB MENU

YOU SIMPLY CANNOT BE IN THE DINING BUSINESS these days and not have a low-carb lineup. Since sub-shop chain Blimpie's introduced its Carb Counter menu in October, sales have kept fattening up, 8% to 10% each month. Mirroring that success, T.G.I. Friday's says its restaurant traffic bumped up 10% for a couple of months after it introduced an officially Atkins-approved menu in December.

12%

The increase in salad orders at U.S. fast-food outlets from 2002 to 2003

Friday's CEO Richard Snead says he came around on Atkins last summer, when waiters at the company's 500 or so U.S. restaurants began to notice a big wave of customers substituting vegetables for potatoes, which left the restaurants holding a surplus of spuds and struggling to fill the side orders. "It didn't take a lot of research to understand that America was under the influence of the Atkins revolution," Snead says. Enter menu items like the Tuscan spinach dip and the tuna-salad wrap. Ruby Tuesday, which was one of the first to start serving Atkins-friendly Splenda on the table next to the traditional Sweet'n Low, Equal and sugar pack-

ets, now has some 40 low-carb items on its revamped menu.

■ PUBLISHING'S PROFIT CENTER

AT ANY GIVEN MOMENT, a quarter of the adult population is on a diet, a figure that has remained fairly steady for decades. Not surprisingly, the publishing world has built a reliable revenue stream serving this market, pumping out titles addressing any and all diet concerns of the day. Book publishers "will jump on any bandwagon," notes Nora Rawlinson, editor in chief of *Publishers Weekly*.

They have truly swarmed this one. More than 140 low-carb books are in print, and 51 more are due out this year, up from just 15 in 1999, reports Simba Information, a publishing-research firm. The crush of new titles exploits every crevice of the low-carb market: *Low-Carb Cocktails, Low-Carb Slow Cooker Recipes* and *Low-Carb Smoothies*. There is *Low-Carb Dieting for Dummies* as well as *The Complete Idiot's Guide to Low-Carb Meals*. It was only a matter of time before a book came along to compare the low-carb diet books. When it did, in mid-January, Jonny Bowden's *Living the Low Carb Life* briefly displaced *The Da Vinci Code* as the best-selling title on BarnesandNoble.com

In all, diet and health books rang up an estimated $500 million in sales last year, and much of that loot was low-carb related. The frenzy continues to be led by *Dr. Atkins' New Diet Revolution,* which has been on the New York *Times* best-seller list for nearly seven years. Even the upstart *South Beach Diet*, which hit print just last year, has spent 53 weeks on the list. Magazines are jumping on the bandwagon too. *Low Carb Energy* will join *LowCarb Living* on newsstands nationwide next month. "No one could have forecast that this cyclone was coming," says Jim Capparell, publisher of *LowCarb Living*. He sat on his idea for nearly a year before acting. "If this is a fad," he adds, "I hope it's as long-lived as low fat, which took 22 years to come and go."

■ DIET INC. DOWNER

THE DIET INDUSTRY IS IN distress. Massive numbers of dieters have migrated to low-carb strategies in the past couple of years, exiting programs that emphasize portion control. The heavyweights of the diet industry, Weight Watchers and Jenny Craig, are feeling the pinch. "Any time there is anything new in the market, it is going to affect clients who want to lose weight quickly," says Cozette Phifer, spokeswoman at Jenny Craig. She concedes that new business is depressed but asserts that the dip won't last long. Both companies say they have refrained from introducing low-carb items because their nutritionists oppose the idea and think it's a fad that will fade. "We believe carbohydrates are an important part of a balanced diet," says Jim Evans, CEO of Jenny Craig.

At Weight Watchers, which is publicly traded, the stock has been sputtering in a strong market since October 2002, and net income has been flat for two years. The firm gets most of its revenue from memberships, which have been flagging, says analyst Kathleen Heaney at the Maxim Group, a New York City brokerage firm. That's temporary, according to Eliot Glazer, vice president of North American marketing for Weight Watchers. "A lot of what is behind low carbs is pseudo science," he says. He reports seeing a flood of disheartened low-carb dieters come to Weight Watchers as "they find they really need help to lose weight."

■ THE BAD-NEWS BEERS

BEER IS WIDELY SEEN AS BAD NEWS FOR anyone counting carbs, which helps explain why beer consumption was down 1.6% last year and why Anheuser is determined to wrest a correction out of Agatston. Interestingly, Anheuser stumbled on the maltose issue when one of its St. Louis—based brewmasters, John Serbia, read Agatston's book before starting the South Beach diet this winter. Serbia ignored the part about abstaining from beer and lost 15 lbs., says Anheuser spokeswoman Katz.

Still, while beer sales have gone flat, volume increased 3% last year for spirits, which generally contain no carbs. Alcohol of any sort is frowned upon in almost every diet because it contains calories and can act as an appetite stimulant. In some cases the body may turn to the more readily available alcohol instead of stored fat to burn as an energy source.

> ## 194
> ### The number of low-carb books that will be in print by year-end, up from 15 in 1999

Despite all that, the spirits industry has made hay with its low-carb status. Distillers, including Bacardi and Diageo, have launched ad campaigns to trumpet their spirits' carblessness. Diageo, which makes Smirnoff, the world's top-selling premium vodka, created the website LowCarbParties.com to tell drinkers how to decarb their cocktails. "The spirit is not the problem," says food and wine expert Ted Allen from *Queer Eye for the Straight Guy*, who helped launch the site. "It's the mixer." Liquor and grocery stores are beginning to carry products like Baja Bob's low-carb margarita mix, which has been sold online and in specialty stores for four years and is now getting space at Meijer and other supermarkets in the Midwest and Northwest. Sales were up 380% last year.

This spirited success spawned the growth of new low-carb beers, which started with phenomenally successful Ultra and now include Coors Aspen Edge and Rolling Rock's Rock Green Light. As a class, these brews are saving the day because "everything else went into the doldrums," says Harry Schuhmacher, editor of the newsletter *Beer Business Daily*. Anheuser attributes its record U.S. beer sales last year (103 million bbl., up 800,000) in large part to Ultra, which was launched in late 2002 and whose sales have more than quadrupled initial projections. "It became the fastest-growing beer brand since Miller Lite was introduced in 1975," says Schuhmacher. The company quietly reformulated its Natural Lite to add to the low-carb train. Promoting low-carb beer got a little trickier this month when the Feds warned against ads portraying these drinks as even remotely healthy.

CAN ANYTHING STOP THE LOW-CARB CULTURE? Not likely anytime soon. It will be years before we have conclusive long-term research on health risks. The arrival of big food companies in this fray means big money is at play and low-carb living will be marketed with a vengeance. The undisputed benefit of low-carb products to diabetics means a durable customer base. And extreme weight-loss methods like having your stomach stapled—though it worked for lovable TV weatherman Al Roker—have proved ineffective for up to 20% of those who tried them. So the fast results and pure simplicity of cutting carbs promise lasting appeal.

That is, until we get sick of it. In the end, the biggest risk to the culture may be the inevitable false or misleading low-carb claims and influx of products that ladle on heapings of calories in exchange for carbs. If enough people are seduced by these foods and fail to lose weight, low carbs will go the way of low fat: a strategy that works when you stick to the rules but fails when marketers rush in with promises no one can keep.

With reporting by Julie Rawe, Alice Park and Daren Fonda/New York; Wendy Cole/Chicago; Jeanne DeQuine/Miami; Rita Healy/Denver; Marc Hequet/St. Paul; Hilary Hylton/Austin; Laura A. Locke/San Francisco; and Sean Scully/Los Angeles

Getting Personal With Nutrition

Some of us have personal trainers, monogrammed towels, vanity license plates, or at least value our "personal" space, but are we ready for "personalized nutrition?"

Well, at least 130 delegates from 17 countries who attended the Second International Conference on Nutrigenomics in Amsterdam, The Netherlands in early November think we might be. A wealth of information about the role of genes in determining our health has become available with the deciphering of the human genome. The concept of "personalized nutrition," or "nutrigenomics" as some scientists call it, takes this information one step further. Personalized nutrition involves the establishment of individual dietary recommendations based on knowledge of nutritional requirements, nutritional status, and each person's unique genetic makeup to potentially reduce risk of disease. Many speakers emphasized that, although this new knowledge is very intriguing, we are still at early points on the learning curve despite the tremendous potential of nutrigenomics.

Shedding Light on the Science

According to Dr. Jose Ordovas of Tufts University, society has often embraced a "one-size-fits-all" approach to current dietary recommendations, such as low-fat and low-cholesterol diets for the entire population. Although this broad approach to recommendations will likely benefit the majority of people, research indicates that a number of complicated genetic factors may minimize the benefits of such dietary changes, potentially harm some individuals, or have no effect for some.

Different species, such as mice and humans, have particular genes in common; however, the genome, or an entire set of genes in a particular arrangement, is unique to each individual. Dr. Ben van Ommen, of TNO Nutrition and Food Research in The Netherlands, stated that it is now possible to determine the sequences of a whole genome and determine how the genes in that genome are expressed; rather than focus on one gene as a single datum point. "Nobody is equal, and neither are our genes, since every gene has at least ten variants," van Ommen said. He also emphasized that nutrition provides more subtle changes to gene expression than do pharmaceuticals.

Robert Kushner, MD, Medical Director of the Wellness Institute at the Northwestern Feinberg School of Medicine and Northwestern Memorial Hospital, shared his perspectives on how physicians may provide information on personalized nutrition to have better quality discussions with their patients. "Nutrigenomics has the potential to spark interest among physicians in seeing that nutritional needs are more clearly determined for individuals," Dr. Kushner stated.

Professor Michael Muller, of Wageningen University in the Netherlands, defined nutrigenomics as an attempt to study the genome-wide influences of nutrition by combining nutrition at the molecular level with genomics. He asked, is it possible that someday we might move from our broad-beam flashlight-approach to adopt more of a fine-tuned laser beam-approach to nutrition recommendations, making them very specific to an individual's needs?

Consumers Lead the Way

The conference featured an impressive array of scientific findings and experts showing great enthusiasm about future possibilities, but what do consumers think about all of this?

Unveiling highlights from a comprehensive, landmark survey of US consumer attitudes toward the broad area of genomics, including nutrigenomics, Christy White, principal of Cogent Research in Cambridge, Massachusetts, indicated that consumers are ready to learn more.

Three-fourths of Americans are interested in obtaining their personal genetic information to identify their risk of diseases like cancer, osteoporosis, and heart disease, and nearly half of Americans are prepared to use diet-related products tailored to their health needs on the basis of their genetic makeup, according to Cogent's October 2003 survey of 1,000 Americans. "Americans are ready and willing to buy products based upon their genetic information, but the science is only in the early stages of being able to deliver," said White. "The good news is consumers aren't looking for complete diet regimens, but for individual approaches and basic recommendations."

The survey reveals that more than 90 percent of Americans are aware of the connection between diet and health, and 71 percent believe that genetics play a crucial role in health

Examining the Ethical Issues of Nutrigenomics

New research designed to help consumers create customized diets on the basis of their genetic make-up could create ethical and legal challenges with serious implications for the scientific and medical communities, according to a panel of international experts.

Dr. David Castle of the University of Guelph presented a paper in Amsterdam, *Nutrition and Genes: Science, Society and the Supermarket*, a joint project of the University of Toronto Joint Centre for Bioethics (JCB) and the University of Guelph philosophy department, the study examines the ethical questions surrounding nutrigenomics, the study of how nutrients and genes interact, and how genetic variations can cause people to respond differently to food nutrients. Castle cautioned against a rush to embrace nutritional genomics before there has been a detailed examination of its moral and ethical implications, backed by national awareness campaigns and public consultations.

The paper, prepared by a nine-member panel of international experts, stops short of prescribing specific ethical guidelines for the development and implementation of nutritional genomics technology. Rather, it is designed to foster public debate, setting out the issues that must be considered as consumers begin customizing diets to prevent and mitigate chronic health conditions. The panel wants input from professional groups, citizens' organizations, and individuals before it issues recommendations. Which it will do in 2004.

Environmental and lifestyle factors are thought to play a large role in the development of many diseases. However, science has determined, for example, that most people's genetic predisposition to cardiovascular disease is dependent upon variations in scores of genes, each of which appears to lead to small increases in susceptibility. As well, it appears that one gene can be involved in a number of conditions. Genetic testing may be able only to indicate an increased susceptibility to cardiovascular disease, rather than the certainty of future disease, the paper says.

The paper identifies the following as principal concerns:

• When is the science strong enough to market genetic tests in a widespread way?

• Who should have access to nutritional genomics information, who should not, and how should improper access be prevented?

• How should nutritional genomics information be delivered to consumers?

• How can society prevent potential nutritional genomics-related inequities, especially those created between developed and developing countries?

• Which nutritional genomics concerns should be the subject of regulation and oversight?

Use of Nutritional Genomic-Related Information

"As more is learned about individual genetic susceptibility to disease, information from genetic tests may become increasingly attractive to outside parties who stand to gain from it," the paper says. "There is a concern that employers or insurers could use genetic information to the unfair disadvantage of some people." Two-thirds of respondents in a 1997 survey said that they would not undergo genetic testing if they thought that health insurers and employers would have access to the results.

One of the most important issues is whether private genetic information should be treated as confidential in nature and not communicated to others without consent. Personal medical information usually remains private, but genetic tests may be relevant to blood relatives. Physicians may therefore face situations in which they must choose between patient confidentiality and providing potentially useful information to other members of the same family.

The main purpose of looking for food-gene interactions is to prevent or reduce the risk of disease; so the sooner useful dietary changes are made, the better the chances of avoiding nutrition-related diseases are. This suggests that testing children early would provide the widest range of health benefits. However, a balance must be maintained between acting in the interests of children before they are mature enough to make decisions and interfering with their right to the confidentiality of their genetic information. "This raises the question of whether the decision to administer a nutritional genomics test to a child falls within the legitimate range of parental discretion," says Dr. Castle.

"The collection, storage, and use of genetic information will be one of the most hotly debated medical issues of the coming decade," says Dr. Abdallah Daar of JCB and director of the Program in Applied Ethics and Biotechnology. "Even at this early stage, scientific progress is outstripping the public's ability to make informed choices about what kind of regulations should be introduced to address ethical and privacy concerns."

For more information go to the JCB Web site (http://www.utoronto.ca/jcb).

throughout life. However, 73 percent are concerned about how personal genetic information would be stored and who would have access to that information (see "Examining the Ethical Issues of Nutrigenomics" above).

In October 2003, the US Senate unanimously passed the Genetic Privacy Bill, which would prevent health plans from providing access to insurance companies on the basis of genetic information and from using such information to underwrite policies. Employers would be allowed to collect genetic information only to determine overall workplace exposures but could not use the information in hiring. Although the

Bush administration supports the bill, the House must still approve it.

Cogent Research also found that consumers most strongly preferred the term "personalized nutrition" with the term "nutrigenomics" being the least-liked term among the terms tested to describe this emerging area. Other terms tested included "nutrigenetics," "individualized nutrition," and "nutritional genomics." Cogent's conclusions on terminology are consistent with research that the International Food Information Council Foundation commissioned Cogent to conduct in December 2002. The findings of Cogent Research are from a broader, syndicated research study on genomics that explored applications including pharmaceuticals, health and beauty products, and nutrition. The study marks one of the largest efforts to understand consumers' acceptance of the use of their genetic information to influence the balance between health and disease.

What will it take to bring the promise of personalized nutrition to reality? Dr. Bruce German of the University of California at Davis painted the big picture for the delegates in Amsterdam. He sees this new knowledge as an opportunity to empower individuals to make informed and personal choices for their diet and lifestyle. According to German, "Scientists can enable the joys of life but not tell people what to do with their lives. We don't want to be the same—we want to be as healthy as we want to be. Success will involve personalizing health and delight simultaneously!"

Reprinted from the International Food Information Council Foundation, (December 2003).

Food, Spirituality, & Mindful Eating

By Mary Kaye Sawyer-Morse, PhD, RD

In this day and age, where there is an abundance of information on diets and dieting, it is interesting to note that Americans seem more disconnected from food than ever. Food is everywhere, and yet our relationship with it can be described as an ongoing struggle reflected by the increasing number of individuals experiencing obesity, overeating, and/or eating disorders.

Food plays a prevalent role in the media and our culture. We are bombarded daily about weight-loss diets, genetically modified or irradiated foods, food-borne illnesses, famine relief, organics, and food-linked health ailments. Most individuals would also view food as a basic tool for survival. Food, therefore, is included in multiple aspects of our culture: body image, entertainment, religious practices, art forms, and myriad social rituals. Somewhere among this cacophony of messages are ideas about our relationships with food and how it supports our general welfare beyond the physical aspects. In other words, what role does food play in our spiritual well-being?

Food and Cultural Traditions

The concept that food choices can impact our spiritual well-being is not new; numerous examples come from a variety of religions and cultures. These various world traditions frequently serve as guides for how to live and denote the connection between food and spirituality. Regardless of personal beliefs about food, these valued traditions encourage us to honor food and consume it with reverence and sincerity. When approached in this manner, food then nourishes both body and soul in a deeper, more satisfying way—a relationship that is difficult to achieve through a fast-food takeout window and a Happy Meal.

Specific cultural examples highlighting the spiritual dimensions of food include how Judaism's dietary laws are designed to honor the sanctity of life that is in both animal and plant-based food and that following the prescribed dietary laws is a reflection of respect for creation.

The concept that food choices can impact our spiritual well-being is not new; numerous examples come from a variety of religions and cultures.

Christians honor the divine by connecting to Jesus Christ through the ceremony of Holy Communion. In this particular ritual, the taking of bread and wine has a significance of something much larger than the rite itself. The ceremony, which invites Christians to experience Jesus' godliness through the ingestion of the bread and wine, nourishes a multidimensional hunger. It might be expressed as an experience designed to nourish not only the physical but also the emotional and spiritual.

Islam also offers an appreciation for the connection between food and spirituality. *Understanding Islam and the Muslims* (Embassy of Saudi Arabia, 1988) states, "The Prophet taught that ... the consumption of wholesome food ... [is a] religious obligation." Specific dietary laws detailed in the Koran ask Muslims to approach food with a heartfelt thankfulness and awareness of God's great gifts. This thankfulness and awareness of God's bounty expressed in food is especially evident during the holy time of Ramadan. During this time, millions of devout Muslims throughout the world fast, observe the scripture, and pray from dawn to sunset. As the Ramadan fast is broken each day after sunset, prayers of appreciation are given for the food and all of life's gifts and blessings.

Another example comes from Buddhism, which maintains that enlightenment or awakening beyond everyday word and thought is our "natural" state. This enlightened

10 Tips to Mindful, Enlightened Eating

1. **Focus on fellowship.** A key aspect to cultural traditions and wisdom is that sharing food is done as part of a community. Dine with others and share your meals with family or friends. Plan to have a least one meal per week where you sit down with others and share what is meaningful to you.

2. **Give thanks.** Express thanks for the food, perhaps with a prayer, if that is your tradition. Acknowledge your connection with all life and the daily gift of nourishment.

3. **Create a ritual.** A ritual can be any practice that connects us with the sacred. Even if your meal is just a sandwich, one way to appreciate and connect with the food is through a ritual that engages all of your senses—sight, taste, touch, and smell.

4. **Grow your own.** Explore the possibility of community gardening, either in an existing space or somewhere new. Working with other people is a great way to stay motivated and get results that would be difficult to achieve alone. If this is not possible, use whatever small space you have—either in the backyard or a container—to grow herbs, decorative and edible vegetables, or flowering fruits. Renew your relationship with all life and connect with the magic of seeds, dirt, and water.

5. **Plan ahead.** Plan to take care of yourself by always carrying fresh water and a healthy snack with you. Avoid making food decisions or doing your food shopping when you are ravenously hungry and will eat anything. Making time for your own needs will provide more energy for your busy day and give you a sense of peace and calm.

6. **Slow down.** Even if you're in a hurry or meeting a deadline while you're eating, pause at least briefly to reflect on the gift of food. Take a few seconds to observe the food and feel what it provides for you. Make a mental checklist of the qualities of the food and how it matches and satisfies your hunger.

7. **Buy local.** Investigate the farmer's markets in your area. The more local the food, the less processing it generally has to go through to get to your table (and often the less chemical spraying, in contrast to out-of-season produce and products shipped from other countries). Talk with your growers and learn who is committed to the idea of healthier foods. They are also a good source of information about what is available in your area.

8. **Share your experiences.** Talk with family, friends, and coworkers about the changes you are making. Encourage them to take time to share meals with you and others important to them.

9. **Connect with the present moment.** Stay in the moment when you eat, shop for, or prepare food. Start with small steps by focusing on the appearance, aroma, or texture of the food. Enjoy the process of creating a nourishing meal.

10. **Go with the flow.** Let these changes occur naturally. Be mindful of what is important to you. Small changes make a difference.

state may be experienced by bringing a mindful, meditative awareness to all aspects of our lives, including food: its selection, preparation, serving, and eating.

There is a common thread—virtually all religions and cultural traditions encourage treating food with reverence and cooking it with love. In addition, many traditions incorporate the idea that food nourishes and restores us on multiple levels. In other words, food and our relationship with it can address physiological problems and deficiencies, unite us with a spiritual dimension, and connect us to a sense of community.

Spirit-Filled Food

Deborah Kesten, in her book *Feeding the Body, Nourishing the Soul: Essentials of Eating for Physical, Emotional, and Spiritual Well-Being* (Conari Press, 1997), describes how food can actually be transformed by love so that it is "infused" with spirit. Her firsthand experience with this process came from spending an evening with

Leonard Laskow, MD, physician and author of *Healing with Love: A Breakthrough Mind/Body Medical Program for Healing Yourself and Others* (Wholeness Press, 1998), who not only explained the method of infusing liquids and food with loving energy but also demonstrated it on that particular evening's meal. Kesten notes that after the "infusion" experiment, the individuals around the dinner table could smell and taste a difference between the "loved" and "unloved" nourishment.

Is this possible? Does what you're thinking and feeling while you are cooking influence the quality of the food? Who knows for sure?

There are, however, hundreds of published studies on the interaction and exchange of awareness between people and plants. A classic example is *The Secret Life of Plants* (Harper & Row, 1972) by Peter Tompkins and Christopher Bird, which gives a variety of demonstrations illustrating how a person's intention—to harm or to care for—affects the plant. Other research detailed in Laskow's *Healing With Love* suggests that plants and food somehow sense and respond to verbal and nonverbal communication from humans.

You may find these ideas extraordinary or perhaps outrageous and unbelievable. Nonetheless, they suggest an interconnectedness of all life. At the very least, by bringing a loving consciousness to food, you connect at a deeper level to the nourishment process. Kesten suggests that you consider creating your own spiritually imbued food and see whether or not you can detect a difference between foods prepared by hand in a conscious, loving manner and those that were not.

Journey to Mindful Eating

It has been a typical, busy day. You managed to drink a cup of coffee before dashing into the early morning staff meeting. Back-to-back patient appointments forced you to skip lunch. Late afternoon finds you at your desk munching on a stale bagel and washing it down with warm orange juice. You're not enjoying the food or even sure if you are hungry, but you know you should eat something.

Sound familiar? How many times have you eaten and then wondered what you had for lunch? Or left the table full, only to find yourself munching your way through the refrigerator one hour later? When you are not mindful and attentive, food and eating become just another activity, an unconscious habit.

Food and our relationship with it can address physiological problems and deficiencies, unite us with a spiritual dimension, and connect us to a sense of community.

The concept of mindful awareness meditation and its application to eating is not specific to any religious practice. Mindfulness may be used at any time, in any setting, with any meal, and involves regarding food and its preparation as sacred. The process requires only your willingness to shift from being on automatic pilot to being fully aware of the moment. Here's how to begin:

Focus

Take several deep breaths and allow yourself to relax into the present moment. When you are rushing, your thoughts and energy are somewhere else. Turn off the television or radio and put away the newspaper. Do not answer the telephone. Rather, focus on maintaining a present-moment awareness throughout the entire meal preparation and consuming process.

Visualize and Plan

See in your mind's eye what you are going to prepare. See each individual food. Focus on the steps you will take to prepare the meal and whom you are preparing it for. As other thoughts enter your mind, simply let them pass and bring yourself back to the meal visualization.

Prepare

Continue your mindful awareness as you prepare the food. Notice the crispness of the vegetables, aroma of the onion, and sizzle in the pan.

Savor

To begin, consider offering a few words of thanks or appreciation for the food. Savor the aroma; chew slowly and experience the variety of flavors. Observe how the food feels in your stomach. Did you eat the right amount for your hunger? After the meal, spend a bit of time appreciating the connection with food and the sense of nourishment eating brings.

What you eat or don't eat is important, but it is not the primary ingredient for mindful eating. The fundamental key to mindful, healthy eating is learning how to change your state of mind. The wisdom of ancient cultures shows that food has always been a tool for spiritual growth and healthy living. Mindful eating provides a template on how to live consciously and with an awareness of how all aspects of life—from food to spirit to community—are connected.

—Mary Kaye Sawyer-Morse, PhD, RD, professional speaker and author, is the owner and education director of The Center for Success, a Texas-based company that provides keynotes, in-service training, and seminars to diverse industries. Her areas of expertise include life-work balance, creating behavior change, women's health issues, and understanding nutrition/health research.

Who's filling your grocery bag?

James E. Tillotson, PhD, MBA

Eight of our largest US food companies sell overwhelming amounts of the snacks that many Americans overeat. In all snack categories—soft drinks, candy, salty snacks, cookies, crackers, ice cream—1 or 2 mega-food companies dominate the market, selling from 50% to 75% of each type of fun food. What effect, if any, does this overarching market concentration have on Americans' obesity?

Nearly two thirds of American adults are overweight or obese, and many of our children are also getting unpleasantly plump. Therefore, it is important to examine all the factors in our food world, including the industry, that could contribute to overeating. In the last column, we saw that a few of the largest food companies—Pepsi, Mars, Coca-Cola, Nabisco, Frito-Lay—have dominant shares of fun-food markets—soft drinks, candy, ice cream, crackers, cookies, and salty snacks. Overwhelming marketing concentration means that these companies have a lot of clout in determining what products and marketing practices rule in the snack categories. Current industry structure and marketing practices deserve a searching look because of the role they *may* play in overeating. Any meaningful analysis must be *based on objective research, not on opinion or emotion*.

Table 1 shows the 8 leading fun-food companies discussed in part 1 of this article, the specific snacks marketed by each, and the estimated combined market share (in either sales or volume) of the 1 or 2 leading companies in each category (candy, carbonated beverages, etc.), as well as each company's total retail sales (2001). Several companies market more than one type of snacks. Some of these companies (Nestle, Unilever, Mars, Kraft, and Kellogg) market a broader range of branded foods than just snacks; others (Coca-Cola, PepsiCo, and Hershey) concentrate their marketing efforts predominantly on snack foods and beverages. Six of the companies are among our 10 largest food companies (sales), and the other 2 are among our 20 largest companies.

If public information is correct, 1 or 2 mega-food companies in each snack category have between 50% and 75% share of the market (based on either dollar or product volume). These are all tasty tempting snacks, which most of us eat in varying amounts. My immediate reaction, on finishing this chart, was to wonder if I had stumbled on one of the leading causes of American obesity.

Then I read a headline about a study by Gladys Block, Professor of Epidemiology and Public Health Nutrition, University of California Berkeley, which read: "Of the food Americans eat, sugary snacks and soda reign supreme over healthier options such as vegetables and fruits."[1] In her analysis of population-based data from the National Health and Nutrition Examination Survey (NHANES) data, she found that on average, *one-third of all Americans' calories* now come from what she defines as "junk food" (with sweets and desserts, soft drinks, and alcoholic beverages supplying many of the calories Americans consume).

One third of all Americans' calories now come from "junk food."

Is that it? Maybe the answer to the obesity problem is to ban, tax, or ration fun foods, and then we will all be svelte. (Except, of course, for those of us who will go to our neighborhood snack speakeasy for our daily fun food fix!). I suppose it's only a natural impulse to blame the marketing efforts of these mega-fun foods, with their outsized market shares and many customers, as "the" problem, simply because they supply so many of the treats we eat so much of so often. However, even 25 or 30 years ago snacks contributed approximately one quarter of all calories in diets, so there are probably other factors involved as well.

In examining the possible causes of heavily eating these leading snacks, we need to remember that we have an inherent liking for sweet, fatty, and salted fun foods (and many that contain alcohol, as well). By catering to this natural taste proclivity, it is likely that eaters will be highly attracted to these manufacturers' treats. Do snacks

Table 1. Major Food and Beverage Companies Selling Snack Categories in the United States

Snacks	Companies	Combined Category Market Share	2001 Sales,* $ Billion
Carbonated beverages	PepsiCo	Approximately 75% volume	26.9
	Coca Cola		20.1
Ice cream	Unilever	Approximately 50% sales	23.8
	Nestle		13.2
Candy	Mars	Approximately 70% sales	15.5†
	Hershey		4.6
Cookies	Nabisco (Kraft)	Approximately 50% sales	33.9
	Kellogg		8.9
Crackers	Nabisco (Kraft)	Approximately 60% sales	33.9
	Kellogg		8.9
Salty snacks	Frito-Lay (PepsiCo)	Approximately 56% sales	26.9
Non carbonated Beverages	PepsiCo	Approximately 75% volume	26.9
	Coca Cola		20.1

Sources: Food Institute, Food Processing, and assorted newspaper articles.
*Total company sales (all products) excluding food/beverage fast-food restaurants and food service subsidiaries.
†Sales for 2000.

produced by megacompanies pose greater risks of overeating just because of these companies' great size? Is the high fun-foods market concentration *alone* a factor in the increased consumption of snacks? *If these companies didn't offer these snacks, wouldn't there be other companies in their place equal in size who would do so?*

I have found no proof that such market concentration, *by itself*, and devoid of other potential advantages, is any more conducive to greater individual consumption than a greater number of medium-sized marketers or even many small companies. *Size alone apparently is not the source of the health problem.*

Are the *megafuns* answering consumers' unfilled natural desires for high levels of foods that contain sweets, fat, and salt that are high in calories, or are they driving consumption beyond people's natural desire levels by some sort of marketing trickery? Are major snack producers creating an *unnatural* demand by tricking our taste buds into overconsuming? Is the latter condition even physiologically or psychologically possible? It is unlikely; *you can't sell people what they don't want to buy.*

Not all people who are obese eat the same foods or even the same commercially prepared food. There are plenty of people who are obese who eat few of the fun foods—soft drinks, candy, salty snacks, ice cream, and fast foods—daily, whereas other people who are equally obese seem to eat nothing but snacks. No question that you can be overweight without fun foods; snacks *aren't the only culprits in obesity.*

Well then, if commercial snack and fun foods are not always a factor in obesity and there is no proof that market concentration, *by itself*, is a factor in increased con-

sumption, then maybe high market share firms are just more adept at catering to people's desires (product, price, and convenience) in snacks, and because of this, people eat a little more of their snacks a lot of the time. The big 8 in snacks didn't get there by just being run-of-the-mill organizations; they got there by being the best in their snack categories over decades. *Plainly and simply, they are better marketers than the other guys!*

We know carbonated beverages have doubled in annual average consumption in recent decades. What caused this to happen? Do we know how much of this increased consumption is the result solely of mega-beverage companies' superior marketing, distribution, and promotional efforts? How much can be attributed to answering unfilled consumer desire for more sweetened drinks? Are the marketers driving the consumer market, or is the consumer market driving the marketers? Are these trends compensated for by decreases in other categories, or is there a net increase overall in calories consumed? *Again, we have no answers.*

Perhaps extreme market concentration of the major snack producers allows for other avenues of influence on consumer consumption, and these, in turn, have an effect on overconsumption of snacks. Here are some, but not all, of the factors that have been suggested and may be involved:

- *Heavy marketing and high profit margins of snack and fun foods.* Industry sources report that among the product mix of these large fun-food companies, food and beverage snacks are commonly their most profitable products. Thus, there is an economic rationale for these companies to place their heaviest marketing emphasis and persuasive skills on their fun-food products. *Suspicion, but lack of proof.*

- *Megacompanies sell more than snack foods alone, so their marketing practices dominate supermarket shelves and consumer purchases.* If we focus our inquiry only on the snacks marketed by these food companies, we limit our understanding of the potential impact that these large companies may be having on Americans' diets. The 8 food and beverage companies listed had an estimated all-product retail sales total of $147 billion (2001), including their top snack brands. Obviously, as shown by their total sales number, the big 8 products in both fun and other types of foods are a significant part of the food purchases of many Americans. *Suspicion, but again lack of proof.*

- *Retail channels demand fun-food giants' products because of consumer demand.* The total US all-products food retail sales (supermarkets, non-food outlets, convenience stores, etc.) were $408.2 billion in 2001. These 8 food-fun giants combined with their other type of food products were apparently the source of 36% of all retail food sales. These mega-8 are a significant source of Americans' food purchases—*one third of all retail sales* (2001). As a result, our supermarkets and other retail outlets may be *required* to preferentially offer their products, both fun and otherwise, to satisfy their customers' everyday product demands. Does the high concentration of major sources of fun foods today in a few megacompanies combined with the broader range of other foods marketed result in retail-purchase condition, favoring purchase and consumption of their snacks?

- *Retailers favor category captains and vice versa.* Do retail channels (supermarkets and other retail outlets) favor these megacompanies because they offer a wider range of foods and thus increased efficiencies for the retail trade in handling and selling both their snack and other food products? Or *do the megas serenade the retailers harder to get what they believe is their rightful Lebensraum of retail shelf space?*

- *Heavy advertising.* Do the economies of scale resulting from market-category consolidation (into a few large companies) result in increased promotional, marketing, and distribution capacities and efficiencies and favor increased sales of the megabrand snacks and fun foods? *The leading snack and fun foods are among our leading advertisers (all-products) and have unbelievably large advertising budgets* (Table 2).

All of these characteristics are structure-related factors of the industry that may result in market conditions (price, product sizes, availability, product shelf space access, pref-

Table 2. Major Food and Snack Companies 2003 Advertising and Ranking

Snack Companies	Us Advertising, $ Millions	Ranking, Top Ten Advertisers
Unilever	1,332	17*
Altria (Kraft)	1,311	18
PepsiCo	1,212	23
Nestle	1,113	27
Mars	813	41
Kellogg	570	57
Coca Cola	473	69
Hershey	NA	†

Source: Advertising Age, June 18, 2004.
* Includes personal care products and food.
†Company not in Top 100 (2003) in advertising spending.

erential product displays) that could be particularly favorable to motivating increased consumer purchase and consumption of snacks. *Suspicion, but lack of proof.*

I pointed out in the first part of this article that in addition to the high market concentration in the fun-food categories, there is wide market concentration throughout the entire consumer food sector; our 10 largest food companies supply more than 40% of each dollar's worth of all food Americans purchase annually at retail; expanding this number to the largest 40 companies, the figure comes up to 80% of all retail food sold. Never in recent times has our nation of some 300 million people been as narrowly commercially sourced by as few food companies.

There could be a silver lining to this market structure. If this high market concentration into megafood firms offers consumers overall the choice of readily available and more balanced dietary choices (in line with the Dietary Guidelines for Americans), this could be a good thing for diet and health.

Today, the prominent business strategy for large food companies is to increasingly concentrate on a limited number of their food brands, where the company's brands are the market leaders or a close competitor to the category leaders, seeking the higher profitably of leading national brands.

This trend has resulted in many large companies getting out of the business of selling low profit-margin commodity-type foods in favor of branded added-valued highly processed foods. For example, companies such as Kraft, Unilever, Nestle, and others have recently discontinued hundreds of second-tier brands, seeking greater overall company profitability.

A cursory search of big-food's product lines today shows a heavy offering of high-caloric-density low-nutrient-density products, as well as other foods of varying degrees of nutritional worth. Moreover, unlike the past, when our largest food firms marketed a broad range of foods, megacompanies today offer a much narrower range of foods. The megacompanies tend to stakeout a more restrictive and a narrower line of products today for all the reasons I mentioned. Then they aggressively market and promote these *fortress brands* because of the competitive advantage such brands offer in the marketplace, as well as the greater profitability that concentrating predominantly on top brands offer.

How about their role in marketing fruits and vegetables? Today, these megacompanies have a negligible market presence (excepting in the fruit-juice beverage categories). The trend in recent years has been for them to divest businesses producing fruit and vegetable products (Birdseye) because of their lower profitability compared to other more profitable leading added-value food products. Some interesting new products are now in place (calcium-fortified orange juice), and others are on the horizon or already doing well in some markets (juices with sterols to lower serum cholesterol). The question is whether consumers will pay for these new bells and whistles.

Bottom Line

The role of our largest fun-food and beverage companies, the 8 giants, and their marketing, their branded snacks, and the resulting structural ramifications not on the market economics but on our overweight problem is far from settled, let alone what to do about if they are proven to be a significant negative factor.

My own personal take, formed by 2 decades in the consumer food industry and my recent time in the academic world studying the food industry, is that megafood companies' activities are certainly not the root cause of the obesity problem. There is a large dollop of personal behavior (*diet, behavior, and physical activity*) and plenty of other environmental factors as well in the causation of obesity.

However, I don't believe that we can let the concentrated structure of the food industry into megafood companies (and also large chain restaurants) totally off the hook. These companies combine their great economic power, marketing muscle, sales strategies, and tasty products to play a dominant role in shaping our daily diets by supplying too many of the discretionary calories we consume.

As a result of this market clout, I believe that there is great likelihood that these few large companies are an important factor in determining what, when, and how much many Americans eat or overeat today. This makes the mega-snack companies among environmental factors suspected as contributing to obesity risk, at least among those who eat a lot of their products. Obesity is similar to cancer in that its causes are complex and multiple and depend on a web of environmental and inborn factors. It follows that tackling this problem must involve the megafood companies as part of the solution. (Could you feed yourself today without these companies?) Therefore, just don't blame them, help fix them!

REFERENCES

1. Yang S. *Nearly One-Third of the Calories in the US Diet Come From Junk Food, Researcher Finds.* Berkeley, Calif: Media Relations; 2004.
2. Block G. Food contributing to energy intake in the US: data from NHANES III and NHANES 1999-2000. *Composition Analysis.* 2004;17:439-447.

James E. Tillotson, PhD, MBA, is currently Professor of Food Policy and International Business at Tufts University. Before returning to the academic world, Dr Tillotson worked in industry, holding various research and development positions in the food and chemical sectors. Correspondence: James E. Tillotson, PhD, MBA, PO Box Ten, Cohasset, MA 02025-0100 (e-mail: james.tillotson@tufts.edu).

Moving Toward Healthful Sustainable Diets

Nutritionists have increasingly been focusing on the challenge of moving consumers toward healthful diets and simultaneously helping them to make the connection between healthy food and a healthy environment. Simply stated, to foster food sustainability, consumers will need to choose minimally processed and minimally packaged foods. In addition, when possible, they should buy locally produced foods to support regional agriculture and local economies, preserve farmland, and use less energy and other natural resources.

BARBARA STORPER, MS, RD

Nutritionists have increasingly been focusing on the challenge of moving consumers toward healthful diets and simultaneously helping them to understand that what's good for their health may well be good for the health of the planet. Promoting food sustainability and ecologic harmony as an essential function of the nutrition professional was first proposed more than 20 years ago by Dr Joan Gussow, Mary Swartz Rose Professor Emeritus of Nutrition Education at Teachers College, Columbia University, and Dr Kate Clancy, Director of The Agriculture Policy Project at the Henry A. Wallace Institute for Sustainable Agriculture. Today, their message falls on receptive ears, as nutritionists better understand the connection between agriculture, the environment, hunger, health, and, ultimately, food security.

Drs Gussow and Clancy first introduced the term "food sustainability" to the nutrition profession in an article published in 1986 by the *Journal of Nutrition Education* entitled, "Dietary Guidelines for Sustainability."[1] They explained how the US Dietary Guidelines, the government's model for promoting health, can also be used as the framework by which nutritionists can promote sustainable diets. The article still serves today as a seminal treatise, calling the profession to promote a diet that is healthy for the individual, the rest of the world, and the planet.

Dr Gussow is still on the forefront of this mission today, promoting the sustainability advantages of "whole foods"—foods that are minimally processed and packaged. Nutritionally, whole foods fit more easily into a healthful diet than their processed and packaged counterparts because they are naturally higher in fiber and lower in fat, sodium, sugar, and additives. Globally, whole foods also bypass the high energy costs of food processing. In general, more profit stays with the farmer, helping farmers to make a livable income, thus staving off the alarming decline of the small and family farm in this country. Last, but far from least, Gussow claims that whole foods taste better, give people more opportunity to prepare them the way they like, and allow people to feel more connected to the food's origin.

> *To foster sustainability, consumers should choose minimally processed and minimally packaged foods and, when possible, buy locally produced foods to support regional agriculture that preserves farmland and is less energy intensive*

What's even better, she proclaims in her newest book, *This Organic Life: Confessions of a Suburban Homesteader*[2] is for people to eat locally produced food, and whenever possible, grow their own. The important current issue, says Gussow, is learning how to produce food for everyone in a way that's sustainable, and we are not doing that. What we are doing, she continues, is overproducing food globally while destroying the environment and our capacity for future food production. Supermarkets "trick" the consumer by selling foods from around the world all year long so that consumers on the East Coast expect summer produce in the winter, such as strawberries in January. The economic and environmental costs associated with these practices, however, are invisible to most consumers.

For Gussow, localization of the food supply remains the optimal approach to foster sustainability. The need to relocalize our food supply is urgent now, according to Gussow, because of the increasing harm caused by agribusiness practices—their emphasis on monocultures (ie, growing single crops over large areas) and their continued dependence on pesticides. She claims that our present agricultural system downplays the health and environmental hazards of pesticides, which are being used today at a far greater rate than when Rachel Carson's[3] *Silent Spring* first exposed their alarming consequences.

SUSTAINABILITY AND MODERN FARMING PRACTICES

Gussow uses the example of a potato to explain why current farming practices are not sustainable. There are 5,000 known varieties of the potato plant. Peruvian Indians in the Andes knew and used 3,000 of them. Yet, today, only 6 are grown commercially in the United States. Why? According to Gussow, it is to meet the demands of a processing industry that requires uniformity. The fast-food industry, in particular, prefers a single variety, the Russet, for its shape. The Russet potato is long enough so that when made into French Fries, the fries can extend beyond the edges of the cardboard container, creating the visual appearance consumers expect. Yet, she claims that limiting a nation's reliance on a few varieties of a crop is precisely what devastated Ireland's economy in the 1840s, when blight struck the two varieties of potatoes on which the entire nation depended for its food supply.

She also argues that monoculture also depletes the soil, creating an increased dependence on fertilizers and pesticides, manufactured from nonrenewable fossil fuels. This overdependence on pesticides, in turn, increases the health problems for growers and consumers of pesticide-ridden produce here and abroad.

Returning to a more locally produced food supply will not only help the environment but also, according to Gussow, make the public more aware of the link between their food and the health and environmental consequences of modern farming methods. Buying locally not only supports small farms and helps to maintain local economies but also helps neighbors stay in business and ultimately promotes sustainable communities.

It is surprising, according to Gussow, that the United States ranks as one of the leading food importers in the world! She believes that emphasizing local agriculture here may also help poor people in other countries who are steadily being pushed off their own lands when large agribusiness firms establish production sites for luxury and out-of-season foods for US tables. Ironically, she notes, the fruits and vegetables we eat out of season are often produced in countries with poor sanitation and questionable hygienic practices. Why eat a fruit from a country where one would not drink the water? Eating locally may offer a safe and healthy alternative to the consequences of a global marketplace.

MOVING TOWARD SUSTAINABLE DIETS

Here are some ways nutritionists can help to promote sustainability:

- Recommend that a certain portion of the weekly grocery money be used exclusively for foods that are produced locally and sold in farmers markets or through farms that establish memberships with local residents.

- Learn about and promote seasonal foods that can be grown locally in the consumer's own region and teach people how to cook these foods—or how to cook at all!

- Have your own backyard garden and encourage public organizations, schools, hospitals, etc, to build community gardens and use the foods grown for feeding programs.

Here are some creative resources nutrition educators can use to promote food sustainability with school-age children:

- LIFE Program (Linking Food and the Environment) a project of Teacher's College, Columbia University promotes the "Food Triangle"—a take-off on the Food Pyramid. Using a triangle, the project staff divide foods into three groups—"plant foods," "animal foods," and "man-made foods"—to help children learn about how their food choices affect their environment and their health. They also use hands-on activities such as gardening, cooking, shopping, composting, and recycling.

- "Earth Friends" is a minidiscovery museum housed at Teacher's College where classes from New York City schools visit and learn about food from farm to table in a series of games, exhibits, and cooking activities. Contact David Russo, Project Coordinator, 212-678-3955.

- "Cookshop" is a classroom curriculum designed by the New York Community Food Resource Center to help students and teachers cook a variety of locally grown wholesome foods that will then be introduced in the school cafeteria. Evaluations show dramatic increases in consumption of these previously unfamiliar foods when students learn about them first in class. Contact Toni Liquori at 212-894-8074 or tliquori@cfrcnyc.org.

- "Close Encounters with Agriculture," a Cooperative Extension Service of the University of Maryland Program links elementary school children with class activities and field trips to agricultural areas to learn about animals, horticulture, and farming.

- "Field to Table," a Cornell University Extension Project helps students to identify and increase their consumption of locally grown fruits and vegetables based on the Northeast Regional Food Guide.

- "From Land to Landfill" is a program developed by nutritionists at Purdue University using a systems approach to integrate health and nutrition into core subject areas.

- "FOODPLAY" is this author's traveling nutrition theater show that tours schools nationally and uses juggling, theater, music, magic, and audience participation to encourage children to make food choices that are good for their health and the health of the planet. Contact Barbara Storper at 800-FOODPLAY or http://www.foodplay.com.

Barbara Storper, MS, RD, is the Director of FOODPLAY Productions, an Emmy Award-winning nutrition media organization that produces national touring school theater shows, video kits, media campaigns, and resources to improve children's health. Ms Storper holds degrees in both journalism and nutrition and has received the first Outstanding Young Nutrition Educator in the Country Award and Media Partnership from the Society for Nutrition Education.

Corresponding author: Barbara Storper, MS, RD, FOODPLAY Productions, 221 Pine St, Florence, MA 01062 (e-mail: barbara@foodplay.com).

REFERENCES

1. Gussow JD, Clancy K. Dietary guidelines for sustainability. *J Nutr Edu.* 1986; 18:1–15.
2. Gussow JD. *This Organic Life: Confessions of a Suburban Homesteader.* White River Junction, Vt: Chelsea Green Publishing Company; 2001.
3. Carson R. *The Silent Spring.* Boston: Houghton Mifflin; 1994..

UNIT 2
Nutrients

Unit Selections

Key Points to Consider

- Calculate the amount of antioxidant vitamins and potassium you consume in one day and compare with your daily requirements.

- Determine the glycemic index of foods you eat in one meal and classify them into high, medium or low glycemic index foods.

- Check out several labels from food containing fats and oils that you eat frequently. Can you tell how much trans-fat each contains?

- Determine the percentage of your average daily calories that is contributed by total fat and saturated fat in 24 hours. What do your calculations tell you about potential health risks?

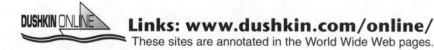 **Links: www.dushkin.com/online/**
These sites are annotated in the World Wide Web pages.

Dole 5 A Day: Nutrition, Fruits & Vegetables
http://www.dole5aday.com

Food and Nutrition Information Center
http://www.nal.usda.gov/fnic/

Nutrient Data Laboratory
http://www.nal.usda.gov/fnic/foodcomp/

NutritionalSupplements.com
http://www.nutritionalsupplements.com

U.S. National Library of Medicine
http://www.nlm.nih.gov

Fish Contamination Resource
www.epa.gov/waterscience/fishadvice/advice.html

This unit focuses on the most recent advances that have been reported on nutrients and their role in health and disease. With the onset and development of new technologies in the area of nutrition, the plethora of information on the role of certain nutrients, and the speed with which information is printed and disseminated, even the professional has a very hard time keeping up with the advances. The media reports any sensational, even erroneous data, which confuses the public and creates many misunderstandings. Preliminary reports have to undergo rigorous testing in animal models and clinical trials before they are accepted and implemented by the scientific community.

Additionally, how individuals will respond to dietary changes will depend on their genetic make-up along with other environmental factors. Thus, the National Academy of Science has a difficult task in establishing the exact amounts of nutrients that will cover human requirements but not create toxicity in the long run for the majority of the population.

The articles of this unit have been selected to present current knowledge about nutrients resulting from state-of-the-art research and controversies brewing at the present time. Articles related to nutrient function and their effects on chronic disease such as cardiovascular disease, obesity, diabetes mellitus and osteoporosis are included.

An area of perennial controversy concerns fats and the types of fat. Americans have focused on single nutrients, attempting to exclude them from food. This has resulted in the proliferation of low-fat products that are not necessarily low in calories. Two articles present current scientific finding about types of fats. Trans fatty acids that arise from food processing, which convert liquid oils to solid margarines, are as harmful to heart health as saturated fat. Current scientific findings on trans-fat are discussed and labeling for trans-fat becomes mandatory by the FDA beginning in 2006. As research evolves, a diet moderate in total fat is advised, especially incorporating omega-3 fatty acids found in fish such as tuna and salmon. Omega-3 fatty acids promote heart health and eye health and have beneficial effects on the immune system. The second article discusses ways to incorporate them in our diet and offers recommendations to prevent methyl mercury toxicity from supplement use and fish consumption.

The importance of vitamins is of great interest to consumers since vitamins have been touted to cure and/or prevent disease. As the baby boomers are aging, diseases that affect their eyes such as macular degeneration and cataracts are on the rise. Several antioxidant vitamins such as vitamins C and beta-carotene and phytochemicals such as lutein and zeaxanthin may have a protective effect.

Even though minerals play major roles in body functions, Americans have less than optimal amounts in their diet. Recent research has unraveled the role potassium plays in reducing blood pressure and thus risk of stroke and the protective effect it has against kidney stones and bone loss. A diet rich in legumes, fish, fruits, and vegetables will result in optimal potassium consumption.

With the rise in obesity and diabetes mellitus in recent years, Americans are going on low-carbohydrate, high-fat and high-protein diets. The misconceptions about carbohydrates and the differences between "good" and "bad" carbohydrates based on the glycemic index and the glycemic load, are explained by Dr. Willett. The food industry as always has been eager to fill consumer demand by developing low-carbohydrate containing products. Added sugars have been decreased and new products are fortified with fiber in form of lignin, arabinogalactosan, gums etc. for weight maintenance, cardiovascular, and gastrointestinal health.

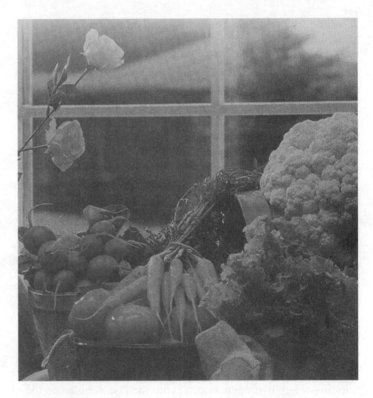

Omega-3 Choices:
Fish or Flax?

What are the health benefits of the fatty acids found in fish and flax?

BY ALISON J. RIGBY, PHD, MPH, RD

Fish consumption has been advocated on the basis of its lean high biological value protein, vitamin and mineral content, and "good" fat value from the omega-3 fatty acids found in fish. The health benefits of eating fish were essentially discovered by epidemiological studies of the Northern Inuit population, who were shown to have reduced rates of myocardial infarction as a result of their consumption of marine omega-3 fatty acids, compared with Western control subjects.[1] European countries have been supplementing their baby formulas for some time with omega-3 fatty acids for brain health. A recent American Heart Association (AHA) Scientific Statement on fish consumption, fish oil, omega-3 fatty acids, and cardiovascular disease amplified the benefits of eating fish and recommended the AHA guidelines of at least two servings of fish per week and the use of omega-3 supplementation for patients with coronary heart disease (1 gram per day) and larger doses (2 grams per day to 4 grams per day) for those patients with hypertriglyceridemia.[2]

REVIEW OF THE OMEGA-3 FATTY ACIDS

The omega-3 fatty acids are polyunsaturated fatty acids (missing many hydrogen atoms), with the last double bond located three carbons away from the methyl end. Eicosopentaenoic acid (EPA), or 20:5n-3, and Docosahexaenoic acid (DPA), or 22:6n-3, are the omega-3 fatty acids found in oily fish, with mackerel, salmon, trout, sardines, and herring being excellent sources. Approximately 1 gram of EPA/DPA can be obtained from 100 grams (3.5 ounces) of oily fish. Although this quantity of EPA/DPA can vary depending upon the degree of oiliness of the fish (Atlantic mackerel = 2.5 grams omega-3 per 100 grams; salmon = 1.2 grams omega-3 per 100 grams;

tuna = 0.5 grams omega-3 per 100 grams; and red snapper = 0.2 grams omega-3 per 100 grams).

The average intake of total omega-3 fatty acids in the United States is approximately 1.6 grams per day (0.7% of energy intake), with actually only 0.1 grams per day to 0.2 grams per day coming from EPA/DHA (the rest from alpha-linolenic acid [ALA]).[2] ALA (18:3n-3) from plant sources can desaturate and elongate in the human body to form EPA and DHA. Sources of ALA include oils from flaxseed, canola (rapeseed), soybean, walnut, and wheat germ, with flaxseed (linseed) being the most abundant source.

HEALTH BENEFITS OF OMEGA-3 FATTY ACIDS

A selection of epidemiological studies with important clinical trials have outlined the benefits of the omega-3 fatty acids.

The Diet and Reinfaction Trial supported the role of fish or fish oil in decreasing total mortality and sudden death in patients with myocardial infarction.[3] The Lyon Diet Heart Study[4] added canola oil as a source of ALA to the diet; the Singh study[5] added fish or mustard oil; and the GISSI-Prevenzione trial[6] added 850 grams to 882 grams of omega-3 fatty acids to a Mediterranean diet for a large 11,324-participant study, resulting in a decrease in mortality for these groups.

In the Cardiovascular Health Study,[7] a population-based prospective cohort study among 3,910 adults, the consumption of tuna and other broiled or baked fish was associated with a lower risk of ischemic heart disease (IHD) death, especially arrhythmic IHD death. In the Nurses' Health Study,[8] the relative risk of total stroke was lower among women who regularly ate fish than among those who did not. A significant decrease in the risk of thrombotic stroke was observed in women who ate fish at least twice per week, compared with women who ate fish less than once per month, after adjustment for age, smoking, and other cardiovascular risk factors.

The omega-3 fatty acids have been associated with having anti-inflammatory, antithrombotic, antiarrhythmic, hypolipidemic, and vasodilatory properties.[9] Some of the health benefits that have been associated with omega-3 fatty acids include the secondary prevention of chronic diseases and an association with the following:

- Inflammatory conditions: Improves rheumatoid arthritis, psoriasis, asthma, and some skin conditions
- Ulcerative colitis and Crohn's disease: Reduces the severity of symptoms
- Cardiovascular disease: Lowers triglycerides and raises high-density lipoprotein cholesterol levels, improves blood circulation, reduces clotting, improves vascular function, and lowers blood pressure
- Type 2 diabetes mellitus: Reduces hyperinsulinemia and insulin resistance
- Renal disease: Preserves renal function in IgA nephropathy; potentially reduces vascular access thrombosis in hemodialysis patients and is cardioprotective
- Mental function: Reduces severity of several mental conditions such as Alzheimer's disease, depression, and bipolar disorder; improvement in children with attention deficit hyperactivity disorder and dyslexia also noted
- Growth and development: Neurodevelopment and function of the brain and also the retina of the eye where visual function is affected

FITTING OMEGA-3 FATTY ACIDS INTO THE DIET

Western diets are characterized by low intakes of EPA and DHA relative to linoleic acid (LA; 18:2n-6) and arachidonic acid (AA; 20:4n-6). The high intake of trans fatty acids in our diets can interfere with the desaturation and elongation of LA and ALA. A high intake of LA leads to decreased production of AA and interferes with the desaturation and elongation of ALA to EPA and DHA. The high intake of LA also promotes a prothrombotic and proaggregatory state, characterized by increased blood viscosity and vasoconstriction, and potentially decreased bleeding time.

The omega-3 fatty acids have been associated with having anti-inflammatory, antithrombotic, antiarrhythmic, hypolipidemic, and vasodilatory properties.

Therefore, the required intake of long-chain polyunsaturated omega-3 fatty acids needed for optimal effects depends on the intake of other fatty acids. The Western diet ratio of omega-6 to omega-3 fatty acids ranges from 20:1 to 30:1[9] and is probably even higher with the increased intake of vegetable oils, historically rec-

ommended as a substitute for saturated fat. The competing omega-6 vegetable oils include corn, safflower, cottonseed, sesame, and sunflower seed oils.

FISH VS. FLAX

The optimal intake of LA compared with ALA appears critical for the metabolism of omega-3 fatty acids. An increase in AA, EPA, and DHA leads to an increase in membrane fluidity, alters the structure of the membrane receptors, and can have other beneficial effects associated with the omega-3 fatty acids. They also play a role in the regulation of cell surface expression, cell-cell interactions, and cytokine release.[10] A ratio of 1:4 (LA:ALA) or less is recommended for conversion of ALA to longer chain metabolites (EPA and DHA).[9] This is an important concept for vegetarians, whose diets are often much richer in LA. The intake of 3 grams per day to 4 grams per day of ALA is equivalent to 0.3 grams per day of EPA with optimal elongation.

The increased consumption of flaxseed, canola, soybean, walnut, and wheat germ oils should be supported. However, ALA does not appear to be comparable with its biological effects, compared with EPA and DHA found in fish oil. It appears that the EPA and DHA from marine oils are more rapidly incorporated into plasma and membrane lipids. Algae and some fungi are also capable of forming omega-3 fatty acids de novo, and the DHA from algae supplements needs to be explored further for the vegetarian.

THE METHYL MERCURY SCARE

A recent local survey in the Bay Area of California found several varieties of fish to contain toxic levels of mercury: swordfish (containing the highest concentration), Chilean sea bass, and ahi tuna. Mercury is the environmental pollutant largely from coal-fired power plants that is at the highest concentration in the large predator fish.

The FDA has an advisory warning that swordfish, shark, king mackerel, and tilefish consumption should be limited by pregnant women and women of childbearing age, and this warning is apparent in many fish markets. Mercury can damage the nervous, cardiovascular, immune, and reproductive systems, and symptoms include tremors, memory loss, and fatigue. Subtle symptoms of methyl mercury toxicity in adults have included numbness or tingling of the hands and feet or around the mouth.

A high dietary intake of mercury from the consumption of fish has been hypothesized to increase the risk of coronary heart disease.

According to the FDA, consumption of fish with methyl mercury levels of one part per million, such as shark and swordfish, should be limited to approximately 7 ounces per week. The FDA states that consumption advice is unnecessary for the top 10 seafood species, which makes up approximately 80% of the seafood market: canned tuna, shrimp, pollock, salmon, cod, catfish, clams, flatfish, crabs, and scallops. The methyl mercury levels in these species are at less than 0.2 parts per million, and not many people eat more than the suggested weekly limit of 2.2 pounds of fish. Canned tuna, which is composed of smaller pieces of tuna, such as skipjack and albacore, typically have lower levels of methyl mercury compared with large fresh tuna, sold as steaks or sushi.

A high dietary intake of mercury from the consumption of fish has been hypothesized to increase the risk of coronary heart disease. In a study that investigated the association between mercury levels in toenails and risk of coronary heart disease among male health professionals with no previous history of cardiovascular disease (40 to 75 years of age), there was no association between total mercury exposure and risk of coronary heart disease.[11] Adjustment with the intake of omega-3 fatty acids did not substantially change the results from this study.

RECOMMENDING OMEGA-3 SUPPLEMENTS

A low rate of coronary heart disease has certainly been shown in fish-eating populations. Studies have highlighted reduced cardiovascular risk with a higher intake of ALA, and the omega-3 fatty acids have also consistently been shown to decrease serum triacylglycerol concentrations in studies in humans. A meta-analysis[12] suggested that dietary and nondietary intake of omega-3 fatty acids reduces overall mortality, mortality due to myocardial infarction, and sudden death in patients with coronary heart disease.

Based on the AHA Scientific Statement, it seems reasonable to recommend at least two servings of fish per week in the diet and the use of omega-3 supplements for patients with coronary heart disease up to 1 gram per day and larger doses (2 grams per day to 4 grams per day) for those patients with hypertriglyceridemia.[2] The exact ratio of EPA:DHA needs to be explored further in clinical trials.

As a cautionary safety note, a dose of 1.8 grams per day of EPA has not been documented as having any prolongation of bleeding time. The use of 4 grams per day has shown increased bleeding time and decreased platelet count, but no overall adverse effects.[13]

A fish oil supplement that is "clean" and has been processed by molecular distillation is important. A good place to start when deciding which brand of fish oil supplement to select is *Consumer Reports* magazine (www.consumerreports.org), which tests the top-selling brands of fish oil capsules. The 16 top-selling brands of fish oil capsules they tested found that the products "all contained roughly as much omega-3s as their labels claimed," and none were contaminated with pollutants.

REFERENCES

1. O'Keefe JH, Harris WS. From Inuit to implementation: Omega-3 fatty acids come of age. *Mayo Clin Proc.* 2000; 75:607–614.

2. Kris-Etherton PM, Harris WS, Appel LJ. Fish consumption, fish oil, omega-3 fatty acids, and cardiovascular disease. *Circulation.* 2002; 106:2747.

3. Burr ML, Fehily AM, Gilbert JF, et al. Effect of changes in fat, fish and fiber intakes on death and myocardial reinfaction: Diet and reinfaction trial (DART). *Lancet.* 1989; 2:757–761.

4. de Lorgeril M, Renaud S, Mamelle N, et al. Mediterranean alpha-linolenic acid-rich diet in the secondary prevention of coronary heart disease. *Lancet.* 1994; 343:1454–1459.

5. Singh RB, Rastogi SS, Verma R, et al. Randomized controlled trial of cardiovascular diet in patients with recent acute myocardial infaction: Results of one year follow up. *Br Med J.* 1992; 304:1015–1019.

6. GISSI-Prevenzione Investigators. Dietary supplementation with n-3 polyunsaturated fatty acids and vitamin E after myocardial infaction: Results of the GISSI-Prevenzione trial. *Lancet.* 1999; 354:447–455.

7. Mozaffarian D, Lemaitre RN, Kuller LH, et al. Cardiac benefits of fish consumption may depend on the type of fish meal consumed: The Cardiovascular Health Study. *Circulation.* 2003; 107(10):1372–1377.

8. Skerrett PJ, Hennekens CH. Consumption of fish and fish oils and decreased risk of stroke. *Prev Cardiol.* 2003; 61(1):38–41.

9. Simopoulos AP. Essential fatty acids in health and chronic disease. *Am J Clin Nutr.* 1999; 70(suppl):560S–569S.

10. Grimm H, Mayer K, Mayser P, Eigenbrodt E. Regulatory potential of n-3 fatty acids in immunological and inflammatory processes. *Br J Nutr.* 2002; 87(1):S59–S67.

11. Yoshizawa K, Rimm EB, Morris JS, et al. Mercury and the risk of coronary heart disease in men. *N Eng J Med.* 2002; 347(22):1755–1760.

12. Bucher HC, Hengstler P, Schindler C, Meier G. N-3 polyunsaturated coronary heart disease: A meta-analysis of randomized controlled trials. *Am J Med.* 2002; (4):298–304.

13. Saynor R, Verel D, Gillott T. The long term effect of dietary supplementation with fish lipid concentration on serum lipids, bleeding time, platelets and angina. *Atherosclerosis.* 1984; 50:3–10.

— Alison J. Rigby, PhD, MPH, RD, is a researcher at Stanford University, where she is currently investigating the use of fish oils in the diet. She also teaches nutrition/dietetics classes at San Francisco State University.

Revealing Trans Fats

Scientific evidence shows that consumption of saturated fat, trans fat, and dietary cholesterol raises low-density lipoprotein (LDL), or "bad" cholesterol, levels that increase the risk of coronary heart disease (CHD). According to the National Heart, Lung, and Blood Institute of the National Institutes of Health, more than 12.5 million Americans have CHD, and more than 500,000 die each year. That makes CHD one of the leading causes of death in the United States.

The Food and Drug Administration has required that saturated fat and dietary cholesterol be listed on food labels since 1993. With trans fat added to the Nutrition Facts panel, you know how much of all three—saturated fat, *trans* fat, and cholesterol—are in the foods you choose. Identifying saturated fat, *trans* fat, and cholesterol on the food label gives you information you need to make food choices that help reduce the risk of CHD. This revised label is of particular interest to people concerned about high blood cholesterol and heart disease.

However, everyone should be aware of the risk posed by consuming too much saturated fat, *trans* fat, and cholesterol. But what is *trans* fat, and how can you limit the amount of this fat in your diet?

What is *Trans* Fat?

Basically, *trans* fat is made when manufacturers add hydrogen to vegetable oil—a process called hydrogenation. Hydrogenation increases the shelf life and flavor stability of foods containing these fats.

Trans fat can be found in vegetable shortenings, some margarines, crackers, cookies, snack foods, and other foods made with or fried in partially hydrogenated oils. Unlike other fats, the majority of *trans* fat is formed when food manufacturers turn liquid oils into solid fats like shortening and hard margarine. A small amount of *trans* fat is found naturally, primarily in dairy products, some meat, and other animal-based foods.

Trans fat, like saturated fat and dietary cholesterol, raises the LDL cholesterol that increases your risk for CHD. Americans consume on average 4 to 5 times as much saturated fat as *trans* fat in their diets.

Although saturated fat is the main dietary culprit that raises LDL, *trans* fat and dietary cholesterol also contribute significantly.

Are All Fats the Same?

Simply put: No. Fat is a major source of energy for the body and aids in the absorption of vitamins A, D, E, and K, and caro-

tenoids. Both animal- and plant-derived food products contain fat, and when eaten in moderation, fat is important for proper growth, development, and maintenance of good health. As a food ingredient, fat provides taste, consistency, and stability and helps you feel full. In addition, parents should be aware that fats are an especially important source of calories and nutrients for infants and toddlers (up to 2 years of age), who have the highest energy needs per unit of body weight of any age group.

While unsaturated fats (monounsaturated and polyunsaturated) are beneficial when consumed in moderation, saturated and *trans* fats are not. Saturated fat and *trans* fat raise LDL cholesterol levels in the blood. Dietary cholesterol also raises LDL cholesterol and may contribute to heart disease even without raising LDL. Therefore, it is advisable to choose foods low in saturated fat, *trans* fat, and cholesterol as part of a healthful diet.

What Can You Do About Saturated Fat, *Trans* Fat, and Cholesterol?

When comparing foods, look at the Nutrition Facts panel, and choose the food with the lower amounts of saturated fat, *trans* fat, and cholesterol. Health experts recommend that you keep your intake of saturated fat, *trans* fat, and cholesterol as low as possible while consuming a nutritionally adequate diet. However, these experts recognize that eliminating these three components entirely from your diet is not practical because they are unavoidable in ordinary diets.

Where Can You Find *Trans* Fat on the Food Label?

Although some food products already have *trans* fat on the label, food manufacturers have until January 2006 to list it on all their products.

You will find *trans* fat listed on the Nutrition Facts panel directly under the line for saturated fat.

How Do Your Choices Stack Up?

With the addition of *trans* fat to the Nutrition Facts panel, you can review your food choices and see how they stack up.

Don't assume similar products are the same. Be sure to check the Nutrition Facts panel because even similar foods can vary in calories, ingredients, nutrients, and the size and number of servings in a package.

How Can You Use the Label to Make Heart-Healthy Food Choices?

The Nutrition Facts panel can help you choose foods lower in saturated fat, *trans* fat, and cholesterol. Compare similar foods and choose the food with the lower combined saturated and *trans* fats and the lower amount of cholesterol.

Although the updated Nutrition Facts panel will list the amount of *trans* fat in a product, it will not show a Percent Daily Value (%DV). While scientific reports have confirmed the relationship between *trans* fat and an increased risk of CHD, none has provided a reference value for *trans* fat or any other information that the FDA believes is sufficient to establish a Daily Reference Value or a %DV.

Saturated fat and cholesterol, however, do have a %DV. To choose foods low in saturated fat and cholesterol, use the general rule of thumb that 5 percent of the Daily Value or less is low and 20 percent or more is high.

You can also use the %DV to make dietary trade-offs with other foods throughout the day. You don't have to give up a favorite food to eat a healthy diet. When a food you like is high in saturated fat or cholesterol, balance it with foods that are low in saturated fat and cholesterol at other times of the day.

The FDA's *trans* fat labeling regulations don't take effect until Jan. 1, 2006, but some manufacturers are already listing the amount of *trans* fat in their products.

Do Dietary Supplements Contain *Trans* Fat?

Would it surprise you to know that some dietary supplements contain *trans* fat from partially hydrogenated vegetable oil as well as saturated fat or cholesterol? It's true. As a result of the FDA's new label requirement, if a dietary supplement contains a reportable amount of *trans* or saturated fat, which is 0.5 gram or more, dietary supplement manufacturers must list the amounts on the Supplement Facts panel. Some dietary supplements that may contain saturated fat, *trans* fat, and cholesterol include energy and nutrition bars.

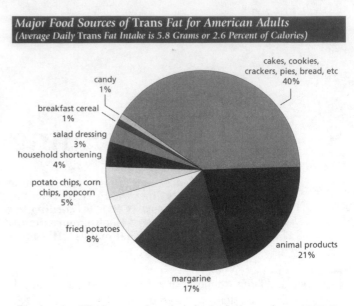

Major Food Sources of Trans Fat for American Adults
(Average Daily Trans Fat Intake is 5.8 Grams or 2.6 Percent of Calories)

- cakes, cookies, crackers, pies, bread, etc 40%
- candy 1%
- breakfast cereal 1%
- salad dressing 3%
- household shortening 4%
- potato chips, corn chips, popcorn 5%
- fried potatoes 8%
- margarine 17%
- animal products 21%

Data based on FDA's economic analysis for the final *trans* fatty acid labeling rule, "*Trans* Fatty Acids in Nutrition Labeling, Nutrient Content Claims, and Health Claims" (July 11, 2003)

Fat Tips

Here are some practical tips you can use every day to keep your consumption of saturated fat, *trans* fat, and cholesterol low while consuming a nutritionally adequate diet.

- **Check the Nutrition Facts panel** to compare foods because the serving sizes are generally consistent in similar types of foods. Choose foods lower in saturated fat, *trans* fat, and cholesterol. For saturated fat and cholesterol, keep in mind that 5 percent of the daily value (%DV) or less is low and 20 percent or more is high. (There is no %DV for *trans* fat.)

- **Choose alternative fats**. Replace saturated and *trans* fats in your diet with monounsaturated and polyunsaturated fats. These fats do not raise LDL cholesterol levels and have health benefits when eaten in moderation. Sources of monounsaturated fats include olive and canola oils. Sources of polyunsaturated fats include soybean oil, corn oil, sunflower oil and foods like nuts and fish.

- **Choose vegetable oils** (except coconut and palm kernel oils) and soft margarines (liquid, tub, or spray) more often because the amounts of saturated fat, *trans* fat, and cholesterol are lower than the amounts in solid shortenings, hard margarines, and animal fats, including butter.

- **Consider fish**. Most fish are lower in saturated fat than meat. Some fish, such as mackerel, sardines, and salmon, contain omega-3 fatty acids that are being studied to determine if they offer protection against heart disease.

- **Ask before you order when eating out**. A good tip to remember is to ask which fats are being used in the preparation of your food when eating or ordering out.

- **Watch calories**. Don't be fooled! Fats are high in calories. All sources of fat contain 9 calories per gram, making fat the most concentrated source of calories. By comparison, carbohydrates and protein have only 4 calories per gram.

To keep your intake of saturated fat, *trans* fat, and cholesterol low:

- Look at the Nutrition Facts panel when comparing products. Choose foods low in the combined amount of saturated fat and *trans* fat and low in cholesterol as part of a nutritionally adequate diet.

- Substitute alternative fats that are higher in mono- and poly-unsaturated fats like olive oil, canola oil, soybean oil, corn oil, and sunflower oil.

Highlights of the Final Rule on *Trans* Fat

- Manufacturers of conventional foods and some dietary supplements will be required to list *trans* fat on a separate line, immediately under saturated fat on the nutrition label.
- Food manufacturers have until Jan. 1, 2006, to list *trans* fat on the nutrition label. The phase-in period minimizes the need for multiple labeling changes, allows small businesses to use current label inventories, and provides economic savings.
- FDA's regulatory chemical definition for *trans* fatty acids is all unsaturated fatty acids that contain one or more isolated (i.e., nonconjugated) double bonds in a *trans* configuration. Under the agency's definition, conjugated linoleic acid would be excluded from the definition of *trans* fat.
- Dietary supplement manufacturers must also list *trans* fat on the Supplement Facts panel when their products contain reportable amounts (0.5 gram or more) of *trans* fat. Examples of dietary supplements with *trans* fat are energy and nutrition bars.

From *FDA Consumer*, September/October 2003. U.S. Food and Drug Administration.

Going Beyond Atkins

[**There's no question that carbs can make you fat.
But are bunless burgers the best alternative?
Here's a healthier, and tastier, way to cut carbs.**]

BY WALTER C. WILLETT, M.D.,
AND PATRICK J. SKERRETT

A middle-aged man, tired of being fat and having trouble losing weight, happens on a low-carbohydrate diet. He tries it for a few months and watches happily as the pounds slip away without the gnawing hunger and cravings that other diets have caused him. He writes a book that is a huge hit with the public, even though the medical establishment scorns it. The book is William Banting's "Letter on Corpulence, Addressed to the Public." It was published in London in 1863.

Imagine Banting's delight if he could listen in on a 21st-century cocktail party. We're still duly obsessed with our corpulence. And thanks to Dr. Robert Atkins, the cantankerous cardiologist who revived Banting's theories in the 1970s, most people now assume that carbohydrates are part of the problem. We don't "diet" anymore. We "go on Atkins," trusting that bunless burgers will do for us what fat-free doughnuts never did. Our faith is not entirely misguided. It's now clear that carb-rich foods can inflate appetite and foster type 2 diabetes, and that low-carb diets promote short-term weight loss. But healthy eating is not quite as simple, or as boring, as living on fat and protein. The truth is, you can have your carbs and eat them, too. You just have to know how to choose them.

When Atkins came out against bread, potatoes and pasta 30 years ago, main-stream nutritionists dismissed him as a crank. Fat was the demon of the day, and carbohydrates were seen as their exorcist. That's still true today, at least according to the poorly built USDA Food Guide Pyramid. But many experts now believe that Atkins was at least half right in condemning carbohydrates. Last year five well-designed clinical trials indicated that low-carbohydrate diets were as good as low-fat diets—and in most cases better—for helping very overweight people shed pounds quickly. Study participants stuck better with low-carb diets than with low-fat diets. And though low-carb dieters increased their fat intake, they didn't suffer harmful changes in blood cholesterol. They enjoyed reductions in LDL (bad) cholesterol and triglycerides (fat-carrying particles associated with heart disease), and increases in HDL (good) cholesterol.

Granted, short-term weight loss is not the best measure of a diet's ultimate value. There is still no clear evidence that Atkins-style diets are better than any others for helping people stay slim, and their broader health effects are still unknown. Will moderately overweight people enjoy the same improvements in triglyceride and HDL levels as the obese study participants? Could the abundant protein in an Atkins-style diet cause kidney damage or bone loss over time? These important questions deserve answers. But the case against carbs doesn't rest entirely on weight-loss trials. Other recent research shows that certain carb-rich foods can cause extreme surges in blood sugar and insulin surges that contribute to weight gain and increase your risk of developing diabetes and heart disease.

The Atkins diet, in its cruder variants, assumes that any food rich in carbohydrates will trigger this toxic cascade. But carbs differ greatly in their potential to do this. The key variable is the glycemic index, a ranking of foods according to how rapidly their sugars are released into the bloodstream. The body converts all digestible carbohydrates into glucose, the sugar that our cells use as fuel. When glucose molecules pass from the gut into the bloodstream, the pancreas releases insulin, a hormone that activates cells to absorb it. Muscle, fat and other cells then sponge the excess glucose from the blood, and insulin levels return to normal. The concept of a glycemic index emerged in the 1990s, when researchers at the University of Toronto showed that some foods (cornflakes or potatoes, for example) raised blood sugar faster and higher than others (oatmeal or brown rice), placing greater demands on the insulin system. That discovery led to an even more useful measurement called glycemic load, developed by a team from

Medium Rare—And Hold the Prions!

Should Atkins fans worry about the recent discovery of mad-cow disease in a U.S. herd? They shouldn't ignore it completely. The prions (infectious proteins) responsible for mad cow can cause a fatal brain disease in people who eat infected animals. The odds of contracting it from any given hamburger are infinitesimal. But if you're concerned, there are steps you can take to lower the risk even further. Some tips:

Skip the head and bones:
Muscle meat is generally safe, but cuts containing nerve tissue are more likely to harbor infectious material. So steer clear of brains, cheeks and cuts that are sold on the bone.

Think twice about sausage:
The machine scrapings used in packaged hot dogs, bologna, salami and meatballs are drawn from numerous animals and may contain spinal tissue.

Consider buying organic:
Beef bearing the USDA ORGANIC label is raised and processed under conditions that minimize the risk of infection.

the Harvard School of Public Health. It takes into consideration both a food's glycemic index and how much carbohydrate the food delivers in a single serving. Most fruits, vegetables, beans and whole grains have low glycemic loads: their sugars enter the bloodstream gradually, triggering only a moderate rise in insulin. But when fruits are squeezed into juices, or grains are pulverized into fine flour, they become the equivalent of sugar water.

"Highly processed grains are the equivalent of sugar water"

After a snack or meal with a high glycemic load, blood-sugar levels rise higher and faster than after a meal with a low load. The insulin needed to stuff all that sugar into muscle and fat cells also blunts the activity of glucagon, a hormone that signals the body to burn stored fuel when blood-sugar levels fall below a certain point. Glucose levels plummet as a result, leaving the brain and other tissues starved for energy. Concentration flags, muscles get shaky and the body perceives an emergency. In search of a quick fix, the gut and brain send out hunger signals long before it's time for another meal. And if you respond to these signals by downing another high-glycemic snack, the cycle repeats itself. The fluctuating sugar levels and elevated insulin levels lead to excessive snacking—and calories.

Foods with a high glycemic load pose another problem for a growing number of Americans. The tissues of people who are overweight or physically inactive resist insulin's signal to pull in glucose from the blood—a condition known as insulin resistance. This keeps blood sugar at high levels for prolonged periods. It also forces the pancreas to produce extra insulin in order to jam glucose into cells. Overworked insulin-making cells can wear out and cease production, leading ultimately to diabetes.

The good news is that you needn't swear off carbohydrates to avoid these problems. The trick is to choose foods with low glycemic loads. As you can see from the table at health.harvard.edu/newsweek, a serving of orange juice has nearly three times the glycemic load (13) of an orange (5), and a serving of cornflakes carries five times the load (21) of a serving of All-Bran (4). Whether you're shopping, cooking or ordering out, it's wise to focus on foods that fall into the low teens and below, and to save those at the high end for the occasional snack or meal. But you don't have to carry a food chart to eat wisely. Here are some rules of thumb for choosing the best carbs:

EAT PLANTS. Eaten whole, most fruits and vegetables have a modest effect on blood sugar and insulin. They also deliver fiber and other healthful nutrients. Starchy vegetables such as potatoes and corn have high glycemic loads, so use them sparingly. And don't count fruit juices as fruit servings. Most fruit juices contain too little fruit, too much sugar and too many empty calories.

BANK ON BEANS. They're an excellent source of protein. They're rich in fiber, vitamins, minerals and other micronutrients. And they generally have a small effect on blood sugar and insulin.

GO NUTS. Almonds, hazelnuts, peanuts, pecans, pistachios and walnuts are great low-carbohydrate alternatives to crackers, chips or pretzels made with refined flour. Walnuts also have heart-healthy omega-3 fats. Keep in mind that at 185 calories an ounce, eating a handful of walnuts a day without cutting back on anything else could make you gain 10 pounds or more during the course of a year.

CHOOSE THE BEST FATS. Fats tend to slow the passage of food from the stomach to the intestine. So eating good fats with a carbohydrate—olive oil with bread, for example—can curb increases in blood sugar. Good fats are unsaturated fats, such as those found in vegetable oils (olive, canola, peanut, corn, soybean), fatty fish, nuts and avocados.

SWITCH TO WHOLE GRAINS. Until the 19th century, humans ate grains either whole or roughly ground. In this form, grains offer a carbohydrate package rich in fiber, healthy fats, vitamins, minerals, plant enzymes and hundreds of other nutrients. Today's refined grains—white bread, white rice and many breakfast cereals—have a higher glycemic load. Fortunately, whole grains are making a comeback. There are at least a dozen options, from brown rice and cracked wheat to quinoa and spelt. Make a habit of starting the day with a bowl of whole-grain cereal. If you're partial to hot cereals, try old-fashioned or steel-cut oats or Kashi. Quick and instant oatmeals are also fine, but they have higher glycemic loads. If you'd rather have cold cereal, the less glycemic ones include

Wheaties, Great Grains, Wheat Chex and Grape-Nuts. And don't give up on pasta. Whole-wheat pasta is now more widely available. If you don't like the texture, try one that is half whole-wheat flour and half white flour.

Can you eat all these carbs and still lose weight? Consider a recent study of overweight teens at Children's Hospital in Boston. One group was assigned to an all-you-can-eat diet that emphasized fruits, vegetables and whole grains, and reduced carbohydrates to about 45 percent of total calories. The other group got the traditional advice for overweight people. Instead of reducing glycemic loads, participants were encouraged to limit overall food intake and reduce fat, so that carbohydrates supplied between 55 percent and 60 percent of calories. The teens on the first diet lost more weight and body fat—and stayed slimmer—than those on the second. But weight control is only one benefit of eating the right carbs. Several large, long-term studies suggest that people who eat two to three servings of whole grains a day are less likely to develop heart disease, diabetes and digestive problems such as diverticulitis and constipation.

Robert Atkins deserves credit for publicizing the perils of refined carbohydrates, but the centerpiece of the original Atkins diet—eating unlimited amounts of beef, sausage, butter and cheese—is a bad idea. Although such a diet may be good for short-term weight loss, it's not a prescription for optimal health. A diet that includes fish, poultry, beans, nuts, fruits and vegetables, whole grains and vegetable oils can work for weight control even as it reduces the risks of heart disease, diabetes and several cancers. In other words, it can bring you greater benefits than any medicine yet invented. It tastes better, too.

Willett and Skerrett are the authors of "Eat, Drink and Be Healthy," published by Simon & Schuster Source. For more information, go to health.harvard.edu/newsweek.

Good Carbs, Bad Carbs

BY RITA SCHEFRIN, MA, RD

The nutrition armies continue to battle, wielding words and theories, each camp claiming it possesses the weapon to win the weight war and promote health. The purported great debate is this: Should we be eating a diet high in protein (often accompanied by high saturated fat) and low in carbohydrate, high in unrefined carbohydrate and low in fat, or should mundane moderation be the maxim? Further, could it be conceivable that there is a reconciling bridge, a common thread, between these three seemingly opposing theories? Such a bridge—increasingly gaining acceptance, though still controversial—exists: the glycemic index and glycemic load.

Glycemic index and glycemic load are two measurements that have been developed to rate the effect of carbohydrate-containing foods on blood sugar, also called blood glucose. Foods containing carbohydrates cause blood glucose to rise. The pancreas responds by releasing insulin into the blood to restore a normal blood glucose level—the higher the rise in blood glucose, the more insulin the pancreas releases into the blood. So, by measuring the effect that a carbohydrate-containing food has on blood glucose, scientists can indirectly gauge the body's insulin response to that food.

One reason that the high-protein camp advises a severe restriction of carbohydrate consumption is to prevent this blood glucose and insulin rise. Now, some scientists who advocate a diet of moderation and those who advocate a diet high in unrefined carbohydrates and low in fat are also advising minimizing this glucose and insulin response, believing that the degree and speed with which a carbohydrate-containing food increases the level of blood glucose and subsequent insulin response may dramatically impact health and weight.

These researchers are recommending restriction or elimination of the carbohydrates that quickly increase blood glucose with a subsequent insulin rush and advocating consumption of the carbohydrates that affect blood glucose more moderately. The carbohydrate-containing foods that produce a small blood glucose rise and subsequent small insulin reaction are those from which glucose is absorbed slowly into our bodies: most fruits, vegetables (nonstarchy), and legumes and many whole, intact grains. The carbohydrate-containing foods that produce a large blood glucose rise and subsequent large insulin reaction are those from which glucose is absorbed quickly into our bodies: refined foods high in starch, including many baked flour products.

What Is a Carbohydrate?

Carbohydrate is an essential nutrient that provides our bodies and brains with the energy needed to function. The National Academies' Institute of Medicine recommends that carbohydrates contribute 45% to 65% of an adult's daily calories.

Carbohydrates are divided into two groups: simple carbohydrates (simple sugars) and complex carbohydrates (starches). Simple carbohydrates are composed of one (monosaccharides) or two (disaccharides) molecules and include glucose (a monosaccharide) also called dextrose, which is found in most plant foods; fructose, or fruit sugar (a monosaccharide), which is found in fruit, some vegetables, honey, and saps; sucrose, or table sugar (a disaccharide), which is also found in honey, maple syrup, fruits, vegetables, and grains; and lactose, or milk sugar (a disaccharide), which is found in dairy products. Fruits, nonstarchy vegetables, and dairy products are simple carbohydrates.

Complex carbohydrates consist of long chains of glucose and are found in grains, such as rice and wheat; legumes (dried beans), such as chick peas and lentils; and tubers, such as potatoes and yams. Glucose is the form of sugar that our bodies use for energy and is the form of sugar found in our blood. After a carbohydrate-containing food is digested and absorbed, the body (liver) converts all of the other forms of carbohydrate in that food to glucose.

Scientists measure carbohydrates in grams. Meats and fats such as oils and butter contain almost no carbohydrates. To learn the carbohydrate content of fruits, vegetables, grains, legumes, and dairy, a table of food values is needed. The following are some examples to keep in mind: one small apple contains approximately 15 grams; one slice of bread contains approximately 15 grams; ½ cup of cooked beans contains approximately 15 grams; 1 cup of milk contains approximately 12 grams; and ½ cup of cooked carrots contains approximately 5 grams.[1] Different fruits and vegetables contain different amounts of carbohydrates. In general, fruits contain more carbohydrates than vegetables, with dried fruits containing the most.

So Simple, Yet So Complex

Today, some experts claim that complex carbohydrates are healthier than simple carbohydrates because complex carbohydrates contain fiber. However, a complex carbohydrate can be refined, such as white breads, white rice, and white flours. These refined complex carbohydrates have had vitamins, minerals, and most of their fiber removed.

Fiber is healthy because it lowers blood cholesterol, aids elimination, is filling, and slows the absorption of glucose into our bodies. Alternatively, simple carbohydrates can be unrefined and contain fiber, such as the simple carbohydrates in whole fruits and vegetables. Instead of "complex," the term to describe the healthier carbohydrates should be "unrefined"—the carbohydrates as they are found in nature, such as fruits, vegetables, legumes, and whole, intact grains.

The Origin of the Theory

Until the early 1980s, scientists assumed that all simple carbohydrates and all complex carbohydrates had the same effect on blood glucose levels. Then, a group of scientists, led by Dr. David Jenkins at the University of Toronto, began questioning this belief and, in order to help people with diabetes, started testing many common carbohydrate-containing foods. The results confirmed their hunches, and the glycemic index was born.

Slow and Steady Should Be the Pace

Why should you care how quickly your body converts carbohydrates to glucose? After eating carbohydrates, which raises blood glucose, the pancreas pours insulin into the blood to restore a normal blood glucose level. Insulin lowers blood glucose by "escorting" glucose from the blood into the cells, where the glucose is used. A rapid rise of blood glucose causes the pancreas to pour out an excessive amount of insulin.

So, what's the problem with high blood glucose and insulin levels? First, they may play a role in the development of heart disease and hypertension (high blood pressure). Another problem may be type 2 diabetes, which has reached epidemic proportions. One theory of the cause of type 2 diabetes is that the pancreas, after years of spewing out insulin, wears out and stops producing insulin. In other words, one of the causes of type 2 diabetes may be an exhausted pancreas, possibly caused by years of overwork due to a diet of high-glycemic-index carbohydrates. In the past, type 2 diabetes occurred mostly in adults, but the number of children with type 2 diabetes is on the rise. Obesity, which has also reached epidemic proportions, may be yet another problem. An abundance of insulin significantly lowers blood glucose (hypoglycemia), causing hunger. Insulin, a fat-favoring hormone, also helps our bodies produce and store fat.

Insulin Resistance and Syndrome X (Metabolic Syndrome)

When the body's cells need more insulin to accept glucose from the blood, that is insulin resistance. This condition overworks the pancreas, forcing it to produce more insulin. The factors that contribute to insulin resistance are obesity, physical inactivity, a diet that promotes insulin production, a diet low in monounsaturated and polyunsaturated fatty acids and high in trans fatty acids, and genetics. In addition to possibly leading to diabetes, insulin resistance may also cause Syndrome X or metabolic syndrome, a cluster of risk factors associated with heart disease: insulin resistance, abdominal obesity, high blood pressure, high blood triglyceride levels, low high-density lipoprotein levels, high blood insulin levels, and elevated fasting blood glucose levels. In *Syndrome X*, author Dr. Gerald Reaven states that approximately 25% to 30% of Americans are insulin resistant and that the high-carbohydrate, low-fat diets are perilous for this population.[2]

Our Paleolithic Past

While most of our stone-age relatives did not live long enough to suffer from any of the chronic diseases that plague us today and that we now believe are at least in part diet-and-lifestyle-related, a look at our ancestral "table" is interesting and perhaps instructive.

In *The Paleolithic Prescription*, Dr. S. Boyd Eaton writes that before the inception of agriculture (8,000 B.C. to 10,000 B.C.), we were hunter/gatherers eating a diet consisting of approximately one-third wild game (according to Eaton, this meat was closer in quality to poultry, fish, and shellfish, having much less total and saturated fat than domesticated meat), with the remaining two-thirds of the diet comprised mostly of a wide variety of fruits and vegetables, with occasional honey. Absent from this diet were grains, dairy (skeletal remains indicate denser bones than we have today, probably due to calcium-rich vegetables and plenty of exercise), legumes, and sugars, such as sucrose and molasses. Even when grains were introduced, they were unrefined—whole and intact.[3]

So, the foods of our ancestors, lacking in refined carbohydrates, did not produce an intense increase of blood glucose with a consequent insulin rush. The diet was "pancreas-friendly." However, as the agricultural age progressed, grains were ground into flours, which became more and more refined until, as is the case of today's white bread and white flour, the fiber almost totally disappeared. Eventually, refined sugars were also introduced.

The Glycemic Index

The glycemic index measures a person's blood glucose response to a carbohydrate-containing food, independent of the number of carbohydrate grams in a portion of that food. The glycemic index is lowest for foods that raise blood glucose levels slowly and moderately; foods with a low glycemic index are converted to glucose slowly because they are slowly digested and absorbed. The glycemic index is highest for foods that raise blood glucose levels quickly and high; foods with a high glycemic index are converted to glucose quickly because they are quickly digested and absorbed. In other words, the harder that your body has to work to convert the starch and sugar in a food to glucose, the lower that food's glycemic index will be. So, anything that slows the digestion and absorption of a carbohydrate-containing food will lower its glycemic index.

The glycemic index of a food is affected by: 1) particle size—larger particle sizes found in stone-ground flour as opposed to finely processed flours slow digestion and lower the glycemic index;

2) soluble, or viscous, fiber—this type of fiber, found in some fruits and vegetables, legumes, oat bran, and oatmeal, slows digestion and lowers the glycemic index; 3) fibrous covering—foods with a fibrous cover, such as beans and seeds, are digested more slowly and have a lower glycemic index; 4) acidity—the acid found in more acidic foods, such as some fruits, pickled foods, and vinegar, slows digestion and lowers the glycemic index; 5) the ratio of different sugars—fructose, for example, has a lower glycemic index than glucose because it is absorbed more slowly since the liver must convert it to glucose; 6) the ease of digestibility of the starch in a food—gelatinized starches and starches with a high amylopectin content are more easily digested and raise the glycemic index; and 7) fat content—fat slows digestion and lowers the glycemic index.

Scientists are now compiling tables of the glycemic index of carbohydrate-containing foods with Dr. Jennie Brand-Miller at the University of Sydney, Australia, who is doing much of the research. (This article cites figures from the book, *The New Glucose Revolution*, by Brand-Miller, Wolever, Foster-Powell, and Colagiuri.)[4] Because the glycemic index is an approximate value, values may differ somewhat from one table to another.

Here is how the scientists unlock the secret: They test foods on volunteers to determine each food's effect on blood glucose. They take a test food that contains carbohydrate, such as a carrot, and compare its effect on blood glucose with the effect of a reference food on blood glucose. They measure the reference and test food's effect on the rise and subsequent fall of a person's blood glucose. The portion size of the reference food and the food being tested must contain identical amounts of available carbohydrates ("available" carbohydrates do not include fiber, a carbohydrate, because the body cannot digest fiber). Usually, the amount of food needed to provide 50 grams of available carbohydrates is used.

To complicate matters, two measurements of glycemic index exist. Some researchers are comparing foods with pure glucose (one reference food), while other researchers are comparing foods with

white bread (the other reference food). Pure glucose is 100% carbohydrates, while white bread is not. (White bread also contains water, protein, fat, fiber, vitamins, and minerals, which add to its weight.) Three tablespoons of pure glucose provides 50 grams of available carbohydrates, and approximately 3½ slices of white bread provides 50 grams of available carbohydrates.

How is this done? A healthy volunteer fasts overnight. The next morning, the volunteer ingests the chosen reference food. He or she drinks either 50 grams of pure glucose dissolved in water or eats enough white bread to provide 50 grams of available carbohydrates. Blood samples measuring the rise and fall of the volunteer's blood glucose are taken several times over the next two or three hours (in people with diabetes). Another day, also after an overnight fast, the volunteer eats a test food—enough to provide 50 grams of available carbohydrates. Again, blood samples are taken over the next two or three hours. The volunteer's response to the reference and test foods are repeated several times, and an average for each is calculated. The reference food receives a value of 100. The glycemic index of the test food is calculated by dividing the volunteer's blood glucose response to the test food by the volunteer's blood glucose response to the reference food (glucose or white bread).

Today, some experts claim that complex carbohydrates are healthier than simple carbohydrates because complex carbohydrates contain fiber. However, a complex carbohydrate can be refined, such as white breads, white rice, and white flours. These refined complex carbohydrates have had vitamins, minerals, and most of their fiber removed.

Because we all respond to a glucose "challenge" a little differently and may respond to individual foods a little differ-

ently, these tests are performed on eight to 10 people. An average is calculated to establish the glycemic index of each food.

You can convert a glycemic index value compared with white bread to a glycemic index value compared with glucose and vice versa. Here is how: With glucose as the reference food, white bread has a glycemic index of 70, or 70%. This means that glucose causes a 30% higher increase of blood glucose than white bread does. Because the reference food gets a value of 100, or 100%, the conversion factor between white bread and glucose is approximately 1.4: $100/70 = 1.43$.

For example, spaghetti has an average glycemic index of 38, or 38%, when compared with glucose. Multiply this glycemic index by 1.4, and you get a glycemic index of 53 when spaghetti is compared with white bread. So, to convert a glycemic index compared with glucose to a glycemic index compared with white bread, multiply the value by 1.4. To convert a glycemic index compared with white bread to a glycemic index compared with glucose, divide the value by 1.4. Because white bread has a glycemic index 1.4 times lower than that of glucose, a test food will have a glycemic index 1.4 times higher when compared with white bread than when compared with glucose.[5] Because the glycemic index numbers differ depending upon the reference food employed, you should always know if glucose or white bread was used as the reference food when looking at the figures.

While the glycemic index is a relative scale, when measured against glucose, a glycemic index less than 55 is considered low, a glycemic index between 55 and 70 is considered intermediate, and a glycemic index more than 70 is considered high.[6]

When measured against white bread, a glycemic index less than 77 is considered low, a glycemic index between 77 and 98 is considered intermediate, and a glycemic index more than 98 is considered high.

The Glycemic Load
The problem with the glycemic index is that the portion size of the test food is the

portion size that contains 50 grams of available carbohydrates from that food. With some foods, however, a portion providing 50 grams of available carbohydrates does not represent an average portion. For example, to analyze the glycemic index of the amount of carrots providing 50 grams of available carbohydrate, 1½ pounds of carrots had to be consumed—not exactly the amount that most people eat at one sitting. The problem then becomes how to measure the effect of a specific portion size on blood glucose.

Enter the glycemic load. Glycemic load is a measure conceived by researchers at Harvard University that takes into account the portion size of food being consumed. To calculate the glycemic load of a portion of food, multiply that food's glycemic index by the number of grams of carbohydrate contained in that portion.

For example, to calculate the glycemic load of ½ cup of boiled carrots, multiply the glycemic index of carrots (49, or 49%, when compared with glucose) by the number of carbohydrate grams contained in ½ cup of carrots, or five grams. The glycemic load for 1 ½ cup of boiled carrots is 2.45 (.49 X 5). (Glycemic load numbers for the same food will differ, depending upon which reference food was used to calculate the glycemic index used.) The glycemic load for one cup of boiled carrots is 4.9 (.49 X 10); 9.8 (.49 X 20) for two cups of boiled carrots; and 14.7 (.49 X 30) for three cups of boiled carrots.

In contrast, consider spaghetti. When measured against glucose, white spaghetti has a glycemic index of 38. One and one-half cups of spaghetti contains 48 grams of carbohydrates. The glycemic load for 1½ cups of the spaghetti is calculated by multiplying .38 X 48, which provides a glycemic load of 18.24. Think about what a 1-cup measuring cup looks like. When you eat spaghetti, do you think that you are eating only ½ cups? Perhaps you are eating 2, 3, or maybe even 4 cups? If you eat three cups, you are eating a glycemic load of 36.48 (.38 X 96). You can see that 3 cups of boiled carrots has a lower glycemic load than 3 cups of spaghetti. So, a food with a higher glycemic index may have a lower glycemic load when portion size is considered.

What glycemic load should we aim for? In *The New Glucose Revolution*, Brand-Miller et al advise that a person eating 250 grams of carbohydrates daily (which translates into 1,000 calories of carbohydrate) averages a glycemic load between 138 and 163, depending upon whether that person's goal is to eat all or only one-half of his or her carbohydrates from low-glycemic-index carbohydrates.[7]

Glycemic Surprises

The glycemic index and glycemic load values for a food are sometimes more different than you might expect. For example, whole-wheat bread made from finely ground, whole-wheat flour has nearly the same glycemic index as refined white bread because the fiber is so finely ground. (But, whole-wheat bread is a better nutritional bet because of its superior vitamin and mineral content.) And, would you believe that the average baked potato has a higher glycemic index than ½ cup of 16%-fat vanilla ice cream? The starch in the potato is swollen, easily digested, and quickly converted to glucose, while the sucrose (a disaccharide consisting of glucose and fructose) in the ice cream is less easily converted to glucose (fructose must be converted to glucose in the liver), and the fat lowers its glycemic index. The glycemic index of the baked potato, when compared with glucose, is 85, while the ice cream has a glycemic index of 38. These numbers translate into a glycemic load of 25.5 for the potato (multiply the potato's glycemic index by the number of carbohydrate grams in one potato, or .85 X 30) and 5.32 (.38 X 14) for ½ cup of ice cream. However, if you eat 1 cup of the ice cream, the glycemic load increases to 10.64 (.38 X 28). And, alas, because of its high-caloric, sugar, saturated fat, and cholesterol content, this lower glycemic index does not make ice cream a food to eat indiscriminately.

Because we eat foods in combination, each meal or snack has its own glycemic index and load. Adding fat or fiber to a meal lowers its glycemic load. For example, juice will probably have a higher glycemic index and glycemic load than the fruit or vegetable from which it was made

because the fiber has been lost; so, adding foods high in soluble fiber such as green, leafy vegetables or broccoli to a meal will lower that meal's glycemic load. Likewise, adding foods high in monounsaturated or polyunsaturated fats such as nuts or oil to a meal is another healthy way to lower a meal's glycemic load.

Be Your Own Detective

Short of testing your own blood glucose—which may not even be accurate because blood glucose response can vary daily—you can get a table of glycemic indexes and loads on the Web or from a book.[8] Or, you can try to be your own detective. If you consistently get hungry ½ hour to 3 hours after eating a certain carbohydrate-containing food, that food may be excessively raising your blood glucose, thus causing an exaggerated insulin response.

What to Eat?

No one can foretell how future nutrition advice might change as knowledge advances. However, the most recent recommendations of the National Academies' Institute of Medicine's Food and Nutrition Board advise that healthy adults eat in percentages of total daily calories a diet of 45% to 65% carbohydrates (with at least 130 grams to avoid ketosis); 20% to 35% fat, limiting saturated fat, cholesterol (animal foods provide almost all dietary saturated fat and all dietary cholesterol), and trans fats (manmade fats, also known as partially hydrogenated fats, found in many commercially processed foods) to the lowest levels possible while maintaining a healthy diet; and 10% to 35% protein (the Recommended Dietary Allowance for protein is 0.8 grams of protein per kilogram of body weight). A healthy diet is rich in fruits and especially vegetables (nonstarchy are low in calories), which provide needed vitamins, minerals, fiber, and phytochemicals (plant substances manifested through the succulent colors of the foods of the plant kingdom that include some of the antioxidants and may protect against disease), and is low in saturated fat, cholesterol, and trans fat. And, studies suggest that whole, intact grains (not refined grains) are protective against diabetes, heart disease, and perhaps cancer.

In his book *Eat, Drink, and Be Healthy*, Dr. Walter Willett, chairman of the department of nutrition at the Harvard School of Public Health and a proponent of the glycemic index and load theories, recommends daily physical activity and weight management as the basis for a healthy lifestyle. For food choices, he advises intact or coarsely ground whole grains; use of monounsaturated oils (such as canola, olive, and peanut oils) and polyunsaturated oils (such as corn, soybean, and sunflower oils); plenty of vegetables; fruits; protein foods that contain less saturated fat than red meat (such as poultry) and that provide beneficial unsaturated fats (such as fish) and are also high in fiber, vitamins, minerals, and phytochemicals (such as beans and nuts); and strict limits on the consumption of foods high in saturated fat (such as butter and red meat) and on foods with a high glycemic index or that produce a high glycemic load (such as refined grains and breads, potatoes, and sweets). Dr. Willett believes that a diet with more than 30% of its calories from fat is fine if the fats are unsaturated and that calcium supplements are the best means of insuring adequate calcium intake.[9]

While some scientists do not accept the glycemic index and load theories, others would advise that most of the carbohydrate-containing foods that you choose have a low glycemic index or that your portion sizes or meals provide a low glycemic load. Brand-Miller, Wolever, Foster-Powell, and Colagiuri believe that only one-half of one's carbohydrates need to come from low-glycemic-index foods.[10] Perhaps individual sensitivity will prove more critical than currently recognized. And, remember: "portion portion"—for weight control, calories (thus, portion sizes) count, no matter what foods are eaten.

—Rita Schefrin, MA, RD, has taught nutrition at Montclair State University. She has a special interest in weight control and has completed the ADA/CDR Certificate of Training in Adult Weight Management program.

Notes

1. American Diabetes Association and American Dietetic Association Exchange Lists.

2. Reaven G, Strom TK, Fox B. *Syndrome X*. New York, N.Y.; 2000.

3. Eaton SB, Shostak M, Konner M. *The Paleolithic Prescription*. New York, N.Y.; 1988.

4. Brand-Miller J, Wolever TMS, Foster-Powell K, Colagiuri S. *The New Glucose Revolution*. New York, N.Y.; 2003.

5. Brand-Miller J, Wolever TMS, Colagiuri S, Foster-Powell K. *The Glucose Revolution*. New York, N.Y.; 1999.

6. Brand-Miller J, Wolever TMS, Foster-Powell K, Colagiuri S. *The New Glucose Revolution*. New York, N.Y.; 2003.

7. Ibid.

8. Brand-Miller J, Wolever TMS, Colagiuri S, Foster-Powell K. *The Glucose Revolution*. New York, N.Y.; 1999.

9. Willett W. *Eat, Drink, and Be Healthy*. New York, N.Y.; 2001.

10. Brand-Miller J, Wolever TMS, Foster-Powell K, Colagiuri S. *The New Glucose Revolution*. New York, N.Y.; 2003.

EYE WISE

SEEING INTO THE FUTURE

By Bonnie Liebman

Eventually, your eyes wear out. First your focus starts to falter. Even middle-aged people who used to have 20/20 vision need glasses to read the fine print.

But that's just the beginning. Cataracts blur the vision of 20 percent of people in their 60s, more than 40 percent of people in their 70s, and nearly 70 percent of those in their 80s.

Worse yet, by age 75, more than one out of four people shows signs of damage to the retina. Degeneration of the macula, the center of the retina, is the leading cause of irreversible blindness in the U.S.

But vision loss isn't inevitable. The right foods, vitamins, and exercise may keep your eyes younger as you age.

Spinach salad or Caesar? Grilled salmon or roast chicken? Nuts or chips? An apple or a doughnut?

It's no surprise that what you eat can inflate your waistline, clog your arteries, and raise your blood pressure. But few people think of their eyes as they scan a menu or pack a snack.

Yet a growing body of evidence suggests that certain vegetables, fruits, fish, nuts, and other foods can protect your vision, while certain fats and baked sweets like cakes, cookies, and pies may blur it. And some sup-

plements may stave off eye damage while others are useless.

The catch is that vision rarely deteriorates in the blink of an eye. To keep seeing clearly, you've got to start early.

Cataracts

At first, it seems like you've got dirty glasses. Colors seem dimmer. Bright lights have a glare. By the time you have a ready-to-be-extracted, or "ripe," cataract, it's almost as though you're looking through a waterfall. (That's what the word "cataract" means.)

What causes the lens to become opaque in places? Researchers aren't sure, but they believe that fibers in the lens play a role.

"The lens continues to lay down new fibers throughout life," says Frederick Ferris III, director of clinical research at the National Eye Institute. "But it can't grow in size because it's stuck inside the eye, so the fibers become more densely packed."

That's one reason people lose the ability to see things that are near as they age, he explains. "The lens loses flexibility so it can't focus up close."

Proteins in the lens are also at fault. "Normally, molecules in the lens keep the proteins separate, in a pattern that allows light through," says Ferris. "But the balance that

keeps the lens clear may tip in the direction of proteins clumping together."

The solution: surgery. Out goes the clouded lens; in goes a clear plastic replacement.

Doctors remove more than 1.5 million cataracts each year in the U.S., at a cost that accounts for more than 12 percent of the Medicare budget.

"Delaying cataracts by 10 years could reduce the number of extractions by half," says Julie Mares, a professor in the department of ophthalmology and visual sciences at the University of Wisconsin Medical School in Madison.

But how? Here's what we know so far.

•**Antioxidant vitamins.** "We have pretty consistent evidence that people who take multivitamins have lower rates of cataract," says Mares.

Researchers believe that oxidation promotes cataracts by damaging the proteins in the lens. "Oxidative stress is high in the eye due to the intense light exposure," explains Mares. And antioxidants seem to protect the lens in animal studies.

But the evidence in humans isn't airtight. In several studies, people who took multivitamins were less likely to get cataracts.[1,2] But in one study, the risk was lower only in people who took vitamin C, not other antioxidants. And the longer they took it, the better.[3]

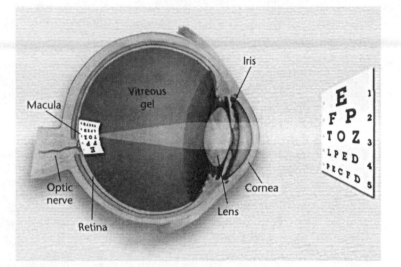

The lens, which focuses light rays onto the retina, is supposed to be translucent. Opaque areas, called cataracts, scatter light and blur vision. When the macula—the center of the retina—degenerates, it blurs the sharp, detailed vision you need to read, drive, sew, etc.

Illustration: adapted from National Eye Institute.

Got a Cataract?

These symptoms of a cataract may also signal other eye problems. Check with your doctor to find out.

- Cloudy or blurry vision
- Colors seem faded
- Glare (headlights, lamps, or sunlight may appear too bright or a halo may appear around lights)
- Poor night vision
- Double vision or multiple images in one eye (this symptom may clear as the cataract gets larger)
- Frequent prescription changes in your eyeglasses or contact lenses

---

"You don't seem to get the benefit until you've taken supplements for at least five years, and we see the greatest benefit in people who've taken them for at least 10 years," says Paul Jacques of the Jean Mayer U.S. Department of Agriculture Human Nutrition Research Center on Aging at Tufts University in Boston.

But that doesn't mean that more is better. While women who got 240 mg to 360 mg a day of vitamin C had

the lowest risk, higher doses didn't cut the risk further.

"That's consistent with our observation that human eye tissues are saturated at intakes of 200 to 300 mg of vitamin C a day," says Jacques.

Still, researchers aren't convinced that vitamin C is a magic bullet. "It's too early to narrow it down to vitamin C," says Mares. "We don't have enough data."

One reason: so far, most evidence that vitamins of any kind keep cataracts at bay comes from studies of people who choose to take supplements on their own.

"We're not sure if people who take multivitamins also eat better and do more physical activity," says Mares, though studies try to account for those and other factors.

To get stronger evidence, researchers have to randomly assign people to take vitamins or a placebo and wait five or 10 years. So far, five out of six of those trials found no benefit from high doses of vitamins.[2]

For example, in the Age-Related Eye Disease Study (AREDS), which followed more than 4,600 people for more than seven years, cataracts were no less common in people who were given high daily doses of beta-

---

Playing the Lutein

If you're looking for lutein-rich vegetables and fruit, here's where to start.

Vegetables and Fruits (1/2 cup cooked vegetable, unless noted)	Lutein + Zeaxanthin (milligrams)
Kale	11.9
Spinach	10.2
Swiss chard	9.6
Collard greens	7.3
Spinach (1 cup raw)	3.7
Peas, frozen	1.9
Broccoli	1.2
Romaine lettuce (1 cup raw)	1.1
Brussels sprouts	1.0
Zucchini	1.0
Asparagus	0.7
Corn	0.6
Green beans	0.4
Iceberg lettuce (1 cup raw)	0.2
Nectarine (1)	0.2
Orange (1)	0.2

carotene (15 mg, or 25,000 IU), vita-

Whose macula is at risk?

Macular degeneration causes no pain. Age is by far the greatest risk factor. Others include:

• Caucasian race
• Family history
• Female gender
• Obesity
• Smoking

min C (500 mg), and vitamin E (400 IU) than in those who got a placebo.[4]

"But both groups were well-nourished," says Jacques. "Two-thirds of the controls were taking Centrum like supplements provided by the investigators." Were the lower doses in an ordinary multi enough to protect their eyes?

Two trials in China suggest that a multivitamin might be enough for people who are undernourished. "In a nutritionally deprived region in China, multivitamins lowered the prevalence of cataract," says Mares. "A supplement containing 120 milligrams of vitamin C and molybdenum did not."

A clearer answer for Americans may come in a nine-year trial testing ordinary multivitamins against a placebo on 1,000 people in Italy, says Mares. "So far, the literature doesn't suggest that taking anything more than a regular multivitamin would be useful."

• **Lutein.** Lutein and its close cousin, zeaxanthin, are pigments found mostly in fruits and vegetables, especially leafy greens like spinach, collards, and kale. (The two are so close that when we say "lutein," we generally mean both.)

In studies that ask people what they're eating and wait to see who gets which disease, lutein seems to help ward off cataracts. "The data from observational studies on cataracts and lutein is quite consistent," says Mares.

In three large studies, people who got the most lutein from their food had a 20 to 50 percent lower risk of getting a cataract or having cataract surgery than people who got the least lutein.[5,6] But exactly how lutein might protect the lens is still fuzzy.

"Lutein and zeaxanthin absorb blue light," says Mares, "but as far as we know, only ultraviolet light is damaging to the lens." So it's too early to say that light at the blue end of the spectrum matters.

"Until we know more, we have to assume that lutein works as an antioxidant," says Jacques.

How much lutein is enough? In studies of more than 36,000 men and 77,000 women, researchers found the lowest risks of cataract surgery in those who consumed about six milligrams (6,000 micrograms) or more a day. "That's well within the range you can get in the diet," says Mares.

For example, men who ate broccoli or raw spinach more than twice a week were about 25 percent less likely to have cataract surgery than men who ate those vegetables less than once a month.[6] Men who ate cooked spinach at least twice a week had about half the risk of surgery, probably because there's more lutein in a typical serving of cooked than raw greens (see "Playing the Lutein").

Corn is rich in zeaxanthin, but it wasn't linked to a lower risk.

• **Overweight.** Most cataracts are either in the inner (nuclear) or outer (cortical) section of the lens. But a cataract at the back of the lens (posterior subcapsular) is the worst.

"Posterior subcapsular cataracts are the least common but the most important because they lead to surgery more frequently than other cataracts," explains Jacques.

Clouding in the back of the lens is most likely to blur vision because that's where light rays are focused into a narrow beam. They're the cataracts that typically cause glare and halos, and they're linked to your waistline.

Seeing AREDS

Do you have macular degeneration that's either intermediate or advanced (not early)?

If so, talk to your doctor about whether to take the high-dose daily supplements used in AREDS—the Age-Related Eye Disease Study: vitamin C (500 mg), vitamin E (400 IU), beta-carotene (15 mg, or 25,000 IU), zinc (80 mg), and copper (2 mg).

Make sure you take *zinc oxide*, because *zinc gluconate* could lead to higher blood levels of zinc. Researchers added the copper because high doses of zinc may interfere with copper absorption.

At high doses, zinc may raise the risk of prostate cancer, lower HDL ("good") cholesterol, and impair immunity. High doses of beta-carotene may increase the risk of lung cancer in smokers. But if your vision is in danger, the benefits to your eyes may outweigh those potential risks.

"Individuals who are overweight tend to have a higher risk of posterior subcapsular cataracts" says Jacques. A supersized belly puts you in greatest jeopardy. Posterior cataracts are roughly twice as common in women with a waist larger than 35 inches than in women with a waist smaller than 31 inches.[7]

"People with diabetes are also more likely to get posterior subcapsular cataracts" says Jacques. What's the link? In both diabetes and obesity, "high blood sugar levels may damage the protein in that part of the lens."

Macular Degeneration

Think of your retina as the film in your (old-fashioned, non-digital) camera. Rods (which handle peripheral and night vision) and cones (responsible for color and sharp vision) convert the image into electrical impulses, which travel to your brain via the optic nerve.

The most sensitive part of the retina is the macula. There, millions of cones are tightly packed to create a high resolution image. It's the macula that can deteriorate with age.

"The cells in your retina—which are there from birth—work very

---

The Bottom Line

To lower your risk of cataracts and/or macular degeneration:

- Don't smoke.
- Eat leafy green vegetables like spinach and broccoli at least twice a week.
- Eat fish at least once a week.
- Take a multivitamin for insurance.
- Lose excess weight.
- Snack on fruits, vegetables, or nuts instead of cookies, cakes, pies, or chips.
- Have a doctor check your eyes after dilating them at least once in your 20s, twice in your 30s, every two to four years between ages 40 and 64, and every one or two years at age 65 or older.
- If you have Intermediate or advanced macular degeneration, talk to your doctor about taking antioxidants or zinc.

---

hard," explains Ferris. "They're among the most metabolically active cells in the body."

And time takes its toll. "The cells accumulate debris over the years, and eventually it catches up with them and they stop functioning properly."

The macula decays in one of two ways. "In dry macular degeneration, cells essentially give up the ghost and die," Ferris explains. "In wet macular degeneration, the cells are sick and crying for help."

The body pitches in by building new blood vessels to nourish the cells. "But this call for blood vessels messes up the job," says Ferris, "because the blood vessels are abnormal and fragile. They can bleed and leak fluid and that causes rapid vision loss."

Doctors can treat the wet type by destroying the new blood vessels

with lasers. There is no treatment for the dry type, which accounts for 90 percent of cases. That's why scientists are so eager to prevent or slow the disease. Some of what they're looking at:

• **Zinc & antioxidant vitamins.** You win some, you lose some. High doses of antioxidant vitamins (C, E, and beta-carotene) didn't prevent cataracts in the Age-Related Eye Disease Study, but they did slow macular degeneration (see "Seeing AREDS," p. 3)." So did a high dose (80 mg a day) of zinc.

"Either antioxidants or zinc made a difference, but the combination worked better than either one alone," says Ferris. Taking both supplements cut the odds that macular degeneration got worse by about 25 percent, but only in people who were at high risk for advanced macular degeneration when the study began.

That's no small potatoes. An estimated eight million people in the U.S. fall into that group.

"If they all took the AREDS supplements, it would prevent more than 300,000 cases of advanced macular degeneration during the next five years," says Ferris. "But that leaves over a million cases still in progress, so we have a long way to go."

How zinc might protect the retina isn't clear, but researchers have some clues. "The epithelial cells that lie under the retina and nourish it have the highest concentration of zinc of any tissue of the body, with the possible exception of the prostate gland," explains Ferris. "And zinc is tied up in many enzymes that may be important in the eye," a number of which act as antioxidants.

But some experts worry that healthy people will start taking high doses of antioxidants and zinc to *prevent* the disease.

"When I talk to people with macular degeneration, they proudly announce that they've told their sons and daughters to take these supplements," says Mares. "So some peo-

ple may be taking boatloads of antioxidants and zinc for decades."

She worries that high doses of antioxidants could interfere with statin drugs like Lipitor and Zocor, and that beta-carotene could raise the risk of lung cancer in smokers.

What's more, she adds, "the long-term use of zinc has been linked with prostate cancer, and AREDS found more urinary tract problems in people who took zinc."

Most of those problems were benign prostatic hypertrophy (enlarged prostate) and urinary tract infections, with only a few prostate cancers—and there were no more cancers in the zinc takers than in placebo takers, says Ferris. So far, only one study has found a higher risk of advanced prostate cancer in people who took zinc for at least 10 years.

Until we know more, says Mares, only people with intermediate or advanced macular degeneration should take high-dose supplements. "We don't know if they're effective in people in the early stages of the disease," she says. (AREDS wasn't large enough to tell.) "And it's unknown whether half of the AREDS doses would be equally effective."

• **Lutein.** It's no surprise that lutein is a prime candidate for chief macula defender. "Lutein is deposited in the retina and concentrated in the macula," says Ferris. In contrast, beta-carotene is nowhere to be found.

And researchers have theories to explain why lutein may help. "Lutein absorbs blue light and it's in front of the cells that develop macular degeneration, so it may lessen the potential for light to cause oxidative or photochemical damage," suggests Mares. "Lutein is also found in the membranes of cells that die in macular degeneration, so it may have an antioxidant role there." Studies show that taking a lutein supplement raises lutein levels in the macula. But so far, they haven't consistently found a lower risk of macular degeneration in people who happen to eat more lutein-rich foods.

"Some studies show a link and some don't," says Mares, possibly because many studies have looked at well nourished populations like nurses, most of whom get sufficient lutein.

The answer may come in a large trial that the National Eye Institute is now planning. "We're still working on the dose," says Ferris, "but it will probably be between six and 15 mg a day."

It's easier to get there with leafy greens than with most supplements. Six milligrams is 24 times more than the 250 micrograms (0.25 mg) you would get in a multivitamin like Centrum Silver.

"Lutein is expensive," says Jacques, "so most supplements have incredibly low amounts compared to what you would get in the diet."

• **Fish, nuts, sweets.** The National Eye Institute's lutein trial will also test DHA (docosahexaenoic acid), one of the two major omega-3 fish oils.

"In AREDS, people who ate fish at least twice a week had a 50 percent lower risk of advanced macular degeneration compared to people who ate no fish," says Ferris.

Results from other studies are similar. For example, when Harvard researchers tracked more than 42,000 women and 29,000 men for 10 to 12 years, those who ate fish one to four times a week had a 23 percent lower risk of macular degeneration than those who ate fish three times a month or less.[9] People who ate fish (mostly canned tuna) more than four times a week had a 35 percent lower risk.

Why single out DHA? "We know that DHA is a very important lipid in rods and cones," says Ferris. "It's

also important in the brain, and the eye is really an outcropping of the brain."

Only one other food seemed to keep macular degeneration from getting worse. Harvard researchers found that patients who ate nuts at least once a week had a 40 percent lower risk of advanced disease than those who never ate them.

In contrast, those who ate baked sweets—like store-bought cakes, cookies, pies and potato chips at least two or three times a day had more than double the risk of people who ate those foods only once every two weeks or so.[10]

Trans fats in the sweets and chips may be to blame, says Harvard researcher Johanna Seddon. But since anyone with eyes also has a heart, they should already be avoiding trans-heavy foods.

• **Obesity.** Can the battle of the bulge turn into a battle for your eyesight? Only a few studies have looked.

Researchers who studied more than 21,000 men in the Physicians Health Study found that obese men had more than double the risk of macular degeneration of men of normal weight.[11]

How fat affects the eyes isn't clear. "It could be an increase in inflammation or an increase in oxidative stress," explains Debra Schaumberg, director of ophthalmic epidemiology at Brigham and Women's Hospital in Boston. Her study found a smaller elevated risk in people who were leaner than in people of normal weight, "but we've had a hard time coming up with a plausible explanation for that."

Extra pounds—especially around the waist—also seem to speed up

damage to the macula. In a study of roughly 260 people who already had early or intermediate macular degeneration, the risk of progressing to advanced disease was double in those who were overweight or obese.[12]

Physical activity appeared to slow the disease's progress, but the study wasn't large enough to say for sure.

Eye Opener

As scientists try to nail down the foods or pills that can protect your eyes, don't forget to bring your blinkers in for a check-up every once in a while.

"Of the four leading causes of blindness—cataracts, diabetic retinopathy, glaucoma, and macular degeneration—all but cataracts can progress without your knowing it," warns Ferris. "The sad part is that by the time you can tell you have them, it's often too late to make a difference."

Anyone older than 60 should have a dilated eye exam. Just getting a new prescription for glasses isn't enough. "You can have good vision and these processes could be rampant," Ferris explains. "Only by looking at dilated eyes can the doctor tell."

Notes

1. *Arch. Ophthalmol. 118:* 1556, 2000.
2. *Nutr. Rev. 62:* 28, 2004,
3. *Arch. Ophthalmol. 119:* 1009, 2001,
4. *Arch. Ophthalmol. 119:* 1439, 2001.
5. *Amer. J. Epidemiol. 149:* 810, 1999,
6. *Amer. J. Gin. Nutr. 70:* 509, S17, 1999.
7. *Amer. J. Clin. Nutr. 78:* 400, 2003.
8. *Arch. Ophthalmol. 119:* 1417, 2001
9. *Amer. J. Clin. Nutr. 73:* 209, 2001.
10. *Arch. Ophthalmol. 121:* 1728, 2003.
11. *Arch. Ophthalmol. 119:* 1259, 2001.
12. *Arch. Ophthalmol. 121:* 785, 2003.

Feast For Your Eyes

Nutrients That May Help Save Your Sight

Research is uncovering yet another reason to eat with health in mind—our eyes. Going beyond the vitamin A in carrots that help us to see well in the dark, other nutrients may protect vision, particularly for aging eyes, including vitamins C and E, beta-carotene, two related carotenoids (lutein and zeaxanthin), zinc, and even certain types of fats.

Age-Related Eye Diseases

Age brings about changes that can lead to two common sight-robbing disorders, cataracts and age-related macular degeneration (AMD).

A cataract is a cloudy area in a part of the eye lens or the entire eye lens that keeps light from passing through the lens. As a cataract develops, it can cause blurred vision, sensitivity to light, increased nearsightedness, and distorted images, eventually causing partial or full loss of eyesight. Cataracts are also associated with diabetes, other systemic diseases, alcoholism, premature birth or birth defects, heredity, smoking, eye injuries, exposure to ultraviolet (UV) rays, and certain medications.

Macular degeneration involves damage to the macula; an area of the retina in the back of the eye responsible for the sharp central vision needed to read, drive, and perform other daily activities. Although the causes of macular degeneration are not known, risk factors include family history, smoking, high blood pressure, high blood cholesterol, and exposure to sunlight.

Visionary Research

Research is shedding rays of hope for individuals suffering from age-related eye disease, and for those at

---

Focus on Food

Although nutrients from supplements may help slow the progression of AMD—mainly for people with intermediate and advanced stages of AMD—data on the benefits of supplementation of these nutrients is still preliminary. A strong body of evidence, however, points to foods that can be consumed to reduce the risk of both AMD and cataracts.

In a study that looked at the intakes of carotenoids and antioxidants from food, people who ate the most antioxidant-rich dark, leafy greens, particularly those rich in lutein and zeaxanthin, had about a 40 percent lower risk of macular degeneration than those who ate the least amount of these vegetables.

The project examined food records and cataract development in women between 50 and 70 years old. The results confirm that antioxidant nutrients, particularly vitamin C, at daily intakes of about three times the Daily Value for vitamin C (60 mg/day), reduced the odds for the development of cataracts by nearly half. With higher intakes, easily attained by five to nine daily servings of fruits and vegetables, the odds were reduced even more.

---

risk of eye disease. Emerging evidence suggests that risk of certain eye changes associated with aging may be reduced by dietary components.

Antioxidant Vitamins and Zinc

The Age-Related Eye Disease Study (AREDS), launched by the National Institutes of Health's National Eye Institute, is an ongoing study aimed at evaluating various combinations of high-dose antioxidant vitamins (beta-carotene and vitamins C and E) and zinc supplements on eye health. One published analysis of a 6-year period in the double-blind study examined these effects on nearly 3,600 people between the ages of 55 and 80. Subjects included men and women with varying macular status ranging from no evidence of AMD in either eye to relatively severe disease in one eye.

Study results related to AMD were impressive, although somewhat limiting. Only individuals with the intermediate and advanced stages of AMD appeared to benefit. Nevertheless, the benefit was such that the study's authors urged high risk individuals with no contraindications such as smoking, to consider taking daily supplements similar to those used in the study: 500 mg vitamin C, 400 International Units vitamin E, 15 mg beta carotene, 80 mg zinc, and 2 mg copper (copper needs are increased with high doses of zinc). The effectiveness and safety of routine use of this regimen by individuals with early AMD or persons at risk for developing AMD remain unclear. It is also important to note that this is a single study and further research is needed.

The high-dose formulations used in the AREDs study had no significant effect on the development or progression of age-related cataracts. Nevertheless, other studies have found that antioxidants have favorable effects, especially vitamin C in larger amounts and for a longer duration (>10 years).

Lutein and Zeaxanthin

The yellow-colored carotenoids, lutein and zeaxanthin, are found in a variety of vegetables, including leafy greens, broccoli, zucchini, corn, peas, and brussels sprouts to name a few. Highly concentrated deposits of lutein and zeaxanthin are also present in the macula. Here they are referred to as macular pigment.

Research has shown that the macular pigment density, or the amount of lutein and zeaxanthin in the macula, appears to be associated with AMD. Dr. Richard Bone, a professor of biophysics at Florida International University, has been studying macular pigments for more than 20 years. In a postmortem study of the eyes of people who had AMD and those who did not, Bone found that those with the highest concentrations of lutein and zeaxanthin had an 82 percent lower incidence of AMD.

Bone and colleagues also studied how lutein and zeaxanthin in the diet affect macular pigment density. "These results suggest an association between dietary intake of lutein and zeaxanthin and macular pigment density," said Bone. "But we don't know yet how much lutein and zeaxanthin are needed to raise the macular pigment density to a protective level." Currently Bone is conducting a dose-response study to determine the appropriate doses.

Dietary Fats

Several studies have hinted at an association between the amount and type of dietary fats consumed and the risk for AMD. Findings from the ongoing Beaver Dam Eye Study suggest that higher intakes of saturated fats and cholesterol may confer an increased risk for AMD.

The high level of polyunsaturated fatty acids in the retina supports the possibility that certain fats may have a protective effect against the development of AMD. Although some results have linked higher intakes of omega-3 fatty acids and fish with a decreased risk for advanced AMD, the majority of population studies have failed to establish a clear connection.

More recently, a case-control population study led by Dr. Johanna Seddon, an eye expert at Harvard University, found that diets high in vegetable (mono- and polyunsaturated) fats were associated with a higher risk for advanced AMD. Although polyunsaturated fats are considered protective against cardiovascular disease, the study's authors suggest that consumption of high levels of unsaturated fats may increase the susceptibility of the macula to oxidative damage. However, an optimal balance of high levels of omega-3 fatty acids (found in fatty fish such as salmon and mackerel) and lower levels of linoleic acid (an omega-6 fatty acid found in various vegetable fats) in the diet appeared to offer a protective effect.

Seeing is Believing

Although some of the results of studies related to the maintenance of eye health through diet are compelling for specific populations, it is too early in the study of nutrition and eye disease to draw general conclusions, advises Julie Mares-Perlman, PhD, associate professor in the Department of Ophthalmology and Visual Sciences at the University of Wisconsin-Madison.

"There are holes in the evidence that need further study," contends Mares-Perlman. As with any research, one or two studies showing a tendency are not enough. "What we do know is that a large body of evidence supports the fact that diet is important in maintaining eye health. How specific nutrients from food or supplements affect the types and stages of eye disease is yet to be defined," she said.

Fortifying with Fiber

Linda Milo Ohr

Dietary fiber has been shown to aid in cardiovascular health, gastrointestinal health, cancer prevention, and weight management. Yet Americans fall short in their consumption of this important nutrient. The American Dietetic Association (ADA) recommends consumption of 20–35 g of dietary fiber/day, but the average American currently eats only 12–17 g. Since about one-fourth of this is soluble fiber, the average American is only consuming 3–4 g of soluble fiber/ day, below the recommended 5–10 g. This is a shame, because a growing body of research supports fiber's various health benefits.

- **Cardiovascular Health.** Soluble fiber has been proven to reduce blood cholesterol levels, thus helping to reduce the risk of heart disease. The heart-health benefits of fiber are acknowledged in the Food and Drug Administration's approved health claim for the relationship between dietary fiber and cardiovascular disease, which is applicable for beta-glucan in oats and psyllium husk.

- **Gastrointestinal Health.** Fiber increases stool weight and improves laxation, maintaining regularity. Dietary fiber also functions as a prebiotic, increasing the number of beneficial microflora in the gut and enhancing the gastrointestinal system and immune system.

- **Weight Management.** Fiber-rich meals are processed more slowly, and nutrient absorption occurs over a greater time period. This aids in the feeling of satiety. In addition, a study on more than 74,000 female nurses in the United States (Liu et al., 2003) showed that those with the greatest increase in intake of dietary fiber gained an average of 1.52 kg less than did those with the smallest increase in intake of dietary fiber. Women in the highest quintile of dietary fiber intake had a 49% lower risk of major weight gain than did women in the lowest quintile.

- **Cancer.** Fiber has been associated with preventing certain types of cancer, such as bowel and breast. A study published last year (Bingham et al., 2003) examined the association between dietary fiber intake and incidence of colorectal cancer in 519,978 individuals age 25–70 years taking part in the European Prospective Investigation into Cancer and Nutrition study. Dietary fiber in foods was inversely related to the incidence of large bowel cancer. The authors concluded that in populations with a low average intake of dietary fiber, an approximate doubling of total fiber intake from foods could reduce the risk of colorectal cancer by 40%.

To obtain these benefits, it is clear that people need to consume more fiber. "Modest increases in intakes of fruits, vegetables, legumes, and whole- and high-fiber grain products would bring the majority of the North American adult population close to the recommended range of dietary fiber intake of 20–35 g/ day," stated ADA in its position on dietary fiber (ADA, 2002). The majority of consumers, however, do not have balanced diets, resulting in inadequate fiber consumption.

This is where fiber-fortified foods can help. Food formulators can use gums, polydextrose, inulin, fructooligosaccharides, and resistant starch to create foods that offer another option for consumers to get more fiber. Here's a run-down of some ingredients that contribute to a food's dietary fiber content.

Inulin

Inulin is a plant-derived carbohydrate with the physiological benefits of soluble dietary fiber. It is not digested or absorbed in the small intestine, but is fermented in the colon by beneficial bacteria. Functioning as a prebiotic, inulin has been associated with enhancing the gastrointestinal system and immune system. In addition, it has been shown to increase the absorption of calcium and magnesium, influence the formation of blood glucose, and reduce the level of cholesterol and serum lipids.

"When used as an ingredient in food products, inulin can be measured and added to foods as a source of dietary fiber," said Bryan Tungland, Vice President of Scientific and Regulatory Affairs at Sensus America, Monmouth Junction, N.J. (646-452-6140)."The entire inulin molecule, due to its solubility in the 80% alcohol step in some older AOAC methods (985.29; 991.43, etc.), has resulted in the requirement to use newer AOAC methods (997.08 and 999.03) to measure the total amount of inulin in a food or food product," he explained. "I should note that the AOAC method 999.03 does not measure fructooligosaccharides (FOS) appropriately and should only be used for inulin of plant origin," he added.

"Using either 997.08 or 999.03 accurately measures inulin's contribution to fiber in various foods," he said. "A total dietary fiber measurement in a food containing inulin can be accomplished by first measuring the food using the standard AOAC method 991.43 and using a specific enzyme to destroy the inulin, and then running the food for total inulin by either of the two specific methods. Totaling the two results provides a measure of the total dietary fiber, including the inulin content."

Sensus America offers *Frutafit®* and *Frutalose®* inulin and FOS for use in a wide variety of foods and beverages. "Many applications of inulin as a health ingredient are related to its properties as a soluble, prebiotic fiber: in developing fiber-enriched and low-carbohydrate foods, improving calcium uptake in the body, and promoting a healthy microflora and immune function in the colon," said Tungland. *Frutafit* inulin, depending on the product of choice, con-

Going with the Grains

Nutritionally speaking, grains are a powerhouse of nutrients. They are a source of fiber, antioxidants, phytoestrogens, and omega-3 fatty acids. Whole grains have been linked to a reduced risk of heart disease and certain forms of cancer, such as lung, colon, and stomach. They have even been linked to aid in weight loss. Here are some nutritious grains to keep an eye on.

• **Amaranth** seed is high in protein (15–18%) and contains respectable amounts of lysine and methionine, two essential amino acids that are not frequently found in grains, according to information from the Wheat Foods Council. It is high in fiber and contains calcium, iron, potassium, phosphorus, and vitamins A and C. The fiber content of amaranth is three times that of wheat, and its iron content is five times more than wheat.

• **Barley** provides soluble fiber that has been shown to improve several cardiovascular risk factors. Kay Behall and colleagues at USDA Agricultural Research Service Diet and Human Performance Laboratory in Beltsville, Md., are investigating whether eating barley and oats can reduce the body's glycemic response and hyperinsulinemia, independent of weight loss.

• **Flaxseed** has been linked to a reduced risk of both prostate and breast cancer. In 2002, researchers from Duke University Medical Center showed that a diet rich in flaxseed appeared to reduce the size, aggressiveness, and severity of tumors in mice that have been genetically engineered to develop prostate cancer (http://news.mc.duke.edu/news/article.php?id=6041). In 3% of the mice, the flaxseed diet kept them from getting the disease at all.

A study in Minnesota among 28 postmenopausal nuns in a convent, chosen primarily because of their strict dietary practices, looked at the effect of flaxseed on breast cancer (Slavin, 2001). Consumption of 5 or 10 g of flax significantly decreased blood levels of certain types of estrogen that may increase a woman's risk of developing breast cancer.

• **Oats** were the subject of a study which found that the risk of obesity is lower for kids who eat oatmeal regularly compared to those who do not. According to the study by researchers from Columbia University and Quaker Oats who presented the results at Experimental Biology 2003, the number of 2- to 18-year-olds who are overweight or at risk of becoming overweight is almost 50% lower in oatmeal-eaters than in children who do not consume oatmeal. In addition, children who eat oatmeal are about twice as likely to meet fiber intake recommendations, with fiber intakes 17% higher than for those who do not eat oatmeal.

• **Rice** is another nutritious grain. One-half cup of cooked white rice provides 0.3 g of dietary fiber, while one-half cup of cooked brown rice provides 1.8 g. The bran layers of brown rice are rich in minerals and vitamins, especially the B-complex group, according to the USA Rice Federation. The protein in rice is considered high quality and well balanced because all eight essential amino acids are present and in proper proportion. Therefore, rice is a unique cereal grain.

tributes at least 90% dietary fiber and as much as 99.5% on a dry-weight basis.

Last year, the Dutch Public Health Ministry approved a "healthy colon" claim for *Frutafit* inulin in breads baked by Bakkerij Veenhuis, a unit of Royal Ahold. The breads are currently marketed in the Netherlands under the brand *Vitaalbrood®*. The claim states that a daily consumption of three slices of the bread with 5 g of inulin/100 g of bread creates a well-balanced intestinal flora composition, which then leads to optimal colon functioning by selectively stimulating the growth of bifidobacteria.

In May last year, FDA stated that it had no objections to the Sensus claim that inulin is Generally Recognized As Safe (GRAS). The U.S. Dept. of Agriculture also approved it for nonstandardized meat applications. "This certainly is an important step in bringing Americans closer to the many physiological and functional benefits that inulin offers," said Tungland.

Another commercial form of an enriched inulin, *Raftilose® Synergy1*, manufactured by Orafti Active Food Ingredients, Malvern, Pa. (610-889-9828). According to Orafti, it has been shown to improve calcium and magnesium absorption in post-menopausal women (www.orafti.com/orafti/OraftiGr.nsf/Home?openform). The study was conducted by Anne Friedlander and colleagues at the Palo Alto VA Health Care System in California. The study involved 15 healthy post-menopausal women and used a randomized crossover design. Calcium and magnesium absorption were measured at baseline and 6 weeks after each treatment period. The study showed that the enriched inulin could enable postmenopausal women to increase both their calcium and magnesium up-take by as much as 20%. Orafti said that this research confirmed previous studies which have shown the positive effects of the ingredient on mineral absorption.

Orafti also offers the *Raftiline®* family, which consists of two main groups of products: those based on native chicory inulin (*ST, ST-Gel*, and *GR*) and those with a longer chain length for high performance applications (*HP, HP-Gel*, and *HPX*). In addition, the *Raftilose* family consists of a group of liquid and powder products composed of oligofructose and the natural sugars glucose, fructose, and sucrose in varying combinations.

Fructooligosaccharides

FOS are natural constituents of a wide variety of fruits, vegetables and grains, and can be produced in commercial quantities. They have shown positive effects on laxation, attenuation of blood cholesterol levels, and blood glucose levels. These prebiotics have found successful use in yogurts, such as *Mountain High Naturally Nutritious Yogurt*, offered by Mountain High, Englewood, Colo. The product contains *NutraFlora®*, a short-chain FOS (*sc-FOS*™) from GTC Nutrition, Golden, Colo. (800-522-4682).

Mountain High states that the fiber enhances calcium absorption. In addition, the company's Web site informs customers that "Scientific studies show that 3 grams of *NutraFlora* dietary fiber per day provide a measurable effect on improving intestinal health." Two 4-oz servings of the yogurt provide 3 g of the dietary fiber.

Colorado-based Horizon Organic also offers *Baby Yogurt* and *Yo-Yo's,* its kids yogurt enriched with the dietary fiber to enhance calcium absorption. The company's Web site states, "As a prebiotic, *NutraFlora* increases the level of good bacteria in your digestive system and promotes overall digestive health."

NutraFlora is 95% pure scFOS, meaning that the molecular structure of the fiber is always glucose terminated (important for beneficial fermentation) and has a chain length no longer than 5. Other forms of FOS may not always be glucose terminated and can have chain lengths up to 10, explained Linda Chamberlain Douglas, Manager of Scientific Affairs at GTC Nutrition. "*NutraFlora* is a prebiotic fiber that consists of a specific, defined composition, so it consistently provides significant health and functional benefits at low doses. It is derived from sugar cane or sugar beets using a natural fermentation process," said Douglas.

The main benefits of scFOS include improving intestinal integrity and function, increasing calcium and magnesium absorption, modulating intestinal immune response, supporting a healthy cholesterol and increasing isoflavone absorption. According to GTC Nutrition, a lowering effect on total and low-density-lipoprotein (LDL)-cholesterol has been demonstrated in people receiving 8 g of scFOS/day. Other studies have shown scFOS to affect the bioavailability of the soy isoflavones genistein and daidzein. For example, in overariectomized mice, scFOS increased the bioavailability of isoflavones, leading to cooperative positive effects on bone mineral density (Ohta et al., 2002).

We believe that in 2004, an increasing number of innovations with scFOS will be realized in the market. In particular, there may be more dairy formulations and nutritional foods, such as bars and shakes, that include prebiotic fiber for its health-enhancing properties," stated Douglas. "Using scFOS in dairy foods presents great opportunity for innovation due to a number of positive synergies, such as increasing calcium absorption. For cultured dairy products, such as yogurt or kefir, the synergy between probiotic cultures and prebiotic fiber results in a maximum potential for optimized health."

GTC also introduced *CalciLife*™ in 2003. This unique ingredient is a combination of calcified sea plants rich in calcium, magnesium, and trace minerals and scFOS. "The trend we are seeing is that food companies are interested in fortifying a variety of foods with calcium and want to increase their ability to make bone health claims by using the calcium–scFOS blend," said Douglas.

Arabinogalactan

Arabinogalactans are water-soluble polysaccharides found in plants, fungi, and bacteria. Dietary intake of arabinogalactans comes from foods such as carrots, radishes, tomatoes, pears, and wheat. Arabinogalactan derived from the larch tree is commercially available as a fiber ingredient and is considered a nondigestible soluble dietary fiber. It is also thought to stimulate the colonic growth of such bacteria as bifidobacteria and lactobacilli.

One commercial form of larch arabinogalactan, *FiberAid*®, from Larex Inc., White Bear Lake, Minn. (800-386-5300), is currently being used in several products on the market as a source of fiber. Affinta, Belmont, MA, sells *Delight-Full*™ snack bars that "help consumers eat less." The bars contain *FiberAid* and other fibers, which, according to the company, are lower-glycemic-index carbohydrates that cause consumers to feel full longer. Each bar offers 2.5 g of dietary fiber. Jamba Juice, San Francisco, Calif., also uses *FiberAid* in the power boost in its smoothies.

Gums

Gums such as guar and arabic also contribute to a food's dietary fiber content. Both provide more than 85% soluble dietary fiber on a dry basis, according to TIC Gums, Belcamp, Md. (800-221-3953).

Guar gum has been shown to provide important health benefits because of its soluble fiber content. Numerous studies have shown that the consumption of guar gum lowers serum LDL cholesterol and triglycerides and increases glucose tolerance. TIC Gums said that in one recent study, rats fed guar gum as a part of their diet showed a 25% decrease in plasma cholesterol. TIC Gums offers *Pretested*® *GuarNT*® *Bland*, which is specially formulated to have low odor properties in addition to its thickening capabilities.

Gum arabic (also known as acacia gum) is derived from the acacia tree. It is water-soluble and contains arabinogalactan. TIC Gums offers an array of *Pretested Gum Arabic* systems to address specific food, beverage, pharmaceutical, and cosmetic functions. Because of its low viscosity, gum arabic can be used to boost fiber levels in a food or beverage without drastically altering the finished viscosity. According to TIC, studies have shown that

gum arabic, as a source of soluble dietary fiber, may provide important dietary benefits such as maintaining healthy LDL and total cholesterol in healthy men, speeding oral rehydration, and acting as a prebiotic.

Another form of acacia gum, *Fibregum*™ has been studied for its bifidogenic properties. It contains more than 80% soluble fiber (AOAC method). According to the supplier, Colloides Naturels Inc., Bridgewater, N.J. (800-872-1850), a single-blind study of ten healthy volunteers studied the bifidogenic nature of the ingredient by measuring its stimulating effect on fecal concentrations of bifidobacteria and lactobacilli. The study was conducted in the Human Nutrition Research Center of Nantes, France, in 1999. An increase in fecal concentrations of bifidobacteria and lactobacilli was observed at both dose levels of 10 and 15 g/ day.

Resistant Starch

Resistant starch from corn functions as insoluble dietary fiber. Depending on how it is processed, it can be labeled as maltodextrin or cornstarch. "The portion of resistant starch that measures as dietary fiber can be included within the total dietary fiber content on the Nutrition Facts box," said Rhonda Witwer, Business Development Manager of Nutrition at National Starch and Chemical Co., Bridgewater, N.J. (800-797-4992). "For instance, the 60% portion of *Hi-maize*™ 260 that measures as dietary fiber is labeled as dietary fiber. We recommend to our customers that our *Hi-maize* branded ingredients be identified as cornstarch (Hi-maize brand) or corn-starch (low glycemic) or simply cornstarch. Our *Novelose 330* is identified as maltodextrin."

National Starch offers *Hi-maize 240* and *260* resistant starch ingredients (previously known as *Novelose 240* and *260*, respectively). As a better-for-you carbohydrate, resistant starch is used to add dietary fiber, lower the glycemic response ("net" carbs) when used as a substitute for flour, improve insulin sensitivity, and promote digestive health in foods. As a prebiotic fiber, resistant starch increases the population of beneficial bacteria within the large intestine and decreases the population of pathogenic bacteria. More than 120 published studies demonstrate the health benefits of resistant starch, ranging from reduced risk of colon cancer, restoring or healing the lining of the large intestine, to positive improvements on insulin sensitivity and the immune system, said Witwer.

For example, a study by Le Leu et al. (2003) showed that resistance starch increased the programmed cell death in intestinal cells damaged by a carcinogen. Once cells within the large intestine are damaged, they can be repaired, be killed, or progress to cancerous growth. This study showed that dietary consumption of the resistant starch increased the body's ability to kill the damaged cells by up to 30%, explained Witwer. The authors concluded that high-amylose starch may protect against the progression of mutated clones.

A human study confirmed systemic benefits from fermentation of resistant starch (Robertson et al., 2003). Two groups of people were fed diets that had the same amount of carbohydrates. The test group received 60 g of resistant starch, and their insulin sensitivity was measured a day later. The group that had consumed the resistant starch had significant increases in insulin sensitivity and lower impact on glycemic response to the test meal. "There is something about the fermentation of *Hi-maize* that impacts the body's metabolism of glucose," Witwer commented. "As reduced insulin sensitivity is a biomarker for Metabolic Syndrome (the combination of risk factors leading to increased risk of heart disease, obesity, cancer and other major health conditions), increases in insulin sensitivity are hugely important. Insulin sensitivity may also contribute to appetite control and weight loss benefits."

Another study (Morita et al., 2003) showed increases in immune biomarkers and a greater capacity of the large intestine to prevent a liver toxin from passing out of the large intestine into the blood and to the liver when resistant starch was ingested. It confirmed that a leaky gut allows toxins to damage other parts of the body and that restoring the health and strengthening the mucosal lining of the large intestine can have systemic health benefits.

Resistant starches can help create foods for the children's and carbohydrate-conscious markets and foods that offer digestive health benefits, said Witwer. For example, adding dietary fiber to white bread gives children who do not like whole-wheat or whole-grain bread another option to obtain fiber's benefits. For the carbohydrate-conscious market, substituting the resistant starch for flour significantly increases the dietary fiber content, lowers the "net" carbohydrate count, and lowers the glycemic response of a baked good, she said. "We have demonstrated

that a bread containing 20% *Hi-maize* lowers the glycemic response in humans by approximately 45–50%. Scientific studies are showing that moderating the glycemic impact of food results in numerous benefits. Greater appetite control is a great benefit for the weight-control market."

Lignins

Plant lignins, which are phytoestrogens, have beneficial effects on heart health, bone health, prostate health, and some forms of cancer. For example, a study by Horn-Ross et al. (2003) linked lignins to a reduced risk of endometrial cancer, the fifth most common cancer among women worldwide. The researchers evaluated the associations between dietary intake of seven specific compounds representing three classes of phytoestrogens (isoflavones, coumestans, and lignins) and the risk of endometrial cancer in a case-control study of women age 35–79. Consumption of isoflavones and lignins, but not coumestans, was associated with a reduced risk of endometrial cancer, particularly among post-menopausal women.

Flaxseed boasts a high concentration of lignins, particularly secoisolariciresinol diglucoside (SDG). In 2002, Acatris Inc., Minneapolis, Minn. (952-920-7700), a division of the Dutch Royal Schouten Group, introduced *LinumLife*™, a concentrated form of flax lignins marketed for prostate health.

This past January, the company added a more concentrated extract, *LinumLife Extra*. It is standardized to contain 20% SDG. The concentrated phytoestrogens in the extract are thought to be capable of balancing natural hormone levels in the body and therefore have a positive role in testosterone production. The extract can be used in capsules or tablets and is also suitable for flax oil enrichment and cosmetic applications. To support existing studies showing the positive effects of flax and lignins on health, Acatris has established a clinical study program to research the extract.

Polydextrose

The polydextrose content of food is measured by AOAC method 2000.11 and can be added to the fiber determined by other methods, according to Danisco Sweeteners, Ardsley, N.Y. (800-255-6837 x2521). The company markets a fiber ingredient, *Litesse*®, manufactured from

polydextrose. According to the company, 17 human, in-vitro, and animal published studies have demonstrated the fiber properties of polydextrose. Its prebiotic effects such as enhancing the growth of bifidobacteria, have been reported with consumption as low as 4 g/day (Jie et al., 2000).

FDA has approved *Litesse* for use in frozen dairy desserts, sweet baked goods and mixes, confections and frostings, salad dressings, gelatins, puddings and fillings, hard and soft candy, chewing gum, fruit spreads, peanut spread, sweet sauces, toppings, and syrups. The ingredient provides just 1 kcal/g; that is 25% of the calories of sugar and 11% of the calories of fats. It is non-glycemic, so it can be incorporated into a wide variety of foods with a reduced glycemic index.

For More Information

There are still more types of dietary fiber that the food industry can utilize in products such as baked goods, pasta, nutrition bars, beverages, and other products. For an extensive listing of dietary fiber types and suppliers, visit www.ift.org and click on the link for IFT's *Nutraceutical & Functional Food Buyer's Guide*, or see the December 2003 issue of *Food Technology*.

REFERENCES

ADA. 2002. Position of the American Dietetic Association: Health implications of dietary fiber. J. Am. Dietetic Assn. 102: 993–1000.

Bingham, S.A., et al. 2003. Dietary fibre in food and protection against colorectal cancer in the European Prospective Investigation into Cancer and Nutrition (EPIC): An observational study. Lancet 361: 1496–501.

Horn-Ross, P.L., John, E.M., Canchola, A.J., Stewart, S.L., and Lee, M.M. 2003. Phytoestrogen intake and endometrial cancer risk. J. Natl. Cancer Inst. 95: 1158–1164.

Jie, Z., Bang-yao, L., Ming-jie, X., Hai-wei, L., Zu-kang, Z., Ting-song, W., and Craig, S. 2000. Studies on the effects of polydextrose intake on physiologic functions in Chinese people. Am. J. Clin. Nutr. 72: 1503–1509.

Le Leu, R.K., Brown, I.L., Hu, Y., and Young, G.P. 2003. Effect of resistant starch on genotoxin-induced apoptosis, colonic epithelium, and lumenal contents in rats. Carcinogenesis 24: 1347–1352.

Liu, S., Willett, W.C., Manson, J.E., Hu, F.B., Rosner, B., and Colditz, G. 2003. Relation between changes in intakes of dietary fiber and grain products and changes in weight and development of obesity among middle-aged women. Am. J. Clin. Nutr. 78: 920–927.

Morita, T., Tanabe, H., Takahashi, K., and Sugiyama, K. 2003. Ingestion of resistant starch protects endotoxin influx from the intestinal tract and reduces D-galactosamine-induced liver injury in rats. J. Gastroenterol. Hepatol., in press.

Ohta, A., Uehara, M., Sakai, K., Takasaki, M., Adlercreutz, H., Morohashi, T., and Ishimi, Y. 2002. A combination of dietary fructooligosaccharides and isoflavone conjugates increases femoral bone mineral density and equol production in ovariectomized mice. J. Nutr. 132: 2048–2054.

Robertson, M.D., Currie, J.M., Morgan, L.M., Jewell, D.P., and Frayn, K.N. 2003. Prior short-term consumption of resistant starch enhances postprandial insulin sensitivity in healthy subjects. Diabetologia. 46: 659–665.

Slavin, J. 2001. Can flaxseed protect against hormonally dependent cancer? Presented at American Chemical Society Div. of Agricultural and Food Chemistry meeting, Chicago, August.

UNIT 3
Diet and Disease Through the Life Span

Unit Selections

Key Points to Consider

- How is the area of nutrigenomics going to help the consumer lessen the risk from degenerative disease?

- Name some factors in the school environment that are going to promote childrens' and adolescents' health.

- What dietary interventions are helpful in the management of diabetes?

DUSHKIN ONLINE

Links: www.dushkin.com/online/
These sites are annotated in the World Wide Web pages.

American Cancer Society
http://www.cancer.org

American Heart Association (AHA)
http://www.americanheart.org

The Food Allergy and Anaphylaxis Network
http://www.foodallergy.org

Heinz Infant & Toddler Nutrition
http://www.heinzbaby.com

LaLeche League International
http://www.lalecheleague.org

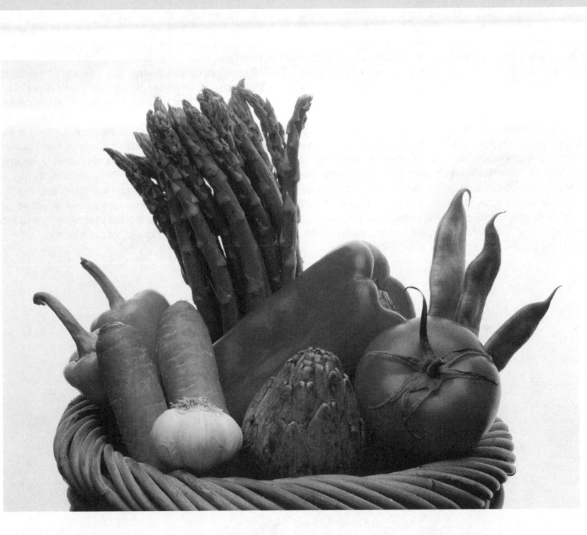

In Ancient Greece, Hippocrates, the father of medicine, stated in his oath to serve humanity that the physician should use diet as part of his "arsenal" to fight disease. In ancient times, the healing arts included diet, exercise, and the power of the mind to cure disease.

Since those times, research that focuses on the connection between diet and disease has unraveled the role of many nutrients in degenerative disease prevention or reversal. But, frequently results are controversial and need to be interpreted cautiously before a population-wide health message is mandated. We have also come to better understand the role of genetics in the expression of disease and its importance in how we respond to dietary change. The decoding of the Human Genome has heralded one of the most crucial medical projects of all time and has improved our understanding of the genetics behind certain diseases. It will help to " fingerprint" people, thus identifying the exact gene that makes a person susceptible to a certain disease. Thus, based on one's genotype, disease risk may be identified and population-wide statements about diet may shift to personal, custom-made diet regimens. This is the emerging science of Nutrigenomics. Additional research about diet and disease has enabled us to understand the importance and uniqueness of the individual (age, gender, ethnicity, and genetics) and his or her particular relation to diet.

With the recent advances in research of phytochemicals (such as flavonoids, carotenoids, saponins, indoles, and others in foods, especially fruits and vegetables) and their potential to prevent disease and increase both quality of life and life expectancy, we are at the zenith of a nutrition revolution. The most prevalent degenerative diseases in industrial countries are cancer, cardiovascular disease, diabetes, obesity, and osteoporosis, which are quickly spreading in developing countries. The number of people with non-insulin dependent diabetes mellitus has increased by 50 percent compared to ten years ago. Phytochemicals that are found in wine, spices, and coffee are presently under study to determine their effects on degenerative diseases. Even though prostate cancer has seen a 20 percent decrease in incidence since the early '90s, it still claims thousands of lives each year. Research on food and supplements that will prevent or arrest prostate cancer is on the rise. Zinc, selenium calcium, lycopene, soy, green tea, and fish diets are examined as possible candidates.

Another risk factor for heart disease is obesity. Eating an excessive number of calories leads to obesity. Animal studies have shown that restricting calories prevents disease and prolongs life. If that also applies to humans, radical changes need to be instituted in American life styles to change food-related behaviors. The recent obesity epidemic has not only affected adults but has also touched children. Approximately 15 percent of children in America between the ages of 6–19 years of age are obese and 30 percent are overweight. Lack of activity and poor dietary habits are the primary contributing factors. Children are not eating enough fruits and vegetables or dairy foods and lack important nutrients for bone growth such as calcium and vitamin D. Children also lack iron and fiber—nutrients crucial for maintenance of body weight and prevention of cardiovascular disease. Food companies have shown interest in collaborating with the American Dietetic Association and the American Academy of Family Physicians to offer healthier choices to children and provide public awareness of healthy eating habits. It has been documented that nutrition affects learning and performance. Even though unhealthy eating habits continue in adolescents, schools have not placed a high priority on student health and nutrition. The important role parents, teachers, and administrators play in developing a food and nutritional policy is crucial. Developing a comprehensive health education program, with nutrition as a major component, should become a standard in middle-school curricula across America. In addition practicing what is preached is important in learning healthy eating behaviors and decreasing chronic diseases.

By the year 2030, twenty two percent of the U. S. population will be composed of people 65 years and older. The elderly are at higher nutritional risk due to a high prevalence of chronic diseases and nutritionally inadequate diets lacking in many vitamins and minerals as well as calcium. Older people should be encouraged to choose foods of high-nutrient density and adequate amounts of protein, calcium, vitamin D, vitamin B12, fiber, and to drink plenty of water. They should be physically active, avoid smoking, limit alcohol consumption, and choose nutritional supplements carefully. Establishment of effective governmental policies are warranted to reduce malnutrition and food insecurity and to prolong independence of the elderly.

DIET AND GENES

It isn't just what you eat that can kill you,
and it isn't just your DNA that can save you—
it's how they interact.

By Anne Underwood and Jerry Adler

JOSE ORDOVAS HAS GLIMPSED the future of medicine, and there's good news for anyone who has just paid $4 for a pint of pomegranate juice. Ordovas, director of the Nutrition and Genomics Laboratory at Tufts University, believes the era of sweeping dietary recommendations for the whole population—also sometimes known as fads—may be coming to an end. Red wine may be better for your arteries than ice cream, but you can't create a diet that's optimal for everyone, Ordovas says—or, to put it another way, even Frenchmen get heart attacks sometimes. Within a decade, though, doctors will be able to take genetic profiles of their patients, identify specific diseases for which they are at risk and create customized nutrition plans accordingly. Some people will be advised to eat broccoli, while others will be told to eat … even more broccoli.

Maybe you have to be a nutritionist to appreciate the beauty of that scheme. The promise of nutritional genomics—a field that barely existed five years ago—is not to overturn a century's worth of dietary advice but to understand on the most basic level how health is determined by the interplay of nutrients and genes. The old paradigm was of a one-way process, in which "bad" foods gave you heart disease or cancer unless "good" genes intervened to protect you. New research suggests a continual inter-

action, in which certain foods enhance the action of protective (or harmful) genes, while others tend to suppress them. This supports what we know from observation, that some individuals are better adapted than others to survive a morning commute past a dozen doughnut shops. Pima Indians in the Southwest get type 2 diabetes at eight times the rate of white Americans. Individuals have widely varying responses to high- or low-fat diets, wine, salt, even exercise. Overwhelmingly, though, researchers expect that conventional dietary wisdom will hold for most people. So keep that vegetable steamer handy.

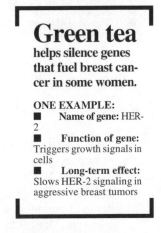

Green tea
**helps silence genes
that fuel breast cancer in some women.**

ONE EXAMPLE:
■   **Name of gene:** HER-2
■   **Function of gene:** Triggers growth signals in cells
■   **Long-term effect:** Slows HER-2 signaling in aggressive breast tumors

The model for nutritional genomics is the work that has already been done on drug-gene interactions. Researchers are starting to unravel the mystery of why a drug may be a lifesaver for one person

while causing a fatal reaction in another, and in a third has no effect at all. Why do a third of patients fail to respond to the antidepressants known as SSRIs, including Prozac, Paxil and Zoloft? The drugs are meant to increase levels of the neurotransmitter serotonin by blocking its "reuptake," or clearance from the brain. Obviously, they can work only if serotonin is being produced in the first place. Last month researchers at Duke University discovered that some people have a variant gene which reduces the production of serotonin by 80 percent—making them both susceptible to major depression and resistant to treatment with SSRIs.

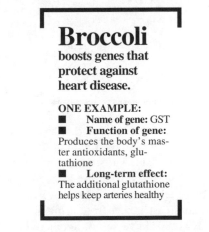

Broccoli
**boosts genes that
protect against
heart disease.**

ONE EXAMPLE:
■   **Name of gene:** GST
■   **Function of gene:** Produces the body's master antioxidants, glutathione
■   **Long-term effect:** The additional glutathione helps keep arteries healthy

But food interactions are usually far more complicated. "Normally, you take one drug at a time and for a limited amount of time," says Dr. Muin Khoury, director of the Office of Genomics and

Disease Prevention at the Centers for Disease Control and Prevention. "If you have a certain genetic variant, you stay away from a particular drug or take a different dose." But nutrients come in bulk, you consume them for a lifetime and you can get them without a prescription, even the Trucker's Pancake Special. Metabolism involves huge numbers of genes interacting in uncountable ways. There are at least 150 gene variants that can give rise to type 2 diabetes, 300 or more that are associated with obesity. Ordovas at Tufts compares the situation to an electrical panel: "We know about certain switches and how to turn them on and off. But in some people, you turn the switch but the light doesn't come on, because there are other switches upstream and downstream that we don't know about yet." It will be years before researchers have a good diagram of the circuit. That hasn't prevented the growth of a fledgling industry in personalized nutritional supplements to treat everything from osteoporosis to obsessive-compulsive disorder. At least one company will even profile your genes to take the guesswork out of choosing makeup.

Soybeans
affect 123 genes involved in prostate cancer.

ONE EXAMPLE:
- **Name of gene:** p53
- **Function of gene:** Kills mutant cells
- **Long-term effect:** A compound in soy increases activity of the p53 gene, helping to block tumor formation

But pieces of the diagram are beginning to emerge. Green tea contains potent antioxidants known to help prevent heart disease and certain cancers, but only some women seem to show a reduction in breast cancer from drinking it. A study at the University of Southern California suggests that part of the reason lies in a gene that produces an enzyme called COMT that inactivates the cancer-suppressing compounds; women with the gene variant that produces a less active form of COMT showed the most benefit from tea.

One interaction that has been studied in detail involves two categories of enzymes known as phase 1 and phase 2. These work in sequence to eliminate certain toxins from the body, such as heterocyclic amines—potent carcinogens that form, infuriatingly, in the tasty crust on broiled meat. Actually, the amines are not inherently harmful; they are dangerous only after the phase 1 enzymes have begun metabolizing them, and before the phase 2s can finish the job. So, obviously, it is desirable to have a balance of the two enzymes. But some people have a variant gene that speeds up the phase 1 enzymes, so they form carcinogens faster than the phase 2s can get rid of them. This gene is found in 28 percent of white Americans, but roughly 40 percent of African-Americans and Hispanics and nearly 70 percent of Japanese-Americans (who, as it happens, have a high rate of stomach cancer). But there are ways to tweak the system: garlic contains nutrients that slow down the phase 1 enzymes, and a substance known as sulforaphane boosts levels of the phase 2s. And sulforaphane is easy to obtain. You get it from broccoli.

Turmeric
suppresses genes that ratchet up inflammation.

ONE EXAMPLE:
- **Name of gene:** Cox-2
- **Function of gene:** Makes inflammatory compounds
- **Long-term effect:** Could help ward off colon cancer and Alzheimer's

"You can see where we're headed. We're starting to take the guesswork out of the things we eat," says Raymond Rodriguez, who heads the Center of Excellence in Nutritional Genomics at the University of California, Davis. One notable case is the gene for a protein known as Apo E, which plays a major role in regulating cholesterol. It has three major variants (or "alleles"), designated E2, E3 and E4, of which E3 is the most common. People with one or two copies of the E2 allele generally have lower-than-average cholesterol, but the E4 variety—an estimated 15 to 30 percent of the population has at least one copy of the allele—is potentially lethal. It increases the risk of diabetes, it raises total cholesterol and it reverses the usual protective effects of moderate drinking. And it vastly increases the risks of smoking. "Smoking is bad for everybody," says Ordovas, "but in a person with E4 it's a total killer. We're not talking about probabilities. It's almost certain you'll get heart disease." But, he adds, E4 is extremely susceptible to environment. The increased diabetes risk is found only in people who are overweight. If you stop smoking, give up alcohol, exercise and eat a diet low in saturated fat, "you can remove *all* the genetic predisposition for heart disease that comes with E4"—not just some, but all of it.

Patients at risk for Alzheimer's may not want to know.

On the face of it, you could make a case for universal screening for the Apo E gene. But we don't do it, and the reasons shed light on the ethical complexities of the field. One reason is peculiar to the Apo E4 allele, which also doubles the risk of developing Alzheimer's. Since there's not much that can be done to prevent it, many doctors are reluctant to give patients this news, and many patients don't want to know it themselves. More generally, there is the danger that insurance companies will discriminate against people with risk factors in their genome. Ruth DeBusk, author of "Genetics: The Nutrition Connection," thinks this concern is overblown, because by and large the risks are spread across the population. "We all have some susceptibilities," she says. "It's not as if one group has all the bad genes and the rest of us are perfect." Susceptibilities, moreover, don't necessarily amount to destiny; perhaps we can figure out what people with the E4 gene should eat to forestall dementia. But Jim Kaput, who founded a genomics-research company, wonders about people who get the correct nutritional advice for their genotype and then refuse to follow it. "Should the insurance company be obliged to pay for their health care, too?"

And—one might ask—what's the point of testing for something if the inevitable advice that comes out of it is to exercise and eat a healthy diet? Didn't we know that already? The answer lies in the "Churchill effect," people's natural inclination to believe that if Winston Churchill lived to 90 on a diet of marrow bones, champagne and cigars, why not them? "People always think the warnings don't apply to them," DeBusk says. "We hope if we can tell them 'Here's what *you're* at risk for,' it will hit home." Conversely, cardiologists now routinely put people on a low-salt diet to control high blood pressure, knowing it doesn't work for as much as half the population. Even if it doesn't work, it can't hurt, and the doctor, after all, isn't the one giving up hot dogs. But, as Dr. Victoria Herrera of Boston University says, telling patients to do something that doesn't work "makes liars out of doctors. We need to make a diagnosis based on genotype, so we can go beyond trial and error."

Not all research in the field is aimed at identifying alleles that differ among individuals. The broader purpose is to understand the interplay of nutrition and genetics. What protects Asians (at least the ones who still live in Asia and eat a traditional soy-based diet) from hormone-sensitive breast and prostate tumors? The most common explanation is that soy contains compounds that bind to estrogen receptors on cells, making them unavailable to more potent hormones. But Rodriguez has identified a soy constituent called lunasin that increases, by his count, the activity of 123 different genes in prostate cells. Among them are genes that suppress tumor growth, initiate the repair of damaged DNA and promote apoptosis, the programmed "suicide" of damaged cells before they begin to multiply. He hasn't been looking for different alleles of these genes, although it's likely they exist and may subtly affect how individuals respond to lunasin. The genetic factors predisposing men to prostate cancer can, in principle, eventually be identified and calculated for each individual. When all is said and done, though, the recommendation will probably stay the same: eat more soy. (And more fresh fruits and vegetables, and less saturated fat … and so on.)

Another compound getting a lot of study is curcumin, the yellow pigment in turmeric, an ingredient in curry spice. Curcumin reduces the action of a number of genes that promote inflammation, which is linked to heart disease, colon cancer and Alzheimer's. "It's probably no coincidence that India has the lowest incidence of Alzheimer's in the world," says Sally Frautschy, a professor of neurology at UCLA, who studies turmeric together with her husband and colleague, Greg Cole. "What I hear from the pharmaceutical industry," says Cole, "is 'What are you trying to do, ruin us?'"

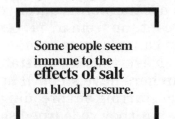

Some people seem immune to the effects of salt on blood pressure.

There's not much chance of that, of course. More likely, nutritional genomics will create opportunities for drug companies to isolate, concentrate, synthesize and improve on the compounds in nature, which they've been doing for a hundred years. What Cole and his colleagues seek is to shed light on the mystery of how the human body has evolved the miraculous ability to overcome, once in a while, the threat posed by the consequences of its own appetites.

PROSTATE CANCER

More Questions than Answers

It's not the worst cancer you can get. The odds of surviving prostate cancer for five years are 98 percent, up from 67 percent in the mid-1970s. That's a higher survival rate than for any common cancer (except non-melanoma skin). After ten years, 84 percent of patients are still alive.

Nevertheless, prostate cancer is a source of immeasurable suffering and loss. And while researchers have stepped up their efforts to find foods or supplements that might keep tumors from starting or spreading, their findings have yet to yield a slam dunk. Here's an A-to-Z guide to what they've learned so far.

Bonnie Liebman

Alpha-Linolenic Acid & Flaxseed

It seems contradictory.

In studies of thousands of men, the risk of prostate cancer is 70 percent higher in those who consume more alpha-linolenic acid, or ALA—an omega-3 fat found in meat, vegetable oils, and other foods.[1] (The body may convert ALA to the longer-chain omega-3s that are found in fish oil.)

"At first we thought that ALA was associated with a higher risk of prostate cancer because men who consumed more ALA also consumed more meat," says Walter Willett, who chairs the nutrition department at the Harvard School of Public Health in Boston. "But now it looks like the ALA in oils like soy and canola are also linked to prostate cancer."

So it seems surprising that flaxseed, one of the richest sources of alphalinolenic acid, lowered PSA levels (from 8.5 to 5.7, on average) in a pilot study of 15 men who were scheduled to have a repeat biopsy.[2] (The men added an ounce a day of ground flaxseed to a lower-fat diet for six months.)

"The findings are conflicting, but people don't eat isolated nutrients—they eat foods," says researcher Wendy Demark-Wahnefried of Duke University in Durham, North Carolina.

"We tested the whole flaxseed, which has a host of nutrients—not just ALA, but lignans, which are fiber-rich plant estrogens."

A recent study at the University of Michigan found that ALA promoted prostate cell growth, she notes. "But that was a study done in cell lines, not in people or even animals. And they used purified ALA, which is devoid of antioxidants and is kept at high temperatures, not ALA as it is found in the body."

Demark-Wahnefried's studies have found that flaxseed slows the growth of prostate tumors in mice.[3] "Those results, plus the slower cancer growth and the drop in PSA we found in men who are flaxseed during the month before surgery, are compelling," she says. "But I wouldn't stand on a soapbox and tell men to eat flaxseed. We first need well-controlled trials to find out if it can help."

She has now started a clinical trial that will give a low-fat diet supplemented with flaxseed to cancer patients who are scheduled to have their prostate glands removed. (Most men have to wait several weeks before the surgery can be performed.)

"Then when the prostate comes out, we can measure the cell proliferation rate," she says. "That's more reliable than measuring PSA."

Demark-Wahnefried suggests several mechanisms to explain why flaxseed might work. "The lignans could be acting like estrogen," which slows prostate cell growth. "Or they could bind to testosterone in the GI tract, just as the beta-glucan fiber in oat bran binds to cholesterol. That would enhance testosterone excretion."

But until more research results are in, it makes sense to avoid too much ALA, especially from concentrated sources like flaxseed oil supplements.

"We found an increased risk of prostate cancer in men who consumed 1.5 grams of ALA a day compared to those who got 0.7 grams," says Ed Giovannucci of the Harvard School of Public Health. Every 1,000 mg of flaxseed in a typical supplement contains roughly 500 mg (0.5 grams) of alpha-linolenic acid.

Until researchers know more, hold off on taking flaxseed oil.

His advice: "ALA is a tough one because we have good evidence that it's beneficial for heart disease, but men can certainly reduce the ALA they consume by eating less red meat." That might protect the prostate without jeopardizing the heart.

Calcium

Calcium is everywhere—fruit juices, breakfast cereals, pancake mixes, and dozens of other foods. You'd never guess that too much calcium may raise a man's risk of prostate cancer. Yet that's what several studies show.[4]

"In earlier studies, we saw roughly four times the risk of advanced prostate cancer only in men who consumed at least 2,000 mg of calcium a day, compared with men who consumed less than 500 mg a day," says Giovannucci.

"But now that we have more precise measurements, we see that the risk is roughly double in men who exceed 1,500 mg," he adds, referring to a new, unpublished study. That's more than the 1,200 mg a day that experts recommend for men, but it's not much more.

How could calcium harm the prostate? Some researchers believe that a high calcium intake lowers levels of vitamin D in the blood. (Taking extra vitamin D doesn't help.) Less D may make it easier for cells to lose their normal structure and to proliferate, two hallmarks of cancer cells.

"That's far from proven," says Giovannucci. "But there's no benefit from getting 1,500 mg or more of calcium a day anyway."

And with the food industry fortifying so many foods with calcium, consuming that much isn't hard. "Ten years ago, it wasn't a problem," says Giovannucci, "but now you can get a lot of calcium from different sources without thinking about it."

Fish vs. Red Meat

Go with surf, not turf.

The Health Professionals Follow-up Study has tracked more than 47,000 men since 1986. Those who reported eating fish more than three times a week had a 44 percent lower risk of metastatic prostate cancer over the next 12 years compared with those who reported eating fish less than twice a month.[5] (Fish oil supplements had no impact on risk.)

Eating more fish may protect the prostate.

It's unclear why fish (a good source of long-chain omega-3 fats) might protect the prostate, while alpha-linolenic acid (a shorter-chain omega-3 fat) might increase the risk.

Fish may appear protective because people who eat more seafood often eat less red meat, which is linked to a higher risk of prostate cancer in some studies.[6] "It's hard to tease that out," says Giovannucci.

If meat does promote cancer, it's not clear how. "It could be related to meat fat, or the nitrites in processed meats, or cooking meat at high temperatures," he explains. "At this point we can't say for sure."

He's more sure about what men should eat.

"Only a few studies suggest that fish may protect against advanced prostate cancer, but it's still prudent to increase fish and to decrease red meat to reduce the risk of heart disease."

Green Tea

American men are three times more likely than Japanese men—and 18 times more likely than Chinese men—to die of prostate cancer. Why?

One theory is that green tea may protect Asian men. When researchers gave green tea extracts—equal to six cups of tea a day—to mice that spontaneously get metastatic prostate cancer, it stopped the spread of cancer cells.[7]

But mice aren't people. "We tested green tea on men with advanced prostate cancer because we had data showing that green tea components were effective in killing prostate cancer cells in the laboratory," explains Aminah Jatoi, an oncologist at the Mayo Clinic in Rochester, Minnesota.

Green tea slowed the spread of prostate cancer in mice, but not men.

Jatoi and other physicians in the North Central Cancer Treatment Group gave six cups of tea a day (each made with one gram of green tea powder) to 42 cancer patients whose PSA levels hadn't dropped despite treatment with hormones.[8] Their PSAs kept rising.

"It's possible that green tea might work at earlier stages," says Jatoi. "But it wasn't effective in patients with advanced cancer."

Since then, a study found that Chinese men who had prostate cancer were less likely to be tea drinkers than men without cancer.[9] But researchers need far more evidence to reach any conclusions.

"It would be wonderful if everything that works in cell lines also worked in people," says Jatoi. "We need more clinical trials to find out."

Low-Fat Diet, etc.

"We put men on a vegan diet of fruits, vegetables, whole grains, beans, and soy products instead of dairy," says Dean Ornish, describing a study he conducted with Peter Carroll and their colleagues at the Preventive Medicine Research Institute in Sausalito and the University of California at San Francisco.

"They exercised three hours a week and did an hour of meditation or other stress-management techniques every day. They also took part in a weekly support group."

Ornish studied 90 men who had chosen to "watch and wait" rather than have surgery or other treatment for their early-stage prostate cancer. After one year, the men on the vegan diet (who were getting 10 percent of their calories from fat) had a small but statistically significant drop in PSA levels, while the control group had a rise in PSA, Ornish reported at a recent scientific meeting. But until the study is published, the results are difficult to evaluate.

"It's encouraging that Ornish saw a drop in PSA," says Mark Moyad, director of complementary and alternative Medicine at the University of Michigan Urology Center in Ann Arbor. "But cancer is difficult to fight, especially when it's aggressive."

When it comes to healthy men, similar but less drastic diet changes had no impact on PSA levels.

In a four-year study of 1,350 healthy men, researchers at Sloan-Kettering Memorial Hospital in New York found that those who ate a low-fat diet (20 percent of calories from fat) high in fiber, fruits, and vegetables had no lower PSAs than those who were simply given a brochure on a healthy diet. [10]

Still, says Moyad, any diet that protects against heart disease is worth eating.

"The worst-case scenario is that you only reduce the risk of the number-one cause of death. We have plenty of men who have beaten prostate cancer only to die of something else. The goal is to live long—not to beat just one disease."

Selenium

The good news: the National Cancer Institute is testing whether selenium (and vitamin E) can prevent cancer in more than 32,000 men nationwide. The bad news: results are not expected until 2013.

Selenium was thrust into the spotlight in 1996 when researchers looked at its ability to prevent recurring skin cancers in the southeastern U.S., where levels of selenium in the soil—and therefore in locally grown foods—are low.

"In the initial report on the study, they found no difference in skin cancer, but they noticed a decrease in prostate cancer incidence," says W. Robert Lee of the Wake Forest University Baptist Medical Center in Winston-Salem, North Carolina.

Since then, other studies have found a higher risk in men with low selenium levels in their blood or toenails. [11]

"Selenium holds the most promise for men who are deficient in selenium," says Lee. "In subsequent analyses of the skin-cancer trial, only those men benefited from selenium." [12]

It's too early to know if Lee is right. But the buzz about selenium may be causing other problems.

"We've got a population of men overdosing on the stuff," says Moyad. Too much selenium is toxic, he points out. "We've seen some men showing up with hair loss and dizziness." (To avoid toxicity, don't exceed 200 mcg a day, the dose used in most studies.)

"Men should have a blood test before they start taking a selenium supplement to see if their levels are low," says Moyad. "Taking selenium without a blood test ignores all we know about the mineral and could be dangerous."

Soy

The soy story is still unfolding.

"Prostate cancer rates are low in Asia, though they're increasing dramatically," says Mark Messina, an adjunct professor at Loma Linda University in California who has consulted for the soy industry.

So far, soy hasn't cut PSA levels in healthy men or prostate cancer patients.

"But we have no large studies in the U.S. because Americans don't eat enough soy." A recent Asian study suggests that soy protects the prostate, he adds. [13]

Without large numbers of soy eaters to track, researchers have instead tested soy—or isoflavones extracted from soy—on PSA levels. (In animal studies, the estrogen-like isoflavones curb the growth of prostate tumors.)

Soy failed to lower PSA levels in three studies on men, and slowed the rise in PSA in a fourth. [14–17]

"So far, it looks like not a lot happens to PSA when people eat soy," says Wake Forest's Lee. Many doctors don't consider a treatment effective unless it lowers PSA levels by at least 50 percent. Smaller changes are difficult to interpret.

"There's no question that if a prostate cancer patient's PSA goes up quickly—say, if it doubles in three to six months—especially after treatment, they're in trouble," Lee explains.

"But if you slow down the doubling time, say, from three to four years to five to eight years, we don't know what that means. It's too much of a stretch to say that PSA doubling time is a surrogate for time to death."

PSA isn't a perfect measure of a cancer's growth, says Lee. "If you do nothing, PSA can sometimes go up or down. For example, bike riding, a biopsy, prostatitis, catheterization, urinary retention, or trauma can raise PSA."

On the other hand, some researchers think that traditional soy foods are worth the gamble. "Soy is heart-healthy and the number-one cause of death in men is heart disease," says Lee.

But there's a catch. "The problem with soy is that people get fixated on bars and pills," says Moyad. "Some bars have 250 calories and some are high in saturated fat. And they may not have the isoflavones and proteins that are in traditional soy foods."

Tomato Sauce & Lycopene

"A new study says men who eat ten pizzas a week are less likely to develop prostate problems," joked Jay Leno in December 1995. "They're more likely to develop size 54 pants."

It's been nearly a decade since Ed Giovannucci and colleagues at the Harvard School of Public Health discovered that men who eat tomatoes at least twice a week have a lower risk of prostate cancer. Dozens of studies followed. [18]

"Researchers recently looked at all the literature and found a 20 percent reduced risk in studies that looked at cooked, not raw, tomatoes," says Giovannucci.

Lycopene may explain why cooked tomatoes seem to be more protective than raw. "One serving of tomato sauce has much more lycopene than a tomato or a glass of tomato juice," says Giovannucci.

Lycopene—the pigment that gives tomatoes, pink grapefruit, watermelon, and guava their red color—is also an antioxidant that's concentrated in the prostate gland. When Giovannucci looked at men who were older than 65 and had no family history of prostate cancer, those with higher blood levels of lycopene had roughly half the risk of getting the disease than those with lower blood levels. [19]

Men who eat tomato sauce at least twice a week have a lower risk of prostate cancer.

"In younger men with a family history, the risk might be more related to genetics," he explains. "But those men comprise only about 10 percent of people with prostate cancer, so lycopene may still be protective for the majority."

It's too early to know, though, whether it's the lycopene or something

The Bottom Line

- Cut back on red meat and shoot for two or three servings of fish a week.
- Try for at least two servings a week of tomato sauce (preferably on pasta or other dishes that aren't smothered in cheese).
- Take a multivitamin with roughly a day's worth of vitamin E (30 IU) and selenium (55 mcg).
- Don't take more zinc than you'd get in an ordinary multivitamin (15 mg).
- Don't assume that more calcium is better. Don't exceed the recommended calcium intakes (1,200 mg a day for men over 50 and 1,000 mg a day for men 50 and under, from food and supplements combined).
- Until researchers know more about alpha-linolenic acid (ALA), avoid flaxseed oil supplements.

else in tomatoes that matters. When researchers recently gave rats a carcinogen, they found fewer prostate tumors if the animals were fed tomato powder, but not if they were fed lycopene.[20]

"We always inferred that lycopene explained the link between tomatoes and prostate cancer," says Giovannucci. "Lycopene may be a factor, but it may also be a marker for something else in tomatoes that's beneficial."

Meanwhile, Aminah Jatoi and North Central Cancer Treatment Group at the Mayo Clinic are testing lycopene in

"The dose—30 milligrams a day—is comparable to a diet with a lot of spaghetti sauce," she explains. In fact, her patients will take their lycopene in tomato sauce.

She expects results in about two years. In the meantime, says Giovannucci, "we don't have enough evidence to recommend that men take lycopene, but we do have enough to recommend that they eat tomato products twice a week."

Just remember that you don't need cheese-heavy dishes like pizza or lasagna to enjoy tomato sauce.

Vitamin E

Vitamin E, once the darling of antioxidant enthusiasts, has lost its luster when it comes to staving off heart attacks. "It's been a bust in studies on more than 55,000 people and cardiovascular disease," notes the University of Michigan's Mark Moyad.

It's too early to say whether the antioxidant will prevent prostate cancer. Most of the promising evidence comes from research in smokers.

"Smokers are notorious for low levels of vitamin E and other antioxidants," says Moyad. "What do you tell a nonsmoking man about vitamin E? No one has any idea what it can do in nonsmokers."

In the SELECT trial, healthy men are taking 400 IU of vitamin E (alphatocopherol) every day for seven to 12 years. That's considerably higher than the U.S. Recommended Daily Allowance (30 IU), or the 50 IU that seemed to cut the risk of prostate cancer in smokers.

High doses may not be harmless, notes Moyad. "They may increase the risk of bleeding in people who take aspirin or other blood-thinning drugs."

Zinc

"Zinc deficiency results in prostate enlargement ... larger supplemental doses, commonly between 50 and 100 mg daily, may help shrink a swollen prostate," says www.doctoryourself.com.

Yet researchers found more than double the risk of advanced prostate cancer in men who got more than 100 mg a day from supplements, compared with those who got less than 25 mg.[21] Either the zinc takers had prostate problems to begin with or zinc damages the prostate.

"Zinc is concentrated in the prostate, so some people say that it's bad if you're not getting enough," says Giovannucci. "But we found an increased prostate cancer risk at intakes well beyond the U.S. Recommended Daily Allowance," which is only 15 mg.

"Zinc is a disaster," says Moyad. "Large doses increase bad cholesterol, decrease good cholesterol, suppress the immune system, interfere with some bone-building drugs, and potentially raise testosterone levels.

"It's the number-one touted product for the prostate, and there's no good evidence for taking it."

Notes

1. *Journal of Nutrition 134:* 191, 2004.
2. *Urology 63:* 900, 2004.
3. *Urology 60:* 919, 2002.
4. *Epidemiol. Rev. 23:* 87, 2001.
5. *Cancer Epidemiol Biomarkers Prev. 12:* 64, 2003.
6. *Cancer Causes Control 12:* 557, 2001.
7. *Proc. Nat. Acad. Sci. 98:* 10350, 2001.
8. *Cancer 97:* 1442, 2003.
9. *Int. J. Cancer 108:* 130, 2004.
10. *J. Clin. Oncol. 20:* 3592, 2002.
11. *J. Nat. Cancer Inst. 96:* 696, 2004.
12. *BJU Int. 91:* 608, 2003.
13. *Cancer Epidemiol. Biomarkers Prey. 12:* 665, 2003.
14. *Cancer Epidemiol. Biomarkers Prev. 13:* 644, 2004.
15. *Journal of Urology 169:* 507, 2003.
16. *Prostate 59:* 141, 2004.
17. *Nutr. Cancer 47:* 111, 2003.
18. *Cancer Epidemiol. Biomarkers Prey. 13:* 340, 2004.
19. *Cancer Epidemiol. Biomarkers Prey. 13:* 260, 2004.
20. *J. Nat. Cancer Inst. 96:* 554, 2004.
21. *J. Nat. Cancer Inst. 95:* 1004, 2003.

From *Nutrition Action Healthletter,* August 2004. Copyright © 2004 by Nutrition Action Healthletter. Reprinted by permission via the Copyright Clearance Center.

COFFEE, SPICES, WINE

New dietary ammo against diabetes?

By Janet Raloff

Non–insulin-dependent diabetes is epidemic in the United States. The potentially deadly disorder afflicts some 16 million people in this country, accounting for 95 percent of all diabetes. The number of people with non–insulin-dependent diabetes is 50 percent greater today than it was just a decade ago. Cardiovascular complications account for half of all deaths among people with this type of diabetes, commonly called type 2, and the disorder is the leading cause of kidney failure, adult blindness, and amputations in the United States. Nationally, medical expenditures associated with treating type 2 diabetes and its complications are about $92 billion per year.

The disease arises when people lose all or part of their sensitivity to insulin, the hormone that normally signals cells to move glucose from the blood into energy-hungry tissues. Because spikes in blood-glucose concentrations can damage the circulatory system and other organs, the long-term health of people with full-blown type 2 diabetes depends upon how tightly they can control their blood sugar concentrations. They do this by making lifestyle changes, such as exercising regularly, losing weight, and choosing certain foods.

People considered to be prediabetic because they have faltering blood sugar control also fare better in the long run if they follow the same lifestyle guidelines.

Restricting intake of sugar and starches is one way that people can maintain moderate blood sugar concentrations. Their diet should include primarily fibrous whole grains that release glucose slowly into the bloodstream (*SN: 4/8/00, p. 236*). That's a tough challenge in today's fast-food world, dominated by refined, highly processed foods.

WHAT A KICK—Though caffeine makes blood sugar concentrations spike, certain trace ingredients in coffee ameliorate that effect. And one study has found that decaf lowers blood sugar.

However, an assortment of new nutrition data may come as unexpectedly sweet news. Researchers are uncovering mechanisms by which a range of dietary agents—including coffee, wine, and cinnamon—appear to restore some of the body's responsiveness to insulin and control of blood sugar. Such changes seem to be transitory, however, so these foods offer no cure for diabetes. But dietary scientists now suggest that regular intake of these foods might slow the disease's onset and reduce its ravages.

COFFEE CLASH Study after study has shown antidiabetic effects of coffee. The March 10 *Journal of the American Medical Association* carries the latest epidemiological evidence—two European studies showing that people who drink 6 to 10 cups of coffee, primarily caffeinated, per day tend to develop type 2 diabetes at lower rates than individuals do who drink 2 or fewer cups a day.

For several years, scientists have been asking what constituent of java works to control blood sugar. Gradually, chlorogenic acids, a relatively minor family of chemicals in coffee beans, have emerged as prime candidates.

Much attention focused on caffeine, which has turned out to have a detrimental effect. Terry E. Graham of the University of Guelph in Ontario and his coworkers recently tested the effect of pure caffeine, caffeinated coffee, and decaf on blood sugar in lean and obese people with and without type 2 diabetes. The amount of caffeine in a mug or two of strong coffee was sufficient to disrupt control of blood sugar for several hours in any of those 67 individuals, says Graham. A paper detailing the 56 nondiabetic volunteers is due out soon in the *American Journal of Clinical Nutrition*.

Giving the volunteers caffeine in plain water followed an hour later by a slug of sugar water induced the highest blood sugar concentrations. The same amount of caffeine delivered in 2 cups of coffee before the sugar jolt raised blood sugar concentrations about 75 percent as much as the pure caffeine did. However, when the researchers gave people two cups of decaffeinated coffee and then the sugar, their blood sugar concentrations were even lower than when they drank plain water before the sugar.

That result suggests that the decaf—and, therefore, some coffee component other than caffeine—has an antidiabetic effect, says Graham.

Last year, Linda M. Morgan and her colleagues at the University of Surrey in England tested nine healthy volunteers. Each made three morning visits to Morgan's lab after fasting overnight. In the lab, they each downed 25 grains of sugar in 2 cups of a beverage. On one morning, they took the sugar in regular coffee; another morning, in decaf; and a third morning, in water. After each sugary drink, they submitted to tests of how much ingested glucose entered their blood during the next 3 hours.

Both coffee types enabled the volunteers to control blood glucose significantly better than they did after drinking the glucose-containing water, the scientists reported in the October 2003 *American Journal of Clinical Nutrition*. Once in the blood, however, glucose that was drunk with caffeinated coffee tended to stay there, as it would in a person with diabetes. The finding is consistent with other studies showing that caffeine can impair insulin's responsiveness to blood sugar.

By keeping the concentrations of chlorogenic acids the same in the decaf and caffeinated coffees, the researchers made sure that those compounds weren't the source of the effect. Earlier studies by the group had shown that low concentrations of chlorogenic acids naturally present in apples attenuated the release of glucose into the blood after volunteers ate the fruit.

Michael N. Clifford, the research team's food chemist, hypothesizes that chlorogenic acids, which are present in far greater concentrations in coffee than in fruit, reduce the efficiency of molecular-scale pumps that move glucose across the walls of cells lining the digestive tract. These acids would thereby tend to keep sugar in the gut and out of the bloodstream, reducing the chances of the high spikes of blood sugar that exacerbate diabetes.

Jane Shearer of Vanderbilt University in Nashville and her colleagues have studied the effects of pure chlorogenic acids, isolated from decaf, on enzymes that regulate the liver's release of glucose. Ordinarily, between meals, the liver sends glucose into the blood to keep it available to tissues. In people with diabetes, the liver inappropriately sends out glucose even after a meal has already boosted blood concentrations of the sugar.

The researchers showed in rats that chlorogenic acids disrupt the liver enzymes' action, bogging down glucose's release into the blood. This helps prevent blood sugar spikes after meals, the researchers reported in the November 2003 *Journal of Nutrition*.

TEA TOO? A few studies have hinted that teas—with their bounty of antioxidants called polyphenols—might also exhibit antidiabetic properties. In the latest such trial, Lucy S. Hwang of National Taiwan University in Taipei measured green tea's effect on insulin action in rats with experimentally induced diabetes.

Hwang's team substituted room-temperature tea for drinking water for half of the animals. After 12 weeks, tea-drinking rodents exhibited improved insulin sensitivity and lower blood-

glucose concentrations during the 2 hours after each meal, the researchers reported in the Feb. 1 *Journal of Agricultural and Food Chemistry*.

In related test-tube studies, the group measured how well fat cells from these animals absorb glucose, an action that in the body would lower blood sugar concentrations. The cells from diabetic rats drinking green tea absorbed more than twice as much of the sugar as did cells from similar animals drinking plain water—indicating, the researchers say, that the tea had indeed improved the fat cells' insulin sensitivity.

Hwang's group has now tested other types of tea. All true teas are made from leaves from the same species of plant. Green tea is unfermented, whereas black and other teas are fermented to various extents.

Like the green tea in the original test, semifermented pouchong tea "significantly increased glucose uptake" by fat ells taken from diabetic animals that drank it, Hwang told *Science News*. However, fully fermented black tea—the favorite of most Western tea drinkers—didn't affect glucose absorption.

Since different teas contain different polyphenols that might underlie the fat-cell response, Hwang's team tested the antidiabetic effects of several polyphenols from the best-performing teas. The most effective turned out to be epigallocatechin gallate, an agent known to have anticancer properties (*SN: 7/23/94, p. 61*). In her lab tests, the compound has "insulinlike activity," Hwang says.

Hwang's team has traced the green tea's antidiabetic attributes to other mechanisms as well. In rats, green tea increased the number of insulin receptors on cells and the blood concentration of a protein—GLUT-IV—that helps move glucose out of the blood and into cells. Moreover, Hwang notes, the tea activated insulin-receptor kinase, an enzyme that makes the receptors available to bind insulin and initiate activity.

SPICE IT DOWN Scientists at the Agriculture Department's Beltsville (Md.) Human Nutrition Research Center have been studying how chromium, which is found in black pepper and some other foods, also boosts the activity of insulin-receptor kinase and related enzymes. Experiments beginning almost a half-century ago showed that chromium supplements can restore blood sugar control to some people and animals with diabetes. The question has been why that is and what might represent effective doses of chromium.

Recent studies have shown that the element chemically alters the cell-surface receptors to which insulin attaches, explains Beltsville chemist Richard A. Anderson. Without chromium, insulin can't dock at the receptors and shepherd glucose from the blood into energy-hungry cells.

When the hormone's job is done, another enzyme switches off the insulin receptor. Chromium also inhibits the shut-off enzyme's action, Anderson says. The element offers dual benefits.

Unfortunately, Anderson observes, the modern diet of highly processed foods is low in chromium. What's more, foods high in sugar stimulate the body to lose chromium.

The formulation of currently available chromium supplements doesn't permit the body to absorb the element efficiently,

Anderson says. However, his team has just received a patent for a new formulation, called chromium histidine, that in human trials results in absorption of about 50 percent more chromium than conventional supplements do, he says.

CINNAMON 'N SUGAR—The same kind of cinnamon that goes into an apple pie can boost insulin activity and blood-glucose control, studies show.

It was during tests of the new chromium supplement that Anderson and his colleagues stumbled onto an entirely different antidiabetes substance in, of all things, apple pie. During the early stages of one study, the researchers were attempting to disrupt some volunteers' blood sugar control by feeding them a low chromium diet that included pie. Surprisingly, these volunteers' blood sugar remained under control. Subsequent test-tube studies showed that cinnamon in the pie was boosting insulin activity, as chromium does, and thus controlling blood glucose. The spice turned out to be the "best thing we ever tested" for that purpose, Anderson says.

Anderson and his colleagues recently studied 60 people with type 2 diabetes. The researchers gave the participants capsules containing either cinnamon or wheat flour. The 30 people getting daily doses of 1, 3, or 6 grams of cinnamon for 40 days experienced an 18 to 29 percent drop in blood glucose, compared with their values at the beginning of the study. A gram of cinnamon is about one-half a teaspoon, says Anderson. Volunteers getting wheat flour for 40 days showed no such benefit.

Cinnamon also improved Study participants' blood-cholesterol and triglycerides concentrations, Anderson's team reported in the December 2003 *Diabetes Care*.

Subsequently, the scientists found that cinnamons active ingredients are polyphenol polymers with insulinlike action. Anderson's team described those experiments in the Jan. 14 *Journal of Agricultural and Food Chemistry*.

Cloves, bay leaves, and other spices show enzymatic effects similar to those of cinnamon, Anderson has found, though none approaches cinnamons potency.

WINE SURPRISE If spices and coffee can help control blood sugar, why not wine? After all, studies have suggested that the alcohol and polyphenols that the beverage contains reduce the likelihood of heart complications among people with diabetes (*SN: 7/24/99, p. 52*). These chemicals might act by increasing cells' insulin sensitivity, reasoned wine biochemist Pierre-Louis Teissèdre of the University of Montpellier in France.

Teissèdre's team separated wine's antioxidant polyphenols from its alcohol. Diabetic mice fed one or the other type of in-

MEDICINAL?—Both the alcohol and polyphenols in red wine offer antidiabetic effects—at least in mice.

gredient showed complementary benefits, the scientists reported in the Feb. 15 *Journal of Agricultural and Food Chemistry*.

For 6 weeks, animals consumed alcohol, polyphenols, both, or neither. The maximum dose was the equivalent, taking body weight into account, of the amount that a person imbibes in three glasses of wine per day. Diabetic animals getting both alcohol and polyphenols controlled their blood sugar after a meal about as well as normal mice did. Mice getting alcohol didn't do quite as well but still had better blood sugar control than did animals getting either the polyphenols only or neither wine ingredient.

The wine components also affected the retarded growth associated with severe diabetes, which prevents cells from accessing the fuel they need to thrive. In Teissèdre's experiment, the mice getting both types of wine ingredients or only alcohol grew larger than did the animals receiving polyphenols only or no wine component.

When receiving both types of wine ingredients, "animals that had been diabetic became nondiabetic," at least temporarily, says Teissèdre. His team envisions developing wines that could be marketed as medicinal beverages—with extra polyphenols for preventing heart disease and fighting diabetes.

CAUTION ADVISED It's still too early to know the medical significance of all these tantalizing new findings, observes endocrinologist Nathaniel Clark of the American Diabetes Association in Alexandria, Va. Some may not hold up in long-term dietary tests in people. Even if they do, he notes, it would be "a tragedy" for people to think that supplementing their diets with coffee, tea, spices, or alcohol could take the place of moderate weight loss, regular physical activity, and restricted carbohydrate intake.

Moreover, Clark cautions, certain of these dietary adjustments shouldn't be adopted without advice from a physician. For instance, the caffeine in 6 to 10 cups of coffee—the amount showing an antidiabetes effect in the recent European studies—might prove too much for people with certain heart problems.

And though the diabetes association currently accepts that a daily serving or two of alcohol can fit into the diet of people with the disease, Clark warns that "the risk of overconsumption of alcohol remains, regardless of any potential benefit."

The bottom line, he says, is that people with diabetes should consider any of the potential new menu changes as an addition to existing dietary, weight-control, and exercise strategies—not as a means to avoid them.

Meeting Children's Nutritional Needs

Linda Milo Ohr

The numbers are all too well known. Nationwide, approximately 30% of children ages 6-19 are overweight and 15% are obese. In addition, 70-80% of obese adolescents become obese adults. This opens up a world of health conditions later in life, such as heart disease, diabetes, and cancer.

Childhood obesity is one of the main concerns when it comes to children's nutrition. Lack of physical activity and poor dietary habits are two overall contributing factors to the problem. Food companies have stepped up to address the growing concern with children's nutrition by offering healthier options and providing public awareness of healthy eating habits.

For example, last year, Kraft Foods, Glenview, Ill., established initiatives to address obesity. In terms of product nutrition, the company stated that it would be determining the levels at which the portion sizes of its single-serve packages would be capped, developing nutrition guidelines for existing and new products, and improving existing products and providing alternative choices, where appropriate. Nabisco 100-calorie packs, a four-item line featuring *Wheat Thins, Chips Ahoy!, Cheese Nips,* and *Oreo* brands, for example, are portion-controlled, single-serve products formulated to have 3 g or less of fat, 0 g of *trans* fat, and no cholesterol. Another new product, *Kool-Aid Jammers 10,* is made with real fruit juice, contains 100% of the daily value of vitamin C, and contributes only 10 kcal/serving.

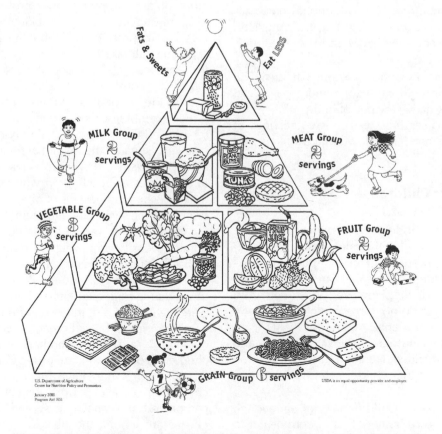

Fig. 1—The Food Guide Pyramid for Young Children is an adaptation of the original Food Guide Pyramid designed to simplify educational messages and focus on young children's food preferences and nutritional requirements.

In October 2003, Quaker Oats, a unit of PepsiCo Beverages & Foods, Chicago, Ill., in collaboration with the American Dietetic Association, introduced a five-step family nutrition program called *Quaker Oatmeal Strive for Five*. The online program teaches parents how to prevent childhood weight gain and obesity by establishing key nutrition habits at home in one month. The program was developed on the basis of a survey of nearly 1,000 ADA-member dietetic professionals who identified acting as a nutrition role model, eating mored whole-grain foods, eating breakfast daily, and understanding portion sizes as top ways that parents can help prevent weight gain and obesity in their children.

In addition to food companies' initiatives, a number of Web sites offer parents and children advice and guidelines on healthy eating.

Kidnetic.com, launched in 2002, is a site for kids 9-12 years old, parents, and health professionals. Games, a frequently asked question section, discussion boards, and recipes are among the many resources available on the site. It is part of an educational outreach program of the International Food Information Council Foundation developed in partnership with several professional associations, including ADA and the American Academy of Family Physicians.

Action for Healthy Kids (www.actionforhealthykids.org) is a nationwide initiative dedicated to improving the health and educational performance of children through better nutrition and physical activity in schools. Guidance and direction are provided by more than 40 national organizations and government agencies, including the American Academy of Pediatrics and the U.S. Dept. of Agriculture's Food and Nutrition Service.

The USDA Food Guide Pyramid for Young Children (Fig. 1) offers basic nutrition guidelines for children ages 2-6 years. They include six daily servings of grains, three servings of vegetables, two servings of fruit, two servings of milk, two servings of meat, and low intake of fats and sweets.

Foods and Nutrients Children Should Be Getting More of

"Balance, variety, and moderation of many foods is the best way for children to get all of their nutrients," said Marilyn Tanner, ADA spokesperson and clinical pediatric dietitian at St. Louis Children's Hospital and Washington University School of Medicine. However, the simple truth is that children of all ages do not have balanced diets and are not getting essential nutrients. According to ADA, intake of several important nutrients, such as calcium and iron, is less than recommended. Here is a rundown of some food groups and nutrients that children should be getting more of:

• **Fruits and Vegetables.** "Children do not eat enough fruits and vegetables," said Tanner. This is detrimental to their diets because these food groups provide fiber, vitamins A and C, B-vitamins, potassium, and complex carbohydrates for energy. Five or more servings of fruits and

vegetables are recommended as part of a healthy diet. According to "State of the Plate," a study published in October 2002 by the Produce for Better Health Foundation, 90% of teen girls and 96% of kids ages 2-12 do not eat five servings per day.

The *5-A-Day for Better Health* program gives Americans a simple, positive message: Eat five or more servings of fruits and vegetables every day for better health. The National Cancer Institute and the Produce for Better Health Foundation jointly sponsor this program. The goal of the program is to increase the consumption of fruits and vegetables in the United States to 5-9 servings every day. In addition, the program seeks to inform Americans that eating fruits and vegetables can improve their health and reduce the risk of cancer and other diseases. It also provides consumers with practical and easy ways to incorporate more fruits and vegetables into their daily eating patterns.

One way to get kids to eat more fruits and vegetables is to make them more fun and portable. According to the State of the Plate study, romaine lettuce and bag lettuce are the only vegetables that Americans are eating more of than before, increasing by an average of two annual servings per person. The bagged salads are more convenient for parents to prepare for family meals. Another example of portability is baby carrots. "Everyone loves these, and they are easy and convenient," commented Tanner.

• **Dairy Foods.** Yogurt, milk, and cheese provide calcium, potassium, phosphorus, protein, vitamins A, D, and B-12, riboflavin, and niacin. USDA recommends 2-3 servings of dairy products daily, but the majority of people only consume half of this. The *3-A-Day* campaign, managed by the American Dairy Association/National Dairy Council, works to promote three servings per day. The program stresses the importance of dairy's role in children's health.

For example, a recent study by Goulding et al. (2004) recognized the importance of milk in children's diets. The study investigated the impact of milk consumption on children 3-13 years old. The investigators compared the fracture histories of 50 children who avoided drinking cow's milk for extended periods of time to a group of 1,000 children from the same city, Dunedin, New Zealand.

"Children who regularly avoided milk had lower bone mineral density and weighed more, two factors that increase fracture risk," said lead researcher Ailsa Goulding of the University of Otago, New Zealand. Nearly one in three of the young milk-avoiders had broken a bone before they were eight years old, frequently from slight trauma such as a minor trip or fall. "Forearm fractures were especially common," said the researchers, concluding that "young children avoiding milk are prone to fracture."

Dairy companies have made innovative strides to increase dairy consumption among children. Flavored milks, carbonated milk beverages, and flavored and colored cheese are among the newest dairy products that make dairy fun for kids. For example, *Raging Cow*™, from Dr Pepper/Seven Up Inc., Plano, Tex., is a five-flavor line of single-serve milk drinks. Chocolate Insanity, Pina Colada

Chaos, Chocolate Caramel Craze, Berry Mixed Up, and Jamocha Frenzy are the five flavors that make milk more exciting. The company's Web site states, "Boring milk needed a kick in the shorts, and with *Raging Cow*, that's just what boring milk got."

• **Calcium.** Because of insufficient dairy consumption, children's diets are lacking in calcium. "Children under 10 need about 900 mg of calcium," said Tanner. "Once they get to the age of 10, they need 1,300 mg of calcium per day."

Information from the *3-A-Day* program states that about 30% of kids ages 1-5 do not get the recommended amount of calcium in their diets; 70% of preteen girls and 60% of preteen boys (ages 6-11) do not meet current calcium recommendations; and nearly 90% of teenage girls and 70% of teenage boys (ages 12-19) do not meet daily calcium recommendations.

Not only is lack of calcium detrimental to children's bone and teeth health, but also recent studies have shown that calcium may play a role in children's weight. Research presented at the Experimental Biology Meeting in April 2003 (FASEB, 2003) suggested that girls who consume more calcium tend to weigh less and have lower body fat than those with low calcium consumption. Researchers at the University of Hawaii at Manoa and Kaiser Permanente Clinical Research Center in Honolulu studied 321 white, Asian, and mixed-ethnicity girls ages 9-14. They found that girls who consumed more calcium on average weighed less than similar girls who consumed less calcium. An increase of one serving of dairy—a cup of milk or a thumb-sized piece of cheese, about 300 mg of calcium—was associated with a 0.9 mm lower skin fold (about half an inch) and 1.9 lb lower weight.

Rachel Novotny, Professor in the Dept. of Human Nutrition, Food, and Animal Sciences at the University of Hawaii, explained that as calcium intake increases, the body increases its ability to break down fat and decreases fat synthesis.

Another study (Skinner et al., 2003) found that higher intake of dietary calcium was associated with lower body fat in young children. The study looked at 52 children ages 2-8 and their mothers. Results showed that dietary calcium and polyunsaturated fat intake were associated with a lower percentage of body fat. Milk and other dairy products were the main sources of dietary calcium in the study, with milk alone accounting for 50% of the total calcium intake.

• **Vitamin D.** This vitamin also is essential for bone health because it helps the body absorb calcium. Vitamin D deficiency largely is to blame for a rise of bone-deforming rickets in recent years among U.S. infants and toddlers, according to the Centers for Disease Control and Prevention.

Research at the University of Maine showed that during the winter, Maine girls are not getting enough vitamin D (Anonymous, 2004). Insufficient levels of vitamin D were detected in nearly half of 24 Bangor-area girls during a three-year study funded by the Maine Dairy and Nutrition Council. The findings worried Susan Sullivan, Assistant Professor of Human Nutrition at the university, because a history of persistent deficiencies of vitamin D could set the stage for osteoporosis later in life.

Infant Nutrition

Newborns and infants have different nutritional requirements than children. If not breastfed, infants' main source of food is formula. Docosahexaenoic acid (DHA), arachidonic acid (ARA), probiotics, and fiber, show promise in benefiting infant health. DHA and ARA are currently used in infant formulas in the U.S., probiotics enhance some formulas in Europe and Japan, and prebiotic fibers are used in some European formulas as well.

• **DHA and ARA.** These two fatty acids are used in infant formulas to improve the visual and brain development of infants. Researchers at the Retina Foundation of the Southwest in Dallas, Tex. (Hoffman et al., 2003), showed that infant formula supplemented with DHA and ARA significantly improved the visual development of infants compared to non-supplemented formula. They studied babies who were breastfed from birth to 4-6 months of age and then randomly weaned. The babies fed the supplemented formula had improved visual acuity at one year of age, compared to the babies fed the nonsupplemented formula after weaning.

"This study demonstrates the continued need for DHA and ARA in the infant diet beyond four months of age to optimize visual development during the first year of life," said lead researcher Dennis R. Hoffman.

• **Probiotics.** Research has shown that probiotics in infant formula may boost the immune system. Scientists at the Pediatric Gastroenterology and Nutrition Unit of Ben-Gurion University in Israel used a double-blind placebo-controlled trial with full term healthy infants between 4-10 months of age (Asli et al., 2003). They randomly received formulas supplemented with either *Bifidobacterium lactis* or *Lactobacillus reuteri*, or the same diet with no probiotics for 12 weeks. Infants fed a probiotics supplemented formula exhibited fewer febrile episodes and fewer gastrointestinal illnesses. They noted that this effect was more prominent in the *L. reuteri* group.

• **Fiber.** Research at the University of Illinois indicated that adding fiber to milk formula may be beneficial on bowel health of infants (Correa-Matos et al., 2003). The study showed that piglets that consumed formula with moderate levels of fermentable fiber tolerated an induced infection by *Salmonella typhimurium* much better than those fed a plain control formula or one with a nonfermentable fiber.

According to the study, diarrhea is a leading cause of morbidity and mortality in infants. The addition of fiber to infant formulas reduces recovery time following pathogenic infection in infants older than six months, but effects on neonates are unknown. The researchers concluded that because fermentable fiber enhanced intestinal function and reduced the severity of symptoms associated with *S. typhimurium* infection, it may be a cost-effective way in which to reduce the severity of pathogenic infection-associated symptoms in infants.

Vitamin D deficiency is most common in post-menopausal women and older Americans. However, Sullivan said, vitamin D intake is critical for children because they add calcium to their bones at a fast pace, maintain those levels into adulthood, then start to lose calcium as they grow elderly.

• **Iron.** "Iron is a part of blood's hemoglobin, which carries oxygen to the cells," Tanner said. "The oxygen helps cells produce energy, without which the body can become fatigued."

Infants need 6-10 mg of iron each day, and children need 10-15 mg. After age 10, children should be getting 15 mg of iron each day. Iron deficiency can be a problem, particularly for girls who experience very heavy periods. In fact, many teenage girls are at risk for iron deficiency because their diets may not contain enough iron to offset the blood loss. Also, teens can lose significant amounts of iron through sweating during intense exercise.

Iron deficiency can lead to fatigue, irritability, headaches, lack of energy, and tingling in the hands and feet. Significant iron deficiency can lead to iron-deficiency anemia.

• **Fiber.** Because children are not consuming five daily servings of fruits and vegetables, their fiber intakes are low as well. To determine how many grams of fiber a child should be consuming each day, it is recommended to add 5 to a child's age in years, said Tanner.

Fiber, especially in cereals, has been linked to the prevention of childhood obesity. A study by Albertson et al. (2003) showed that children who frequently consume cereal are less likely to be overweight. Cereal eaters were found to have a lower body mass index (BMI) and a higher nutrient intake than infrequent or non-cereal eaters.

The study, which included 603 children ages 4-12 years, examined the relationship between cereal consumption habits and BMI of school-aged children. The investigators concluded that children who consumed eight or more servings of cereal within a period of two weeks had significantly lower BMIs compared to the children who consumed fewer servings during that same time. Statistically, nearly 80% of the children who frequently consumed cereal boasted an appropriate body weight for their age and gender.

"For an average 10-year-old boy, the decision to eat cereal or not can equate to about a 12-pound difference," said G. Harvey Anderson, Professor of Nutrition at the University of Toronto and coauthor of the study. The authors also found that cereal consumption benefited the children in the study who were at risk of being overweight. Children of this age group who ate cereal lowered their risk to 21.3%.

Another study (Quaker Oats, 2003) showed that the risk of obesity is lower for children who eat oatmeal regularly compared to those who do not. The percentage of children 2-18 years old who are overweight or at risk of becoming overweight is almost 50% lower in oatmeal eaters than in children who do not consume the fiber, according to the study, which was funded by Quaker Oats.

In addition, the study found that children who eat oatmeal are about twice as likely to meet fiber intake recommendations—fiber intakes were 17% higher than for those who do not eat oatmeal.

The findings of the study were presented by researchers from Columbia University and Quaker Oats at Experimental Biology 2003.

"This study found that children and teens who consumed higher intakes of dietary fiber had lower BMI levels or less body fat," said Christine Williams, Professor of Clinical Pediatrics and Director of the Children's Cardiovascular Health Center at Columbia University. "Our data further suggests children who have diets rich in high-fiber foods, such as oatmeal, as early as age two could help them prevent obesity throughout their lives."

Suggestions for Food Manufacturers

When it comes to formulating food for children, Tanner stressed the importance of portion sizes, in addition to important nutrients, in her suggestions for food manufacturers:

• **Reduce portion size.** "Sell items in smaller packages. For example, lose the "grab bag" and go back to the 25-¢ ½-oz bag," she said. "Also consider smaller beverage containers."

• **Replace candy with fruit.** "A prepackaged lunch does not need candy to sell," she said. "Replace the goop with fruit. There are healthy options—the challenge is to keep them preserved so they are tasty and the fruit is fresh."

• **Add vegetables.** "Help make veggies cool. They have a great taste and are good for you, but for some reason the "not so cool" connection is there. Advertising speaks volumes!

• **Provide lower-fat, yet tasty options.** "The bottom line is that kids will not eat anything if it does not taste good."

REFERENCES

Albertson, A.M., Anderson, G.H., Crockett, S.J., and Goebel, M.T. 2003. Ready-to-eat cereal consumption: Its relationship with BMI and nutrient intake of children aged 4 to 12 years. J. Am. Dietetic Assn. 103: 1613-1619.

Anonymous, 2004. Umaine study: Teenage girls lacking in vitamin D. Univ. of Maine News press release, Jan. 29. www.umaine.edu/news/020204/GirlsVitaminD.htm.

Asli, G., Alsheikh, A., and Weizman, Z. 2003. Infant formula supplemented with probiotics reduces gastrointestinal infections' rate in day care infants. Presented at Ann. Mtg., Am. Pediatric Soc., May. www.reuteri.com/eng/sidor/studies/scientific_posters/stage2.pdf.

Correa-Matos, N.J., Donovan, S.M., Isaacson, R.E., Gaskins, H.R., White, B.A., and Tappenden, K.A. 2003. Fermentable fiber reduces recovery time and improves intestinal function in piglets following Salmonella typhimurium infection. J. Nutr. 133: 1845-1852.

FASEB 2003. Adolescent girls who consume more calcium weigh less. Press release. Fed. of Am. Socs. for Exp. Biol., www.eurekalert.org/pub_releases/2003-04/foasagw033003.php.

Goulding, A., Rockell, J.E.P., Black, R.E., Grant, A.M., Jones, I.E., and Williams, S.M. 2004. Children who avoid drinking cow's milk are at increased risk for prepubertal bone fractures. J. Am. Dietetic Assn. 104: 250-253.

Hoffman, D.R., Birch, E.E., Castaneda, Y.S., Fawcett, S.L., Wheaton, D.H., Birch, D.G., and Uauy, R. 2003. Visual function in breast-fed term infants weaned to formula with or without long-chain polyunsaturates at 4 to 6 months: A randomized clinical trial. J. Pediatrics. 142: 669-677.

Quaker Oats. 2003. Study reveals oatmeal can play role in preventing childhood obesity. Press release, www.quakeroats.com/qfb_News/PressRelease.cfm?ID=201.

Skinner, J.D., Bounds, W., Carruth, B.R., and Ziegler, P. 2003. Longitudinal calcium intake is negatively related to children's body fat indexes. J. Am. Dietetic Assn. 103: 1626-1631.

The Role of the School Nutrition Environment for Promoting the Health of Young Adolescents

In spite of obesity and other nutrition-related health problems of young adolescents, middle schools have not put student health or the school nutrition environment very high on the priority list.

By Mary Kay Meyer, John Marshak, & Martha T. Conklin

While there is a growing emphasis on increasing middle grades students' achievement, nutrition has long been recognized for its impact on student success. What is really going on nutritionally at the middle level that is affecting the well being of students? To help answer this question, school superintendents and principals were asked to describe the practices they observed on a daily basis. Though some exceptional practices were found, overall the picture painted by the participants was bleak.

Participants confirmed the students' frequent consumption of foods such as pizza, chicken nuggets, hamburgers, French fries, tacos/burritos, chips, candy, and carbonated beverages during the school day. All of these foods would be classified as high fat or high sugar. It has been said that choices lead to behaviors, behaviors lead to habits, and habits lead to a way of life. Today, the health of adolescents and the adults they will become is critically linked to the health related behaviors they choose to adopt. The nutritional adequacy of students' diets does affect students' learning and performance today and will affect the health of the adults they will become.

A close relationship between nutrition and learning has been well established (Galler, Ramsey, Solimano, & Lowell, 1983; Murphy, Wheler, Pagano, Kleinman, & Jellinek, 1998; Pollitt, Leibel, & Greenfield, 1981; Pollitt, Lewis, Garza, & Shulman 1982; Scanlon,1989; Simeon, & Granthom-McGregor, 1989; Wahlstrom & Begalle, 1999). Chronically undernourished children are more likely to become sick, miss classes, and score lower on tests (Centers for Disease Control, 1997). Recent statistics show that the percentage of children meeting the recommended number of food group servings was 14% for fruit, 17% for meat/meat substitutes, 20% for vegetables, 23% for breads/grains, and 30% for milk. Girls ages 14 to 18 have especially low intakes of fruits and dairy products. More than two-thirds of females ages 14 to 18 exceed the recommendations for intake of total fat and saturated fat, but even greater percentages of children exceed these recommendations than among other age/gender groups. Children's diets are high in added sugars. For all children, sugars contribute an average of 20% of total food energy. Children are heavy consumers of regular or diet soda. Overall, 56% to 85% of children consume soda on any given day. Teenage males were especially heavy consumers of soda, with more than one-third consuming more than three servings a day (United States Department of Agriculture, 2001).

These trends have contributed to several serious diet-related concerns. The percentage of young people who are overweight has more than doubled in the past 30 years (Centers for Disease Control, 1997; United States Department of Agriculture, 2001). One of the most serious aspects of overweight and obesity in children is Type II diabetes. Type II diabetes accounted for 16% of the diabetes in children in 1994, up from 4% in 1992. Overweight adolescents are more likely to become overweight adults, with increased risk of developing heart disease; stroke; gallbladder disease; arthritis; and endometrial, breast, prostate, and colon cancer (U.S. Dept. of Health and Human Services, 1988).

Middle school students spend up to one-third of their days in the school environment and are greatly influenced by what they experience during these hours.

Adolescents' eating behavior is influenced by personal characteristics and environmental factors in the home, school, and the community (Bandura, 1986; Gillespie, 1981). These factors are composed of the objective and subjective culture of their behavior settings (Klepp, Wilhemsen, & Andrews, 1991). The objective cultures are the tangible effects of the environment and subjective cultures are the norms, attitudes, and learned values from family and peers (Triandis, 1972). Middle school students spend up to one-third of their days in the school environment and are greatly influenced by what they experience during these hours.

In today's school environment many tangible elements such as a la carte foods, vending machines, and snack bars compete with creating a nutrition environment that encourages healthy eating behaviors (Story & Neumark-Sztainer, 1999). Cullen, Eagen, Baranowski, Owens, and de Moore (2000) found that fifth-grade students who ate only meals from a snack bar consumed significantly less total fruits, juices, and vegetables than fifth-grade students who ate school meals. Wildey, Pampalone, Pelletier, Zive, Elder, and Sallis (2000) reported that in middle schools where school stores were available, 88.5% of inventory items were high in fat and/or sugar. Because of the limited research in assessing the nutrition environment in schools, coupled with the concern for the growth and development of children in middle grades, a research study was conducted throughout the country to identify the nature of the nutrition environment in the middle grades from the principals' and superintendents' points of view and to determine which elements of a school's nutrition environment these school administrators considered most relevant to students' health and well-being.

Method

Focus groups were used to explore the context for promoting healthy eating behaviors among students within the middle school environment. Focus groups allowed researchers to explore the socio-environmental, behavioral, and attitudinal dimensions of this issue without imposing predetermined boundaries. The *Focus Group Kit* developed by Morgan and Krueger (1998) was used as the basis for developing the research design. Dr. Richard Krueger, University of Minnesota, served as a consultant on the project.

The focus group sessions were held at three sites throughout the United States: Kansas City, Missouri; Las Vegas, Nevada; and Reston, Virginia. Participants included principals and superintendents from a nine-state radius around each location.

They included 17 school principals and 9 superintendents. Of the 26 participants, 17 had more than 17 years of experience and only three had less than five years of experience. The school system size of participating districts ranged from 267 to more than 131,000 students in middle grades. The percentage of students receiving meal assistance ranged from 6% to 69% free and from 3% to 22% reduced.

Figure 1

School District Characteristics of Participants in the Middle Grade Nutrition Environment Study (N=25)

Characteristic	Number of Participants
Schools participating in the federally funded breakfast program	23
School districts in which food service personnel are involved in nutrition education in the middle grades	8
School districts in which nutrition is included in the curriculum in middle grades	25
School districts in which a comprehensive health curriculum that includes nutrition is offered in middle grades	18
School districts which the school board had a policy concerning contracts with vendors for food/drink items	19
School districts serving middle grades with vending machines All buildings Some buildings No buildings	13 10 3
School districts serving middle grades with school sponsored stores All buildings Some buildings No buildings	5 7 14

Results

A la carte items were sold in 17 of the participating school districts. The most frequently sold a la carte items were pizza, French fries, and chips. The most frequently identified items sold in vending machines and school-sponsored stores were soda, candy, sports drinks, chips, cookies, and flavored water. This is consistent with Wildey and associates (2000) who reported that items sold in middle school stores were high in fat and sugar. Figure 1 shows additional school district characteristics.

Most school administrators did not think the environments in middle grades schools were conducive to healthy eating habits. Vending machines and a la carte sales of unhealthy food items received much discussion. One of the first questions asked participants was, "When you think of a school environment that promotes healthy eating behaviors, what comes to mind?" Participants mentioned healthful food choices, friendly staff, time to eat, low-fat foods, absence of vending machines, and a relaxed cafeteria environment as important. Several responses from participants concerned whose responsibility providing such an environment should be.

"It is the responsibility of the school to make sure what they do serve the children is healthy."

"School food service directors to superintendents and everyone between should be involved."

Participants were asked to identify five qualities they thought were essential to a school's nutritional environment. The most often given responses were an attractive dining environment, time to eat, friendly staff, taste of the food, and menu choices.

Another question posed to participants was, "When you consider all of the things that you have to contend with (administration, management, security, serving meals, day-to-day operations), where do you place the school's nutritional environment in your list of priorities? The average score for this question for all groups was 2.9 on a scale of 1= low to 7= high. When asked, "What would it take to move this rating to a higher priority?" numerous participants answered "time." Other responses included awareness, administrative support, vision for the school, and "When it becomes my responsibility."

The major barriers to having a good nutrition environment in middle grades identified by school administrators were:

- **Funding**

  Funding in various forms was the most frequently mentioned barrier in each focus group: "time, long lines, and the physical plant itself … when you have an environment that is very inviting and conducive for students to come in, it helps with participation. If you had enough money to do this, it would be a dream cafeteria." Another participant's expression of the need to improve capital funding for the cafeteria: "I think it's the money. … I really do, it's the simple matter of where are you going to put your priorities." This quotation addresses the importance of other issues, such as improving test scores, over building healthy eating habits in setting the budget priorities. "We have a 1965 budget with 2000 needs." Many participants expressed the need for the revenue generated by the sales of the less nutritious products to supplement the budget. No longer did they think it was just nice to have extra funds from vending and snack bar sales, but it has become a necessity to fund any number of essential needs.

- **Attitudes of parents and students**

  "It is the parents' attitudes that spill over to students' attitudes." "Eat junk at home; eat junk at school."

- **Outside influences**

  One of the greatest outside influences discussed was the media. "We have Channel 1 News every morning and between the news segments, soft drink and fast food hypes are on."

- **Peer pressure**

  "We had the best food going, but the kids would not eat it because it wasn't cool. … We had to work to make it cool."

- **Lack of vision**

  "I think you have to have a vision of what you want for your nutritional program for your kids in your school and you use the same process that you use with everything else to get it done."

- **Lack of knowledge**

  "Major barriers are people based … from a knowledge position … because if I think, or the board thinks, or the community thinks that it is extremely important, the money will come from somewhere."

- **Inequity among free, reduced, and paying students**

  In some locations there is a social stigma associated with having to eat in the "regular" lunch line. Not all schools have been able to overcome the difficulties of differentiating between those students on free and reduced priced meals and those who are not. Therefore, students who qualify for free and reduced meals often choose not to eat.

- **Food preparation and limited choices**

  Limited choices were a concern. Participants frequently characterized the food as poor quality, greasy, tasting artificial, and lacking visual appeal.

- **Lack of commitment**

  Participants did not think that school districts acknowledged the importance of nutrition.

The topic of mixed messages generated great discussion in all groups. Included in the mixed messages being sent in the schools concerning nutrition were, vending machines and what is stocked in them, what is sold at concession stands, candy sales being used for fund raisers, teachers giving candy as classroom incentives, and serving hamburgers, corn dogs, and French fries in the cafeteria. "We are doing it. I am just as guilty. After a state exam we give all our kids chocolate chip cookies and donuts."

One of the two closing questions asked participants was, "Of all the things we have discussed, what is the most important?" Three themes consistently arose: involvement, funding, and vision.

"It was nice to hear that we all believe that all kids need to eat."

"We need more impact, communication, involvement at all levels from the superintendent down."

"You have to be a change agent in your school because no one else is going to do it."

"Money dictates what we do or don't do for kids, and I think that is a really sad scenario."

Conclusion and Application

Recently legislation has been introduced to regulate the sale of foods of minimal nutritional value in our nation's schools. Legislation will not solve the problem. Many states currently have such laws that are ignored by school administrators. Local school districts, communities, parents, educators, and school administrators must work together to eliminate the barriers to a healthy nutrition environment in our middle grades. School administrators can lead the challenge by ensuring that financial decisions do not undermine nutrition goals. This will not be easy and may necessitate making hard decisions about funding.

School administrators also can initiate the organization of a school health or nutrition advisory committee that includes teachers, parents, students, as well as the community. These stakeholders should also be involved in developing food and nutrition policy. These policies may involve questioning a decision to allow exclusive contracts with the large beverage companies.

Greater efforts should be made to ensure students have enough time to eat. It is critical for the health and well-being of our adolescents to receive proper nutrition. They cannot be expected to accomplish this when cafeterias are over crowded and it takes as much as 20 minutes of a 25 minute lunch period to be served. The physical environments of the cafeteria should allow students a pleasant and stress free environment for consuming the nutritious meals they need to nourish their bodies to allow them to better assimilate the knowledge gained through their classroom experiences.

Vending machines should be stocked with healthful snacks and beverages and the sale of high-fat and high-sugar snacks should be eliminated totally from middle school campuses. More healthful snack items such as baked chips, trail mix, dried fruit, low fat cookies, and 100% fruit juices should replace the high-fat and high-sugar items. Fund raisers should focus on non-food items. Raffles and silent auctions could replace the sale of candy and cookies as fund raisers for school organizations.

A comprehensive health education program with nutrition as a major component should be the national standard for middle school curriculum. Classroom and physical education teachers, food service managers, and other staff should work together to ensure the flow of nutrition throughout the curriculum.

Schools are in a unique position to promote healthful food choices and help assure appropriate nutrient intake of our young adolescents, as well as reinforce nutrition education and provide opportunities for students to practice healthful food choices. School administrators hold the keys to success. They must initiate and support efforts to provide a number of elements necessary to create a healthy environment for our young adolescents. But, it will take all involved parties working together to make this happen. One participant in the focus group research stated it best when he said, "When it becomes a priority, it will get done."

Acknowledgment

This article was written by the National Food Service Management Institute-Applied Research Division, located at The University of Southern Mississippi with headquarters at The University of Mississippi. Funding for the Institute has been provided with Federal funds from the U.S. Department of Agriculture, Food and Nutrition Services, The University of Mississippi. The contents of this publication do not necessarily reflect the views or policies of The University of Mississippi or the U.S. Department of Agriculture, nor does mention of trade names, commercial products, or organizations imply endorsement by the U.S. Government.

References

Bandura, A. (1986). *Social functions of thought and action: A social cognitive theory.* Englewood Cliffs, NJ: Prentice Hall.

Centers for Disease Control and Prevention. (1997). *CDC's guidelines for school health programs: Promoting lifelong healthy eating.* Atlanta, GA: Author.

Cullen, K. W., Eagen, J., Baranowski, T., Owens, E., & de Moore, C. (2000). Effect of a la carte and snack bar foods at school on children's lunchtime intake of fruits and vegetables. *Journal of the American Dietetic Association, 100,* 1482–1486.

Galler, J. R., Ramsey, F, Solimano, G., & Lowell, W. E. (1983). The influence of early malnutrition on subsequent behavioral development: Degree of impairment in intellectual performance. *Journal of the American Academy of Child Adolescent Psychiatry, 22,* 8–18.

Gillespie, A. (1981). A theoretical framework for studying school nutrition education programs. *Journal of Nutrition Education, 13,* 150–152.

Klepp, K., Wilhemsen, B. U., & Andrews, T. (1991) Promoting healthy eating patterns among Norwegian school children. In D. Nutbeam, B. Haglund, P. Farley, & P. Tillgren (Eds.), *Youth health promotion from theory to practice in school and community* (pp. 137–156). London: Forbes Publishers.

Morgan, D. L., & Krueger, R. A. (1998). *The focus group kit.* Thousand Oaks, CA: Sage Publications.

Murphy, J. M., Wheler, C. A., Pagano, M., Kleinman, R. K., & Jellinek, M. S. (1998). The relationship between hunger and psychological functioning in low-income American children. *Journal of the American Academy of Child Adolescent Psychiatry, 37,* 163–170.

Pollitt, E., Leibel, R., & Greenfield, D. (1981). Brief fasting, stress, and cognition in children. *American Journal of Clinical Nutrition, 34,* 1526–1533.

Pollitt, E., Lewis, N., Garza, C., & Shulman, R., (1982). Fasting and cognition. *Journal of Pediatric Research, 17,* 169–174.

Scanlon, K. S. (1989). *Activity and behavioral changes of marginally malnourished Mexican pre-schoolers.* Unpublished master's thesis, University of Connecticut, Storrs Connecticut.

Simeon, D. T., & Granthom-McGregor, S. (1989). Effects of missing breakfast on the cognitive functions of school children of different nutritional status. *American Journal of Clinical Nutrition, 49,* 646–653.

Story, M., &. Neumark-Sztainer, D. (1999). Competitive foods in schools: Issues, trends, and future directions. *Topics in Clinical Nutrition, 15*(1), 37–46.

Triandis, H. (1972). *The analysis of subjective culture.* New York: Wiley-interscience.

U.S. Department of Agriculture. (2001). *Foods sold in competition with USDA school meal programs. A report to Congress.* Washington, DC: Author. Retrieved June 2001 from `www.fns.usda.gov/cnd/Lunch/Competi.../` `competitive.foods.report.to.congress.html`

U.S. Department of Health and Human Services. (1988). *The Surgeon General's report on nutrition and health* (HHS Publication 88-50210). Washington, DC: U.S. Government Printing Office.

Wahlstrom, K. L., & Begalle, M. S. (1999). More than test scores: Results of the universal school breakfast pilot in Minnesota. *Topics in Clinical Nutrition, 15,* 17–29.

Wildey, M. B., Pampalone, S. Z., Pelletier, R. L., Zive, M. M., Elder, J. P., & Sallis, J. F. (2000). Fat and sugar levels are high in snacks purchased from student stores in middle schools. *Journal of the American Dietetic Association, 100,* 319–322.

Mary Kay Meyer is a research scientist at the National Food Service Management Institute, Division of Applied Research at the University of Southern Mississippi, Hattiesburg. E-mail: mk.meyer@usm.edu

John Marshak is an assistant professor of educational leadership at the State University of New York at Cortland.

Martha T. Conklin, formerly of Southern Mississippi University, is an associate professor at Pennsylvania State University, University Park.

UNIT 4
Obesity and Weight Control

Unit Selections

Key Points to Consider

- As the incidence of obesity increases, how can it best be prevented?

- What are some of the causes behind a person becoming obese?

- What sort of health risks can result from some of the most popular weight-loss methods?

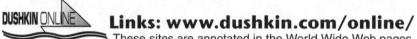 **Links: www.dushkin.com/online/**
These sites are annotated in the World Wide Web pages.

American Anorexia Bulimia Association/National Eating Disorders Association (AABA)
http://www.nationaleatingdisorders.org/

American Society of Exercise Physiologists (ASEP)
http://www.asep.org/

Calorie Control Council
http://www.caloriecontrol.org

Eating Disorders: Body Image Betrayal
http://www.bibri.com/home/index.htm

Shape Up America!
http://www.shapeup.org

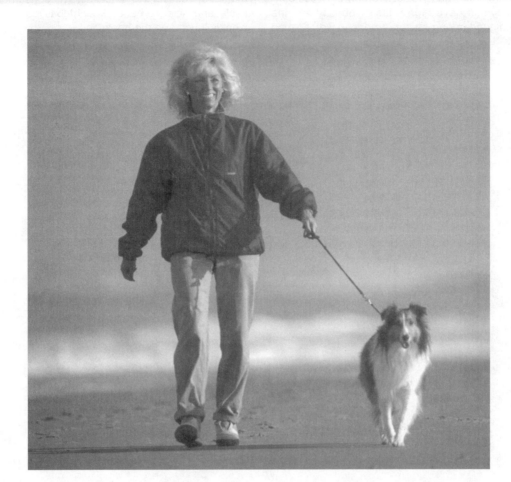

Overweight and obesity have become epidemic in the United States during the last century and are rising at a dangerous rate worldwide. Approximately 5 million adults are overweight or obese according to the new standards set by the U.S. government—using a body mass index (BMI) of 30 to 39.9. Reports suggest that by the year 2050, half of the U.S. population would be considered obese. This problem is prevalent in both genders and all ages, races, and ethnic groups. Twenty-five percent of U.S. children and adolescents are overweight or at risk, which emphasizes the need for prevention—as obese children become obese adults. The catastrophic health consequences of obesity are heart disease, diabetes, gallbladder disease, osteoarthritis, and some cancers. The cost for treating this degenerative disease in the United States is approximately $100 billion per year.

Even though professionals have tried hard to prevent and combat obesity with behavior modification, (a healthy diet, and exercise), it seems that these traditional ways have not proven effective. In a society where fast-food eateries are the mainstay of meals; where "big," including food servings, is better; where there is a universal reliance on automobiles; and where the food industry is more interested in profit than in the health of the population—we should not be surprised that obesity has become an epidemic. Dr. J. Tillotson examines the powerful influence of a

few mega food companies on the food choices of Americans. They spend millions of dollars in advertising fast foods loaded with simple sugars and saturated fat. Their aggressive advertising coupled with food accessibility and large portion size has created the "obesigenic" characteristics of our environment whose interaction with genes resulted in the obesity pandemic. Other obstacles to maintaining a healthy diet are the lack of promoting healthy food, its low accessibility, and expense. More recently, scientists have reported that fat is a dynamically active endocrine organ that releases hormones and inflammatory proteins that may predispose a person to chronic diseases including heart disease. Thus, there is a great need for a multifaceted public-health approach that would involve mobilization of private and public sectors. It should focus on building better coping skills and increasing activity. Inclusion of health officials, researchers, educators, legislators, transportation experts, urban planners, and businesses—which would cooperate in formulating ways to combat obesity is crucial. A sound public health policy would require that weight-loss therapies have long-term maintenance and relapse-prevention measures built into them. Healthy People 2010 is the U.S. government's prevention agenda designed to ensure a high quality of life and reduce health risks. One of the 28 areas it focuses on is overweight and obesity. Its main objectives are to reduce the proportion of overweight and obesity of children, teens and adults to 15 percent and increase the proportion of adults who are at a healthy weight. Twice as many teens from poor households are overweight in comparison to those from middle-to high-income households. Women with less education and lower incomes have high rates of obesity and the rates of obesity are higher among African American women than Caucasian. Gender differences in the incidence of obesity have been observed in Hispanics and African Americans with 80 percent greater in women than men. A plethora of diet books in the market are selling like hotcakes. The consumer looking for a reliable and science-based weight-loss book should beware of what is lurking on the bookshelf.

How We Grew So BiG

Diet and lack of exercise are immediate causes— but our problem began in the Paleolithic era

BY MICHAEL D. LEMONICK

IT'S HARDLY NEWS ANYMORE THAT Americans are just too fat. If the endless parade of articles, TV specials and fad diet books weren't proof enough or you missed the ominous warnings from the National Institutes of Health, the Centers for Disease Control and Prevention and the American Heart Association, a quick look around the mall, the beach or the crowd at any baseball game will leave no room for doubt: our individual weight problems have become a national crisis.

Even so, the actual numbers are shocking. Fully two-thirds of U.S. adults are officially overweight, and about half of those have graduated to full-blown obesity. The rates for African Americans and Latinos are even higher. Among kids between 6 and 19 years old, 15%, or 1 in 6, are overweight, and another 15% are headed that way. Even our pets are pudgy: a depressing 25% of dogs and cats are heavier than they should be.

And things haven't been moving in a promising direction. Just two decades ago, the incidence of overweight in adults was well under 50%, while the rate for kids was only a third what it is today. From 1996 to 2001, 2 million teenagers and young adults joined the ranks of the clinically obese. People are clearly worried. A TIME/ABC News poll released this week shows that 58% of Americans would like to lose weight, nearly twice the percentage who felt that way in 1951. But only 27% say they are trying to slim down—and two-

thirds of those aren't following any specific plan to do so.

It wouldn't be such a big deal if the problem were simply aesthetic. But excess poundage takes a terrible toll on the human body, significantly increasing the risk of heart disease, high blood pressure, stroke, diabetes, infertility, gall-bladder disease, osteoarthritis and many forms of cancer. The total medical tab for illnesses related to obesity is $117 billion a year—and climbing—according to the Surgeon General, and the *Journal of the American Medical Association* reported in March that poor diet and physical inactivity could soon overtake tobacco as the leading cause of preventable death in the U.S. And again, Americans recognize the problem. In the TIME/ABC poll they rated obesity alongside heart disease, cancer, AIDS and drug abuse as among the nation's most pressing public health problems.

So why is it happening? The obvious, almost trivial answer is that we eat too much high-calorie food and don't burn it off with enough exercise. If only we could change those habits, the problem would go away. But clearly it isn't that easy. Americans pour scores of billions of dollars every year into weight-loss products and health-club memberships and liposuction and gastric bypass operations—100,000 of the latter last year alone. Food and drug companies spend even more trying to find a magic food or drug that will melt the pounds away. Yet the nation's collective waistline just keeps growing.

It's natural to try to find something to blame—fast-food joints or food manufacturers or even ourselves for having too little willpower. But the ultimate reason for obesity may be rooted deep within our genes. Obedient to the inexorable laws of evolution, the human race adapted over millions of years to living in a world of scarcity, where it paid to eat every good-tasting thing in sight when you could find it.

Although our physiology has stayed pretty much the same for the past 50,000 years or so, we humans have utterly transformed our environment. Over the past century especially, technology has almost completely removed physical exercise from the day-to-day lives of most Americans. At the same time, it has filled supermarket shelves with cheap, mass-produced, good-tasting food that is packed with calories. And finally, technology has allowed advertisers to deliver constant, virtually irresistible messages that say "Eat this now" to everyone old enough to watch TV.

This artificial environment is most pervasive in the U.S. and other industrialized countries, and that's exactly where the fat crisis is most acute. When people move to the U.S. from poorer nations, their collective weight begins to rise. As developing areas like, for example, Southeast Asia and Latin America catch up economically and the inhabitants adopt Western lifestyles, their problems with obesity catch up as well. By contrast, among people who still live in conditions most like those of our distant Stone Age ancestors—such as the

Kids Twenty years ago, 5% of American kids were overweight; **today 15% are, and another 15%** are headed that way • In 1969 **80% of kids played sports every day;** today 20% do • By 17, a child has spent **38% more time in front of the TV** than in school

Cost **Americans spend $117 billion** a year on obesity-linked illnesses • **Diet and poor exercise** trail only tobacco as a cause of preventable death • Half of all obese adults have **hypertension**

Maku or the Yanomami of Brazil—there is virtually no obesity at all.

And that's almost certainly the way it was during 99.9% of human evolution. For most of the 7 million years or so since we parted ways with chimps, life has been very harsh—"nasty, brutish and short," in Thomas Hobbes' memorable phrase. The average life expectancy was probably well under 30. But much of that dismal brevity can be chalked up to accidents, infections, traumatic childbirth and unfortunate encounters with saber-toothed cats and other such predators. If a Cro-Magnon, say, could get past these formidable obstacles, he might conceivably live into his 60s or even longer, with none of the obesity-related illnesses that plague modern Americans.

United States Of Obesity

Weight is not evenly distributed in the U.S. The highest concentration of obese Americans forms a wide belt across the southern states

Our earliest ancestors probably ate much as their cousins the apes did, foraging for fruits, shoots, nuts, tubers and other vegetation in the forests and savannas of Africa. Because most wild plants are relatively low in calories, it took constant work just to stay alive. Fruits, full of natural sugars like fructose and glucose, were an unusually concentrated source of energy, and the instinct to seek out and consume them evolved in many mammals long before humans ever arose. Fruit wasn't always available, but those who ate all they could whenever it was were more likely to survive and pass on their sweet tooth to their progeny.

Our love affair with sugar—and also with salt, another crucial but not always available part of the diet—goes back millions of years. But humanity's appetite for animal fat and protein is probably more recent. It was some 2.5 million years ago that our hominid ancestors developed a taste for meat. The fossil record shows that the human brain became markedly bigger and

more complex about the same time. And indeed, according to Katherine Milton, an anthropologist at the University of California, Berkeley, "the incorporation of animal matter into the diet played an absolutely essential role in human evolution."

For starters, meat provided a concentrated source of protein, vitamins, minerals and fatty acids that helped our human ancestors grow taller. The first humans were the size of small chimps, but the bones of a *Homo ergaster* boy dating back about 1.5 million years suggest that he could have stood more than 6 ft. as an adult. Besides building our bodies, says Emory University's Dr. S. Boyd Eaton, the fatty acids found in animal-based foods would have served as a powerful raw material for the growth of human brains.

Because it's so packed with nutrients, meat gave early humans a respite from constant feeding. Like lions and tigers, they didn't have to eat around the clock just to keep going. But more important, unlike the big cats, which rely mostly on strength and speed to bring down dinner, our ancestors depended on guile, organization and the social and technological skills made possible by their increasingly complex brains. Those who were smartest about hunting—and about gathering the plant foods they ate as part of their omnivorous diets—tended to be better fed and healthier than the competition. They were thus more likely to pass along their genes.

The new appetite for meat didn't mean we lost our passion for sweets, though. As Berkeley's Milton points out, the brain's growth may have been facilitated by abundant animal protein, but the brain operates on glucose, the sugar that serves as the major fuel for cellular function. "The brain drinks glucose 24 hours a day," she says. The sugars in fruit and the carbohydrates in edible grains and tubers are particularly good sources of glucose.

The appetite for meat and sweets were essential to human survival, but they didn't lead to obesity for several reasons. For one thing, the wild game our ancestors ate was high in protein but very low in fat—only about 4%, compared with up to 36% in grain-fed supermarket beef. For another, our ancestors couldn't count on a steady

supply of any particular food. Hunters might bring down a deer or a rabbit or nothing at all. Fruit might be in season, or it might not. A chunk of honeycomb might have as many calories as half a dozen Krispy Kreme doughnuts, but you might be able to get it once a year at best—and it wouldn't have the fat.

Beyond that, hunting and gathering took enormous physical work. Chasing wild animals with spears and clubs was a marathon undertaking—and then you had to hack up the catch and lug it miles back to camp. Climbing trees to find nuts and fruit was hard work too. In essence, early humans ate what amounted to the best of the high-protein Atkins diet and the low-fat Ornish diet, and worked out almost nonstop. To get a sense of their endurance, cardiovascular fitness, musculature and body fat, say evolutionary anthropologists, look at a modern marathon runner.

That was the condition of pretty much the entire human race when anatomically modern humans first arose, between 150,000 and 100,000 years ago, and things stayed that way until what some anthropologists have called humanity's worst mistake: the invention of agriculture. We now had a steady source of food, but there were downsides as well. For one thing, our ancestors began gathering in much larger population centers, where bacteria and viruses could fester. Small bands of hunter-gatherers can spread disease only so far, but the birth of cities made epidemics possible for the first time.

Nutritionally, the shift away from wild meat, fruits and vegetables to a diet mostly of cultivated grain robbed humans of many of the essential amino acids, vitamins and minerals they had thrived on. Average life span increased, thanks to the greater abundance of food, but average height diminished. Skeletons also began to show a jump in calcium deficiency, anemia, bad teeth and bacterial infections. Most meat that people ate came from domesticated animals, which have more fat than wild game. Livestock also supplied early pastoralists with milk products, which are full of artery-clogging butterfat. But obesity still wasn't a problem, because even with animals to help, physical exertion was built into just about everyone's life.

That remained the case practically up to the present. It's really only in the past 100 years that cars and other machinery have dramatically reduced the need for physical labor. And as exercise has vanished from everyday life, the technology of food production has become much more sophisticated. In the year 1700 Britain consumed 23,000 tons of sugar. That was about 7.5 lbs. of sugar per capita. The U.S. currently consumes more than 150 lbs. of sweetener per capita, nearly 50% of which is high-fructose corn syrup that is increasingly used as a sugar substitute. Farmers armed with powerful fertilizers and high-tech equipment are growing enormous quantities of corn and wheat, most of which is processed and refined to be tastier and more convenient but is less nutritious. They are raising vast herds of cattle whose meat is laden with the fat that makes it taste so good. They are producing milk, butter and cheese by the tankerload, again full of the fat that humans crave.

And thanks to mass production, all that food is relatively cheap. It's also absurdly convenient. In many areas of the U.S., if you had a craving for cookies a century ago, you had to fire up the woodstove and make the dough from scratch. If you wanted butter, you had to churn it. If you wanted a steak, you had to butcher the cow. Now you jump into the car and head for the nearest convenience store—or if that's too much effort, you pick up a phone or log on to the Internet and have the stuff delivered to your door.

Unless you make a determined effort, you'll probably choose the path of least resistance. Evolving during a time of scarcity, humans developed an instinctive desire for basic tastes—sweet, fat, salt—that they could never fully satisfy. As a result, says Rutgers University anthropologist Lionel Tiger, "we don't have a cut-off mechanism for eating. Our bodies tell us, 'Fat is good to eat but hard to get.'" The second half of that equation is no longer true, but the first remains a powerful drive.

This doesn't necessarily mean we're doomed. There's no doubt that the obesity epidemic is real and our collective health has been getting progressively worse. Indeed, says Yale public-health expert Dr. David Katz, "today's kids may be the first generation in history whose life expectancy is projected to be less than that of their parents."

There's plenty of reason for hope. Researchers are hard at work trying to understand the basic biochemistry of hunger and fat metabolism; policymakers are pushing for better labels and nutritional information; school boards are giving their cafeteria menus a closer look and reconsidering vending-machine contracts with makers of sugary soft drinks; urban planners are rethinking our cities and towns to get us out of the car and onto our feet; Americans in record numbers are putting themselves on low-carb and low-calorie diets; and more and more foodmakers are beginning to see increased awareness of the obesity epidemic not as a threat but as a business opportunity. It's too soon to tell if it's working, but there's at least one hopeful sign. For the first three quarters of 2003, there was no increase in obesity among adult Americans, according to preliminary data from the National Health Interview Survey.

Campaigns against smoking and drunk driving have raised the national consciousness about these public-health issues dramatically. There's no reason to think an anti-obesity campaign can't do so as well—as long as everyone involved acknowledges that the problem is real and that solving it will be as hard as anything we've ever done. After all, it's not easy to fight millions of years of evolution.

— **Reported by David Bjerklie/New York**

Pandemic Obesity

What is the solution?

"What is the practical solution to the obesity problem?" is the perceptive question I was recently asked by Linda Hirsh, Field Producer for the *Peter Jennings' Show*. She was preparing a television show on the American obesity problem for fall viewing on ABC. This column looks at whether there is a practical solution yet, and, if there is, what is it? Here goes!

James E. Tillotson, PhD, MBA

In this series on our pandemic obesity, we've seen how certain of our agricultural and industrial policies have had the unintended and unforeseen consequences of increasing overweight and obesity. I have argued that our government's present nutrition policies are a dismal failure because more of us are fat than thin by a wide margin. Health professionals don't have anything to crow about either. The 1990s were supposed to be *the* nutrition decade. Nutrition and nutritionists were at center stage in print, media, and talk shows, and the public was captivated by various diet crazes. However, it was in the 1990s that we reached new highs in fatness as a nation.

We should have called the 1990s the decade of Great Expectations or Great Illusions, not the Nutrition Decade. The high hopes that the nutrition community shared for improving American diet and health with the passage of the Nutrition Labeling and Education Act in 1990, with its required nutritional labeling of all packaged foods, was misguided. Belatedly, nutritionists discovered that most people, including nutritionists, rarely used nutrition fact labels. Much of what Americans eat doesn't have a nutrition facts label; we rely increasingly on *unlabeled* ready-to-eat foods and, as the fast-food ads say, "lovin' it!"

What is the problem? The ultimate problem, of course, is obesity, but why do we have a problem in solving the pandemic obesity?

A few weeks ago when reading *Advertising Age*, I saw an item that helped me crystallize the problem we face between environmental factors and individual behavior as they relate to obesity. The article showed how immense the problem is as we try to rein in Americans' ravenous eating.

It was *Advertising Age*'s yearly summary of the Top 200 Megabrands—ranked by spending on US measured

total advertising spending (television, radio, magazines, newspapers, etc) in 2002.[1] This shouldn't be confused with total company advertising spending; rather, it is the total advertising spending muscle put behind a company's individual brands, such as Gillette shaving products, Ford cars, Kodak film, Hallmark cards, Clorox detergent, as well as food brands, such as Coke beverages, Campbell's soup, KFC restaurants. These advertising dollar numbers are a better measure of effective firepower aimed at consumers to buy a product than companywide spending. These are real purchase-motivating dollars put behind a specific consumer product.

> **The 1990s were to be the nutrition decade, but they should have been called the Great Illusions.**

I did a little arithmetic with the list of the 200 top brands and counted that 25 (12.5%) were food brands (Figure 1). Of these 25, 9 were the nutritionists *enfant terrible* fast-food chains (McDonald's, Burger King, KFC restaurants, etc.), 6 beverage companies (Budweiser, Coca Cola, Pepsi, etc.), 5 cereal and bakery companies, and 5 miscellaneous companies (soup, gum, dairy brand, diet drink, etc.). Certainly, the most highly promoted foods don't constitute a balanced diet.

The total spending for these 25 food brands came to $4.71 billion for total measured media spending in 2002, ranging from $548.2 million down to $95.8 million for a dairy brand. Remember, this is advertising for a single consumer item, not total company advertising. In adver-

Twenty-five brands were food and beverage products.

Among these 25 brands:
9 fast-food chains
6 beverages (beer and soft drinks)
5 cereal and bakery products
5 miscellaneous (soup, gum, dairy, diet drink, and packaged food brand)

Spending for these 25 brands ranged from $95.8 to $548.2 million for measured US ad spending (television, newspapers, magazine, etc)

Total ad spending for 25 brands was $4.71 billion.

Figure 1. Top 200 megabrands. Ranked by US measured advertising spending, 2002.
Source: *Advertising Age*, July 21, 2003.

Table 1. 2002 Top Five Fast-Service Chains (U.S. Co-Owned Units)

Chain	Co-Owned US Units	Share of US System, %
1. Starbucks	3,312	74
2. McDonald's	2,102	16
3. Pizza Hut	1,760	23
4. Jack in the Box	1,517	81
5. KFC	1,284	24
Total US units	**9,975**	

Source: Food Marketing Institute, Technornic, Inc.

Table 2. 2002 Top Five Fast-Service Chains (US Franchised Units)

Chain	Franchised US Units	Share of US System, %
1. Subway	14,521	100
2. McDonald's	11,389	84
3. Burger King	7,422	92
4. Pizza Hut	5,839	77
5. Taco Bell	4,881	79
Total US units	**44,052**	

Source: Food Marketing Institute, Technomic, Inc.

tising at this level, these companies are exercising their constitutional right of commercial free speech. These food products are the on-again off-again darlings of the financial sector. However, they make up a lot of the firepower behind high-caloric eating for already-hefty Americans.

Advertising in this league is the "go-the-for-gut, anything-that-gets-by-the-FTC" type of advertising that is designed by highly creative people in leading ad agencies. The agencies are in a constant war with other agencies to attract the high-roller, big-spending, prime-time, fast-food chain advertisers. Of course, the advertisements are successful at getting consumers into fast-food outlets. The chains spending the advertising dollars also get the sales numbers. If advertising didn't work, why would they spend all that money? Besides being perfectly legal, this is a necessary expenditure for any fast-food player in the American economic system. This is the reality of the business situation.

Let's dig a bit deeper with the fast-food marketers in this high-advertising group of companies. Checking with the Food Marketing Institute on leading fast-food chains, I looked at who had the largest total numbers of fast-food individual restaurants for the top 5 fast-food chains in the United States for 2002.[2] To get the total number of outlets, I first looked at the co-owned outlets (Table 1) and then at franchised units (Table 2). This gave me 2 lists of 5 fast-food chains on each list.

There were 2 chains represented on both lists (McDonald's and Pizza Hut) of the total 10 chains shown in the 2 lists, for a total of 8 different fast food chains in the 2 lists (Subway, McDonald's, Burger King, Pizza Hut, Taco Bell, KFC, Jack in the Box, and Starbucks). I dropped Starbucks from my calculations, because it is mainly a coffee chain and not a full eatery. This left me with a list of the leading 7 fast-food chains in restaurant numbers in the United States.

Then I cross-checked these 7 chains with my list of the 9 fast-food chains among the top 200 megabrands advertisers (McDonald's, Burger King, Wendy's, KFC, Subway, Taco Bell, Pizza Hut, Domino's Pizza, and Arby's). As expected, 6 big advertising-spending fast-food" restaurants were on my list of 7 outlet chains, spending a total of $1,675.7 million in 2002 (Table 3).

I understand that it is common for the fast-food outlets in this top tier to sell, at a minimum, more than $1 million worth of food a year. Therefore, these 6 top fast-food chains in outlet numbers (49,198 in 2002), with their franchisers, sell a minimum of approximately $50 billion of fast-food a year, spending $1.68 billion on advertising! Just these 6 fast-food chains, based on US Department of Agriculture estimated total US away-from-home sales in 2002 of $425.5 billion, sell Americans 11.8% of this type of food! (The advertising effectiveness of their commercial messages to potential customers is demonstrated by an industry study for the third quarter of 2003, showing that 8 fast-food television commercials were among the top 20

Table 3. 2002 Top Fast-Service Chains in Units Versus Advertising Brand Spending

Chain	Total US Units	Total Advertising Spending, $ Million
1. Subway	14,521	218.7
2. McDonald's	13,491	546.2
3. Pizza Hut	7,599	154.1
4. Burger King	7,422	336.3
5. Taco Bell	4,881	195.8
6. KFC	1,284	224.6
Unit total	**49,198**	**Total 1,675.7**

Source: Food Marketing Institute, Technomic, Inc.

most remembered commercials of all advertised products by polled viewers.)[3]

In short, they have a powerful influence on the American diet.

Now remember, there is no required nutritional labeling here. I don't remember seeing any mention of this type of food in official government advisories. Plus the advice I receive on fast foods from my "card-carrying" nutrition associates runs the gamut from "avoid" to "take in small doses," just like Victorians' views of sex! This is interesting but not likely to be easy to follow in today's American lifestyle, given the realities of our current food supply.

Why do we have a problem in solving the obesity problem?

Remember—in the real world, fast-food restaurants account for 74% of the average 206 meals purchased at commercial establishments for those both eaten out and taken home to eat by Americans last year.[4] That's what is going on in the 277,208 such fast-food restaurants in the United States! This feat is possible, according to Technomic Inc, the well-respected food consulting group, because out ready-prepared food production system has now reached 1 fast-food outlet for each 1,000 Americans, up from 1 in 1,400 people in 1990 and 1 in 2,000 in 1980.[4] There may be more fast-food restaurants than churches!

This is based on only advertising spending and outlet numbers of these 6 leading fast-food chains. Regarding their influence on the diet, you must consider that their

food is inexpensive, great tasting, available everywhere at all hours, and usually in shiny clean surroundings, catering to people's eating desires. These chains are doing just what they should be doing as marketers in the American economy—satisfying their consumers' wishes and desires.

Speaking of marketing, these chains have crack marketing professionals, designing hard-charging, volume-increasing, total-marketing plans, using all the advances available in modern marketing, based on cutting-edge social and motivation psychologies—branding, endorsements from sports heroes and movie characters (Disney figures), deals (dollar deals and give aways), product placements, etc. Nothing illegal or out of the ordinary in consumer marketing here, but again, the unforeseen and unintended consequences that are present throughout our pandemic obesity problem. Remember, this is only one part of one food sector (fast food); similar cases of hard selling are replicated many times throughout our present $920 billion consumer food market. Do we have anything in our current arsenal of public health options to counter such overwhelming marketing power?

What should we do?

To start, can you rationally imagine, except in some Walden Pond or 19th-century Utopia, that Americans wouldn't always use fast-food feeding in some manner. Under our constitutionally protected free speech (commercial free speech), fast food will always be over-aggressively promoted with our brand of capitalism. Will it result in any other social order?

Remember that consumers who are entering these fast-food outlets everyday do so by free choice—with all the other places to eat they pick this type of restaurant. The numbers show they return again and again. The food, price, quality, and convenience squarely fit their daily needs! Also by now, every American has a fair idea that big-time eating of fast food leads to big middles. Yet, the number of people eating fast food increases every year, especially if you include the new fast casuals![5]

Fast-food chains have grown and prospered since the 1950s. This was during the same period when nutrition made its largest advances in understanding diet and health relationships! Has nutritionists' hectoring of the public about fast-food eating done much good in reducing obesity rates?

Currently, the courts and Congress don't look as if they will make fast-food illegal or sue the chains out of existence as happened with cigarettes! Public-opinion surveys show that many Americans don't want the government telling them what to eat, unless it is for their children. A recent study by Euro RSCG Tatham Partners, an international marketing group, reported that some 90% of Americans polled believed that they are personally responsible for their weight condition and are not blaming fast foods.[6]

> *Fast-food chains have grown and prospered since the 1950's, the same period during which nutrition made its largest advances.*

After the lack of progress on agricultural subsidies and tariffs at the World Trade Organization meeting at Cancun, Mexico, do you expect US agricultural policy to change much in the immediate future?[7] Cheap food is here to stay! Do you want our free-enterprise capitalistic food system to change, given its overall net benefits?[8] Do you think we can prevent innovation in the supply chain like that which gave rise to fast-food restaurants?

What is the practical solution to our "lard" problem? I ask my students, but they don't have any answers either, and this is discouraging because they are our human seed corn.

Bottom Line

Are those of us who are food and nutrition professionals and members of relevant industries, whom society expects to solve the obesity problem, stuck in our ruts? Are we like poor wretches caught up in other compulsive behaviors, such as addiction to drugs, liquor, and gambling? Is overeating a compulsive behavior, too? If so, we need new thinking and insights to alter overeating and to overcome the blocks in our thinking.

It is time to admit publicly that we don't have a solution to the pandemic obesity problem, given the social, economic, legal, and political factors and restraints we have surrounding the food-supply system today. All of us—health professionals, government representatives, industry leaders, politicos, activists, media types, and others—have to admit that we are whistling in the dark and don't have a clue as to what to do. We don't have the collective will to give up our present vested potential solutions to seek new understanding, new approaches, and new ways to solve the obesity problem probably from new sources and players.

I believe that the solution will come from what Joseph Schumpeter, the great philosopher/economic thinker, called *creative destruction*. Society, through "waves of innovations," seeks to renew itself through innovation by throwing out the old for the new.[9] To begin, we must imagine some approaches to feeding and eating beyond current fast-food menus that will appeal to the public organoleptically, economically, speedily, and socially but without all the obesity negatives.

Or should we seek new strategically based public-health policies, adequately funded and driven by a unified enlightened government regime that works to positively influence Americans' diets? However, do we have the collective will? Do we have the ability to motivate necessary public interest to get the bucks to do the job? Do we?

REFERENCES

1. AdAge special report: megabrands. *Advertising Age.* July 21, 2003, S-2.
2. Top spots: fast-feeders top Q3 charts. *Advertising Age.* October 27, 2003, 12.
3. The Food Institute. *Food Institute Report.* September 1, 2003, 4.
4. Sloan EA. What, when, and where Americans eat. *Food Technol.* 2003;57:48.
5. Tillotson JE. Fast-casual dining. Our next eating passion? *Nutr Today.* 2003;38:91–94.
6. Big business: the obesity industry. *The Economist.* September 27–October 3, 2003, 64.
7. Tillotson JE. Pandemic obesity: agriculture's cheap food policy is a bad bargain. *Nutr Today.* 2003;38:186–190.
8. Tillotson JE. Pandemic obesity: time for a change in economic and development politics affecting the food industry? *Nutr Today.* 2003;38:242–246.
9. Heilbroner RL. *The Contradictions of Joseph Schumpeter, The Worldly Philosophers: The Lives, Times and Ideas of the Great Thinkers.* 6th ed. New York: Simon & Schuster, Inc.; 1980.

James E. Tillotson, PhD, MBA, is currently Professor of Food Policy and International Business at Tufts University. Before returning to the academic world, Dr Tillotson worked in industry, holding various research and development positions in the food and chemical sectors.
Corresponding author: James E. Tillotson, PhD, MBA, PO Box Ten, Cohasset, MA 02025-0100 (e-mail: james.tillotson@tufts.edu).

A Call to
ACTION

Seeking Answers to Childhood Weight Issues

To solve the current obesity dilemma, more attention should be focused
on increasing children's activity levels.

BY CAROL M. MEERSCHAERT, RD, LDN

One morning, I grabbed a cup of consciousness (or espresso roast coffee) and headed to the computer. In my e-mail inbox was one of those "words of wisdom" letters titled "People Over 35 Should Be Dead." Being older than 35 myself, the heading quickly woke me from my morning stupor.

The e-mail read: "Those of us who were kids in the 1940s, 1950s, 1960s, or even maybe the early 1970s probably shouldn't have survived. We ate cupcakes, bread and butter, and drank soda pop and Kool-Aid with sugar in it, but we were never overweight because we were always outside playing. We would leave home in the morning and play all day, as long as we were back when the street lights came on. We did not have PlayStations, Nintendo 64, X-Boxes—no video games at all—no 99 channels on cable, videotape movies, personal computers, or Internet chat rooms. We had friends! We went outside and found them."

As a dietitian, parent, and lover of physical activity, this message struck home. We have struggled to find the answers to the complex issues of childhood overweight prevention and treatment, and there, suddenly, the answer seemed to be staring at me from my inbox.

You all know the statistics on overweight: Currently, 64% of the adult population—or 123 million people—is either overweight or obese. The rate has doubled in children and tripled in adolescents since 1980. Approximately 15% of children and teens are overweight. The problem of overweight/obesity in America costs $117 bil-

lion annually and accounts for at least 14% of deaths in the United States, or some 300,000 premature deaths each year. As professional nutritionists, you also know that weight control is the time-honored balance of caloric intake and expenditure. So how do we help overweight children deal with this problem? How do we help prevent other children from becoming overweight?

> Could it be that a large decrease in physical activity, not changes in caloric intake, is responsible for increases in childhood obesity rates since 1980?

While everyone agrees that children should be encouraged to eat a healthful diet, weight-loss diets are not the answer. The National Institutes of Health-funded Growing Up Today Study examined a cohort of children who are offspring of the Nurses' Health Study II participants. These children were followed for three years, and those who were on weight-loss diets gained more weight relative to predicted body weight than the nondieters. Binge eating was also associated with dieting to control weight.[1] The authors concluded that for many adolescents, chronic dieting is not only ineffective, but it also may promote weight gain.

In an earlier study, Field and colleagues found that dieting among teens did not necessarily lead to lower caloric intake, nor was dieting restricted to girls who were overweight. Sadly, 50% of the girls who were below the national age-standardized 15th percentile for body mass index (BMI) reported their ideal weight as less than their current weight.[2] Emphasis on thinness and dieting seems to backfire.

A prospective, three-year study of female students in grades 7 to 10 found that restrained eating, body dissatisfaction, drive for thinness, self-induced vomiting, laxative use, diet pill use, and alcohol use significantly increased, while attitudes about physical appearance and self-concept significantly decreased among frequent dieters compared with nondieters.[3]

What about the energy expenditure side of the energy balance equation? A group at Brigham and Women's Hospital in Boston examined a nationwide cohort of 6,149 girls and 4,620 boys aged 9 to 14. They found that in both boys and girls, a one-year increase in BMI was larger in those who reported more time with TV and videos. Larger increases in BMI were also seen among girls who reported higher caloric intakes and less physical activity.[4]

Lisa Sutherland, PhD, RD, research assistant professor of nutrition at the University of North Carolina at Chapel Hill, studied national health data on adolescent obesity, calorie intake, and physical activity from 1980 to 2000. To determine overweight in children, she used National Health and Nutrition Examination Survey II and III and 1999 Centers for Disease Control and Prevention (CDC) data on BMI. Calorie intake was determined using the Nationwide Food Consumption Survey (NFCS) and the Continuing Survey of Food Intake by Individuals from the U.S. Department of Agriculture. Physical activity was determined by examining data from the Youth Risk Behavior Survey, CDC.[5] The result was that in people aged 12 to 19, obesity rose 10% during that time frame; calorie intake rose a mere 1%; and physical activity fell a substantial 13%.

Could it be that a large decrease in physical activity, not changes in caloric intake, is responsible for increases in childhood obesity rates since 1980? Decreased physical activity has an impact on adolescent overweight. Sutherland concluded that both sides of the energy equation need to be addressed when creating community, state, and federal programs and policy that address childhood obesity.

A National Bureau of Economic Research paper by Lakdawalla and Philipson gives compelling evidence that technological change has induced weight gain by making people more sedentary.[6] They argue that 60% of the weight gain seen in the U.S. population may be due to factors such as declining physical activity from technological changes. When was the last time your kids shoveled the driveway? Hung clothes on a clothesline? Chopped wood for the woodstove? Waxed the floor?

A National Association for Sport and Physical Education survey found that 81% of adults said they believe daily physical education should be mandatory in schools. Surprisingly, Illinois is the only state that requires daily physical education classes for students in grades kindergarten through 12. The California Education Code mandates physical education for all students in grades 1 through 9, but only one additional year in the four years of high school. In contrast, Colorado and South Dakota do not have any mandate for physical education at any grade level. The result is that grade school children are now 24% more active than high school students. Schools struggle to meet the demands of state education initiatives and federal initiatives such as "No Child Left Behind," so physical education and recess get squeezed out of the school day.

When trying to solve the puzzle of increasing childhood overweight, ponder this: In my elementary school, we had recess three times per day. In my son's school, they get one 15-minute recess after lunch. I walked to school; now my children take a bus. According to the CDC, 85% of children's trips to school are by car or school bus, and only 13% are on foot or by bike. Does your community have bike racks and sidewalks? Crossing guards? Sutherland suggests that nutrition professionals get active in community programs, creating links with parents to increase opportunities for children to be active. She is currently a coinvestigator in the National Evaluation of the Walk to School Project. This critical evaluation seeks to understand how and why the program works and to identify parent and child barriers that prevent walking or biking to school. (To learn more, check out the CDC Kids Walk to School Program at www.cdc.gov/nccdphp/dnpa/kidswalk.)

American children do not walk as much as others. Susan D. Vincent, PhD, from Brigham Young University used pedometers to measure walking and showed that Americans walked less than their Swedish or Australian counterparts. Swedish boys, for instance, took as many as 18,346 steps per day, Australians took 15,023, and Americans took 13,872 steps.[7]

> Schools struggle to meet the demands of state education initiatives and federal initiatives such as "No Child Left Behind," so physical education and recess get squeezed out of the school day.

Often, tight budgets are the scapegoat for cutting physical education, sports, and other opportunities for kids to get active. However, a Harvard School of Public Health survey of 1,002 adults presented at their Spring Obesity conference found that 76% of adults would support measures such as offering more physical education classes and educating parents about healthful eating and exercise, even if it meant higher taxes. Further, 42% would pay $100 more per year in taxes to support these kinds of efforts.

Physically active children gain more than just weight control. A California Study matched scores from the spring 2001 administration of the Stanford Achievement Test, Ninth Edition (SAT-9), with results of the state-mandated physical fitness test, known as the Fitnessgram, given in 2001 to students in grades 5, 7, and 9. Reading and math scores were matched with fitness scores of 353,000 fifth-graders, 322,000 seventh-graders, and 279,000 ninth-graders. Higher achievement was associated with higher levels of fitness at each of the three grade levels measured. The relationship between academic achievement and fitness was greater in mathematics than in reading, particularly at higher fitness levels. Students who met minimum fitness levels in three or more physical fitness areas showed the greatest gains in academic achievement at all three grade levels.

How can nutrition professionals get more information to get more involved?

• Visit www.cdc.gov/mmwr to read a report on how your state measures up. The CDC, in the August 15, 2003, issue of MMWR, "New Physical Activity Measures include Lifestyle Activities, Behavioral Risk Factor Surveillance System 2001" provides baseline data nationally and for each state and U.S. territory based upon the measurements used for 2001.

• The California Department of Education (www.cde.ca.gov/cyfsbranch/lsp/health/pecommunications.htm) has recommendations on physical education for teachers, students, and their families.

• Check out www.presidentschallenge.org, a new interactive Web site to help all Americans build a regular physical activity routine. This Web site tracks progress toward earning presidential awards for active lifestyle and physical fitness.

• Download or order materials from the VERB Campaign (www.cdc.gov/youthcampaign/materials/index.htm) to increase physical activity. The materials feature campaign materials for use with 'tween audiences, including posters, stickers, and temporary tattoos that organizations can order free of charge.

• The CDC also has free brochures to help increase physical activity among elementary and middle school-aged children. The parents' brochure is available in English and Spanish versions at www.cdc.gov/healthyyouth/physicalactivity.

• Learn about the National School Fitness Foundation (www.cdc.gov/youthcampaign/materials/index.htm), a public, nonprofit organization, founded in March 2000 to fight childhood obesity and inactivity. Their Leadership in Fitness Training (LIFT) program offers aerobic and strength training equipment, computerized assessment kiosks, curriculum, and complete faculty training and certification to schools. As of September 2003, the LIFT Program was being utilized by students in more than 450 schools in 18 states (www.nsff.net).

• Use the tools found on www.kidnetic.com, a healthy eating and active living Web site designed for kids aged 9 to 12 and their families to inspire them to move toward healthier lifestyles. Kidnetic.com is also a resource for health professionals and educators to use when working with patients and students. Kidnetic.com is the initial program element of ACTIVATE, an educational outreach program of the International Food Information Council Foundation developed in partnership with the American Academy of Family Physicians, American College of Sports Medicine, American Dietetic Association, International Life Sciences Institute Center for Health Promotion, and National Recreation and Park Association.

References

1. Field AE, et al. *Pediatrics*. 2003;112(4):900-906.

2. Field, et al. *J Am Acad Child Adolesc Psychiatry*. 1993;32(6):1246-1252.

3. French SA. *J Adolesc Health*. 1995;16(6):438-447.

4. Berkey CS, et al. *Pediatrics*. 2000;105(4):E56.

5. Centers for Disease Control and Prevention. National Center for Chronic Disease Prevention and Health Promotion. Youth Risk Behavior Surveillance System, 2001.

6. Lakdawalla D, Philipson T. The Growth of Obesity and Technological Change: A Theoretical and Empirical Examination NBER Working Paper No. w8946. May 2002.

7. Medicine and Science in Sports and Exercise. August 2003. Available at: http://www.ms-se.com

---

—Carol M. Meerschaert, RD, LDN, is a freelance writer in Falmouth, Me.

Social Change and Obesity Prevention

Where Do We Begin?

Obesity in the United States has reached epidemic proportions in both adults and children. Multi-factorial causes are responsible, including social, economic, and other environmental forces acting on a susceptible genetic heritage. Halting and reversing the epidemic will require multi-factorial solutions, including implementing cognitive coping strategies and mounting an effective social change movement.

John C. Peters, PhD

Dramatic increases during the past 2 decades in the prevalence of overweight and obesity in the United States have prompted medical and public health officials to declare the situation epidemic. Rising obesity rates have also fueled alarming increases in type 2 diabetes in children and adults, projecting a tremendous toll on health and quality of life and an escalating financial burden to individuals and society.[1-5]

Historically, the first response to an epidemic is to find and isolate the causal agent, and then strategies can be put in place to stem the outbreak and prevent future incidents. What is the cause of the obesity epidemic? Can we isolate the offending agent(s) and eradicate the problem? Can we inoculate the population against further attack?

There is an emerging scientific consensus that the recent rise in obesity is a function of multi-factorial causes, reflecting an interaction between our susceptible genetic heritage and an environment that promotes excessive food consumption and a sedentary lifestyle.[6,7] Our human ancestors developed multiple and redundant biologic systems that encouraged us to eat when food was available and conserve energy when expending it was not required to meet basic survival needs. It is no wonder that in our age of relative food abundance and accessible high-technology machines, people are eating more, moving less, and gaining weight.

Obesity and Our Environment

It is easy to identify characteristics of our everyday environment that promote eating … from the ready accessibility of food in virtually every locale to large portions and aggressive advertising. Today, food is inexpensive and it takes little time or energy to prepare it for consumption. Thanks to technological advances in food production, stabilization, and preparation, "fast" food is available at home, at school, in the workplace, and in restaurants and other venues throughout our communities. Literally centuries of efforts to create a world in which food availability, cost, and convenience are no longer problems have finally paid off.

However, there are new problems. In addition to the seemingly constant pressure to eat, the temptation or even the requirement to be sedentary is a defining feature of our modern lifestyle—in schools, on the job, and at home. In the most sought-after high-paying jobs, people are essentially paid to be sedentary, spending hours in front of a computer screen managing and transacting business with the click of a mouse. Outside of work we can conduct most aspects of daily business without ever having to step out of our cars. Never has going to the bank, picking up a prescription, or getting dinner been easier or taken less physical exertion. Leisure time entertainment has become increasingly sedentary and ever more attractive, with hundreds of television channels to watch, movies to rent, and electronic games to play. We have engineered the need for physical activity out of our lives to a large extent. Just a few decades ago, physically active jobs were typically low paying and less desirable. Ironically, more and more of us now pay to be physically active, as evidenced by the dramatic growth of the health club market.[8]

As our technological prowess grew and our lifestyle priorities changed, we built our communities to reflect these evolving preferences. Land use and community design changed dramatically in ways that now make it difficult to adopt a more physically active lifestyle, even if this became a priority.[9] For example, traditional early 20th-century neighborhood design followed a characteristic grid pattern in which there were many intersections and few major thoroughfares.[9] It was easy to walk to school; the park, the grocery store, or the beauty salon. Doing business on foot was as safe and convenient as relying on the automobile.

Contemporary neighborhoods are characterized by a more amorphous design, with few intersections and large multilane thoroughfares.[9] Because of land costs in suburban America, new schools are often built miles from population centers so that walking or riding a bike is not an option. Sidewalks are absent from many neighborhoods, making even casual physical activity a safety risk. We have constructed the modern world to best suit conducting our lives from the comfort and safety of our chairs, couches, and automobiles. Inadvertently, we have nearly eliminated the single largest source of physical activity (energy expenditure involved in moving our bodies) from our traditional human existence—walking.

It is easy to find what appear to be important factors in the causal chain leading to obesity. Are these features of our food and physical activity environment the root causes of obesity, or are they merely symptoms of deeper sociocultural issues? Clearly, no one set out to make the American public obese. The myriad businesses that promote food consumption and physical inactivity are not purposefully targeted at making people gain weight. So what is driving the epidemic?

Sociocultural Drivers of Obesity

One could argue that these "obesigenic" features of our environment arose and evolved to meet the demands of a population that was seeking the proverbial American dream. Who *wouldn't* want abundant food that was convenient, tasted great, and was inexpensive? Who *wouldn't* want a subsistence that didn't require hard physical exertion? Who *wouldn't* want wide access to affordable and enjoyable entertainment?

In the tradition of our ancestors, most of us toil to make a better life for our children, to make life easier in every way, so future generations can be as happy and productive as possible. Individuals and society have benefited enormously from the technological advances that have transformed the food supply, the workplace, and our community and home environments. Standards of living for most people have never been higher. The food is less expensive, more convenient, and tastes better than ever. We don't have to do hard physical labor on the job, but there have been unintended consequences of achieving this once only-imagined American dream.

Prominent among them is the ever-accelerating pace of our modern globally connected "electronic" lives. "Keeping up" not only eliminates the time we would otherwise spend preparing wholesome nutritious meals and enjoying physical activity but also adds stress to our lives, reducing sleep and making us vulnerable to eating as a way to medicate the stress. To top it off, a multitude of sedentary entertainment options help us cope with the strain brought about by life in the fast lane.

All of these environmental features and adaptive behaviors provide immediate gratification and are strong drivers of the choices we make every day about what and how much to eat and how much physical activity in which to engage. However, in our quest for the American dream, we haven't taken time to examine the long-term health consequences on body weight and chronic disease of these short-term benefits. The question is: now that we are beginning to recognize these unintended consequences and confront the problem … what do we do about it?

The underlying cultural, economic, and social drivers that shaped our current environment are so complex and interrelated that changing the environment will be a long-term process—but it is one that can begin today. Although there is a natural tendency to search for the single cause or "villain" in the obesity epidemic, this will be essentially impossible to do retrospectively, and finding someone or something to blame will not solve the obesity crisis. Rather, we must embark on two parallel efforts: First, we need to mount a concerted social change movement to create a future state in which healthy lifestyle behaviors are socially normative behavior. Second, we need to provide people with better tools to support cognitive management of body weight within the prevailing environment—before the future state becomes a reality.

The solution: two parallel efforts—a social change movement to create socially normative healthy lifestyle behaviors and tools to help in cognitive management of body weight.

Building for Social Change

What will this take? There are numerous examples of previous successful social change campaigns, including the recycling movement, smoking cessation campaigns, and the move toward routine seat belt use.[10] These movements shared many common features, including a definition of the crisis in immediate terms relevant to individuals, eg, "how will this affect me personally" a strong science base, and the importance of a solution that was economically feasible and sensible. Although there is currently much media attention on the obesity epidemic, recent surveys show the average consumer does not place this at the top of his or her list of personal concerns.[11]

Perhaps one way to highlight the immediacy and personally threatening nature of the crisis is to highlight the externality of this issue. That is, to show how unhealthy lifestyle choices by one individual may have a negative effect on others—without their consent. The turning point in the movement to provide wide availability of smoke-free environments was driven by the release of the secondhand smoke report in the mid-1980s, which showed that one person's decision to smoke can have a negative health effect on nonsmokers via secondhand smoke.[10] This was seen as a violation of personal liberty, one of the strongest values in America. One could apply the same logic to eating and physical activity health behaviors. For example, among participants in a group health insurance plan, those making healthy lifestyle choices and consequently spending less on healthcare are effectively subsidizing other consumers who may not be making healthy choices and consequently cost the insured group more money. If this situation were made clear to those in the group making healthy lifestyle choices, they might be inspired to drive a campaign for change—tied to our American values of personal liberty and fairness/justice.

Build in immediate benefits for healthy choices to reinforce them

---

In the end, a successful social change movement will require cooperation among all sectors of society—public and private. Creating and sustaining a future state in which the prevailing environment supports healthy eating and physical activity behaviors will require institutionalizing incentive systems that provide people with immediate benefits for "doing the right thing." Years of public health and behavioral research has shown that few people will change these immediately rewarding behaviors based solely on the long-term promise of better "health."[12–14] In our current environment and social system, there are essentially no short-term incentives to maintain healthful eating and physical activity patterns. Instead, health behaviors must come from within the individual—supported by a level of self-actualization that is likely present in only a minority of the population. Because the immediate benefits of eating too much and moving too little are strongly reinforced by our biologic predisposition (eat when food is available and rest when

you can), the incentives (and possibly disincentives) for alternative behaviors will have to be strong and compelling.

Building Better Coping Skills

Comprehensive social change will take time, yet the obesity epidemic is worsening rapidly. We need to provide people now with better tools to use in their day-to-day lives to combat weight gain. In the current environment, we can no longer rely on our body's inherent physiology to manage body weight—we will need to exert cognitive control over the current environmental pressures to eat and be sedentary.[15] Current diet and physical activity guidelines are difficult to implement for many people. For example, although the current guidelines recommend a certain number of servings of specific food types and so many minutes of physical activity per day, how many people can or do keep cumulative track of their progress toward these goals during the day. Most of us don't carry food diaries to log our servings of fruits and vegetables or stop watches to log the number of minutes we spend in various activities. Furthermore, most people don't know how to equate the energy value of food and physical activity, so they do not have the knowledge or skills to balance energy intake and energy expenditure. Finally, the diet and physical activity goals set by public health authorities may be scientifically sound and appropriate, but for many people, starting from where they are, these targets may seem too high and too far out of reach to even begin contemplating change.

As a nation, we need to set more realistic goals for combating obesity. *Healthy People 2010* set as a goal to reduce obesity prevalence to 15%[16]—we are now at more than 30%[17] and rising! A more realistic goal might be to simply stop any further excess weight gain in the population—among adults and children. Over time, this would lead to reductions in population obesity prevalence as our youth would not join the ranks of the overweight when they became adults—but what about adults who are already overweight and obese? Stopping further weight gain alone could have tremendously positive benefits for health and healthcare costs.[18] Furthermore, even if we were to focus on reversing established obesity, we have had little success in doing so with individually focused treatments thus far,[19, 20] and there are no proven effective population-based solutions.

Better coping skills and more realistic targets for decreasing overweight are needed

---

To stop weight gain, we need to provide people with simple tools to better cope within the current environment—actionable solutions that can help them balance energy in and energy out. Increasing lifestyle physical activity would seem to be a promising approach to helping manage energy balance, because it is easy to monitor using readily available technology and can be related to the energy value of food. A recent report shows that the median weight gain of the US population is approximately 2 lb per year.[7] A positive energy balance of 100 kcal/day can explain the weight gain of 90% of the population. Simply eating less and moving more in some combination adding up to 100 kcal/day could stop weight gain in 90% of the population.[7] On the physical activity side of the equation, walking 2,000 additional steps (almost a mile) each day would burn the entire 100 kcal. In addition, taking 100 calories out of daily food intake would be equally accessible using simple strategies such as like food substitution (eg, using a reduced-fat or reduced-calorie option) and portion "right-sizing."

Cutting back a little on eating or increasing energy output by 100 calories a day would help a lot

---

Using a combination of both strategies would offer consumers the most flexibility and choice—as long as we can keep it simple and consumers can easily keep track. Monitoring the extra steps (walking) is easy using inexpensive electronic pedometers and can be an easy first step toward implementing a strategy to stop weight gain.[21] Framing the problem and the solution in these terms—small steps can have a big impact—might seem less daunting for individuals and the population as a whole, and it offers hope that making progress in combating obesity may be surprisingly within our reach.

As an example of this approach—simple steps to better health—is a new national initiative called America on the Move (**www.americaonthemove.org**). Sponsored by a nonprofit public-private organization, the Partnership to Promote Healthy Eating and Active Living, America on the Move (AOM) promotes a simple and fun way for people to begin the process of adopting a healthier lifestyle. Based on the analysis showing that weight gain could be prevented by a reduction in positive energy balance of only 100 calories per day,[7] AOM emphasizes making small daily changes in eating and walking that can fit with peoples' hectic lives. As a start, the initiative encourages people to take 2,000 more steps per day than they take currently (monitored by a pedometer) and to reduce food intake by 100 calories. The program was successfully pilot tested in Colorado, showing that these goals are easily achievable by the majority of participants.[21] AOM was launched nationally on the Internet in July 2003 and is currently being implemented into communities via a network of state affiliates. Ongoing research (J.O. Hill, personal communication) is

showing that once people reach these initial goals, their confidence and self-efficacy increase and they often go beyond to achieve more challenging health behavior goals. Importantly, AOM is working with both the public and private sectors, including the retail and food industries, to provide incentives and other support in work sites, schools, restaurants, businesses, and communities for people to engage in these healthy behaviors.

Solving the obesity crisis facing the nation today will likely take generations. Obesity is a multifaceted problem that will require multifaceted and comprehensive solutions. It will take time to generate the political will to begin changing the systems and institutions and social values that support the current environment and that, in effect, reward people for practicing behaviors that promote obesity. It will take time before we find affordable and sustainable ways of engaging and rewarding people to "do the right thing" from a purely personal health perspective. It will take time for society to evolve so that leading a healthy active lifestyle becomes "normative behavior" and, thus, becomes self-sustaining. As a society, we will succeed in bringing about these changes because we must—we can't afford not to. In the meantime, we should all be working to inspire our families, friends, and communities to take those first small steps that can have a big effect. After all, you have to start somewhere.

Notes

1. McGinnis JM, Foege WH, Actual causes of death in the United States. *JAMA*. 1993;270:2207–2212.
2. Allison DB, Fontaine KR, Manson JE, Stevens J, VanItallie TB. Annual deaths attributable to obesity in the United States. *JAMA*. 1999;282: 1530–1538.
3. Sturm R, Wells KB. Does obesity contribute as much to morbidity as poverty or smoking? *Public Health*. 2001;115:229–235.
4. Ford ES, Williamson DF, Liu S. Weight change and diabetes incidence: findings from a national cohort of U.S. adults. *Am J Epidemiol*. 1997;146:214–222.
5. Wolf AM, Colditz GA. Current estimates of the economic cost of obesity in the United States. *Obes Res*. 1998;6:97–106.
6. Hill JO, Peters JC. Environmental contributions to the obesity epidemic, *Science*. 1998;280:1371–1374.
7. Hill JO, Wyatt HR, Reed GW, Peters JC. Obesity and the environment: where do we go from here? *Science*. 2003;299:853–855.
8. Sturm R. The economics of physical activity: societal trends and rationales for interventions. *Am J Prev Med*. 2004. In press.
9. Saelens BE, Sallis JF, Frank LD. Environmental correlates of walking and cycling: findings from the transportation, urban design, and planning literatures. *Ann Behav Med*. 2003;25:80–91.

10. Economos CD, Brownson RC, DeAngelis, MA, et al. What lessons have been learned from other attempts to guide social change? *Nutrition Reviews*. 2001;59:S40–S56.

11. Lee T and Oliver JE. Public opinion and the politics of America's obesity epidemic. Available at: `http://ksgnotesl.harvard.edu/Research/wpaper.nsf/rwp/RW P02-017?OpenDocumen`. Accessed March 3, 2003.

12. Hill JO, Goldberg GP, Pate RR, Peters JC. Summit on promoting healthy eating and active living: developing a framework for progress. *Nutr Rev*. 2001;59:S4–S6.

13. Wetter AC, Goldberg GP, King AC, et al. How and why do individuals make food and physical activity choices? *Nutr Rev*. 2001;59:S11–S20.

14. Booth SL, Sallis JF, Ritenbaugh C, et al. Environmental and societal factors affect food choice and physical activity: rationale, influences and leverage points. *Nutr Rev*. 2001;59:S21–S39.

15. Peters JC, Wyatt HR, Donahoo WT, Hill JO. From instinct to intellect: The challenge of maintaining health weight in the modern world. *Obesity Reviews*. 2002;3:69–74.

16. U.S. Department of Health and Human Services. *Healthy People 2010: Understanding and Improving Health and Objectives for Improving Health*. Washington, DC: Government Printing Office; 2000.

17. Flegal KM, Carroll MD, Ogden CL, Johnson CL. Prevalence and trends in obesity among US adults, 1999–2000. *JAMA*. 2002;288: 1723–1727.

18. Willett WC, Manson JE, Stampfer MJ, et al. Weight, weight change, and coronary heart disease in women. Risk within the "normal" weight range. *JAMA*. 1995;273:461–465.

19. Wing RR. Behavioral interventions for obesity: recognizing our progress and future challenges. *Obesity Res*. 2003; 11:3S–6S.

20. Lowe MR. Self-regulation of energy intake in the prevention and treatment of obesity: Is it feasible? *Obesity Res*. 2003;11:44S–59S.

21. Wyatt HR, Peters JC, Reed GW, et al. Using electronic step counters to increase lifestyle physical activity: Colorado on the move. *J Physical Activity Health*. 2004. In press.

John C. Peters, PhD, is the Head, Nutrition Science Institute, and Associate Director of Food and Beverage Technology, Procter and Gamble, Cincinnati, Ohio.

Correspondence: John Peters, PhD, Procter and Gamble, 11810 Miami River Rd, Room 1D32A, Box 742, Cincinnati, OH 45252 (e-mail: Peters.jc.1@pg.com).

FAT
More than just a lump of lard

"For many years, fat was viewed as a balloon that fills up when you eat more food and burn fewer calories and is deflated when you eat less food and burn more calories," says Jeffrey Friedman of Rockefeller University in New York.

"With the discovery of leptin and subsequently other molecules, it's pretty clear that fat is an endocrine organ that plays a dynamic, active role."

Scientists are scrambling to figure out exactly how fat cells influence our ability to lose or gain weight, play a key role in the immune system, and increase the risk of heart attacks, diabetes, and other diseases. And they're learning that not all fat is equally harmful or tough to lose.

To researchers, that extra bulge around your waist isn't a roll of flab, it's a cutting-edge science lab.

The breakthrough came in 1994.

That's when Jeffrey Freidman's research team at Rockefeller University discovered leptin, a hormone secreted by fat cells that controls fat stores and much more.

"It's not at all surprising that fat isn't passive," says Friedman. "Much of our survival depends on our ability to get nutrition just right, so there are a lot of signals in a complex network designed to do just that."

For example, if a woman has too little body fat to successfully carry a baby to term, her fat cells may signal her brain to stave off pregnancy.

For most of human history, though, survival meant avoiding starvation, not a supersized belly. Unfortunately—at least for people who are tempted with food every time they walk (or, more likely, ride) to a shopping mall, gas station, drugstore, or movie theater—our bodies are set up to deal with scarcity, not abundance.

"The body has lots of ways to respond to overindulgence," says exercise physiologist Cris Slentz of Duke University. "They're all the result of too much food and too little activity."

Swollen Fat Cells

When we eat more calories than we burn, the body converts most of the excess to fat. Where does the fat go? "It's got to be stored somewhere," says Slentz.

First, so much gets stuffed into our fat cells (also called adipose cells) that they swell. That's problem No. 1.

Fat cells secrete more than a dozen proteins that trigger changes throughout the body. And when fat cells expand, they release more of some proteins and less of others. For example:

• **Leptin.** "People originally were taken by the notion that leptin might be the cure for obesity," says cell biologist Philipp Scherer of the Albert Einstein School of Medicine in New York.

Leptin sends signals to tell the brain whether to boost or curb appetite. "The more fat in the body, the more leptin that circulates," explains Scherer.

In theory, extra leptin should rein in appetite and burn more calories. But so far, it doesn't appear to be the anti-blubber drug of our dreams.

Swallowing leptin in a pill doesn't help the overweight because, like any other protein, it gets digested in the gut before it reaches the bloodstream. And even if leptin is injected, it doesn't curb appetite and burn more calories.

"People who are obese are not sensitive to leptin," explains obesity expert Samuel Klein of Washington University in St. Louis. They have plenty, but they don't respond to it.

"It's possible that leptin may help maintain weight loss after people lose excess weight," says Klein, but it's too early to know.

Meanwhile, leptin can work against the dieter. Lose enough weight and your fat cells shrink, which means they release less leptin.

"When leptin levels drop, the brain sees that as evidence of starvation and it causes you to be hungry," says Scott Weigle, professor of medicine at the University of Washington School of Medicine in Seattle.

It's a Catch-22. "Leptin levels fall as you lose weight, and that tends to promote weight gain because the fall is a stimulus to eat more and burn less," says Friedman.

Burning fewer calories makes it harder to lose weight. "The tragedy is that when you reduce the number of calories you take in, you become much more efficient at using them," says Scherer. "Once you get off the diet, you're still using calories efficiently, so people gain so much back that they often overshoot their original weight."

<table>
<tr><td>

Leptin

Gain weight and your fat cells release more leptin. In theory, that should make you eat less and burn more calories. But the fatter you get, the less your leptin works. When you lose weight, your fat cells release less leptin. That makes you eat more and burn fewer calories, which makes it tougher to keep the weight off.

Adiponectin

This "good guy" hormone enables insulin to hustle sugar from the bloodstream into your body's cells, where it's stored or burned for fuel. The more fat you have, the less adiponectin your fat cells secrete.

Ghrelin

When you lose weight, your stomach (not your fat cells) releases more ghrelin, which makes you hungry and makes it tougher to keep the weight off.

Inflammatory Proteins

Fat cells release proteins (like interleukin-6 and tumor necrosis factor-alpha) that cause low-level inflammation throughout the body. Inflammation can rupture the plaques that clog arteries, leading to a heart attack or stroke.

</td></tr>
</table>

• **Adiponectin.** "Larger fat cells are associated with insulin resistance," says Klein. And adiponectin—a protein secreted by fat cells—helps explain why.

Insulin admits blood sugar into the body's cells, where it's stored or used as fuel. Many overweight people produce plenty of insulin, but the hormone loses its punch. This "insulin resistance" can lead to high blood sugar levels and raises the risk of heart disease even if it doesn't cause diabetes (see "Insulin Alert").

"The more fat you have, the less adiponectin your fat cells produce," says Scherer, who discovered adiponectin.

Adiponectin is low in anyone who's overweight, but it's especially low in people who are insulin resistant, which suggests that it makes the body responsive to insulin.

"Adiponectin is a good-guy hormone," says Weigle.

So far, no one has tried to inject adiponectin into people, but even if they could, it would mostly affect insulin resistance, not spare tires.

• **Inflammatory Proteins.** The larger your fat cells, the more they stir up the immune system. "Fat cells put out cytokines like interleukin-6 and especially tumor necrosis factor-alpha," says Slentz. "They increase inflammation."

The inflammation is too subtle to cause a fever, pain, or any other sign of trouble. But it's still insidious.

"Inflammation causes the plaques that clog arteries to begin rupturing," says Slentz. "That's when people have heart attacks."

All the Wrong Places

Once your fat cells are stuffed to the brim, then what?

"There's only room for about 1.2 micrograms of fat per cell," says Klein. "The cells get bigger, but not huge. They don't get big enough to store, say, three micrograms of fat."

Cells that can't get any bigger do what anyone looking for more storage space would do. "If people continue to consume more calories than they burn, they make more fat cells," says Scherer.

People used to think that only babies could make new fat cells. "There was a notion that if you gain too much weight in the first two or three years of life, you would be fat for life," says Scherer. "Now that notion has been dispelled."

In fact, a chubby teenager is more likely than a chubby toddler to become an obese adult.

That's good news for parents of young children, but bad news for everyone else.

"Now we know that people can make new fat cells at any age," says Scherer. "And while loading up a fat cell with more fat is quite reversible, once you make more fat cells, they're going to be around for a very long time."

"The half-life is probably at least a year, but I think it's longer," he notes. "Once you've accumulated a number of fat cells, they may be there to stay. If you put yourself on a diet, you primarily reduce the amount of fat stored in a cell," not the number of fat cells.

And in many people, even new fat cells aren't enough to store the excess fat. So it starts going places that it's not supposed to, like the liver, muscles, and maybe the pancreas.

"In muscle, you can see fat cells interspersed between muscle cells," says Scherer. "It looks like the white veins that you see in a marbled steak."

That misplaced fat seems to lead to insulin resistance. "People with diabetes have low-density muscle because so much fat is stored there," says Slentz.

Endurance athletes are an exception, he adds. They store fat in their muscles without any apparent harm.

But for most people, says Klein, "the more fat we store in muscle, the liver, and the heart, the more abnormalities we see in those organs."

Gut Issues

Dumping fat into fat cells is less harmful than stashing it in muscles, the heart, and other organs. But *where* those fat cells are also makes a difference.

People who gain weight around the middle (so-called "apples") have a higher risk of heart disease and diabetes than people who gain weight in the hips and thighs ("pears"). Men are more likely to be apples. Younger women are usually pears, but move closer to apples as their weight shifts after menopause.

"Premenopausal women put fat on their thighs or the backs of their arms," explains Slentz. "Those are good places to store it because it doesn't cause insulin resistance." (Women may beg to differ, of course.)

Insulin Alert

If you have any three of these five risk factors, you probably have the metabolic syndrome (also known as the insulin resistance syndrome), which raises your risk of heart disease and diabetes. The underlying cause: too much weight and too little exercise.

1. Abdominal obesity	Women: more than 35-inch waist
	Men: more than 40-inch waist(*)
2. Triglycerides	150 or higher
3. HDL cholesterol	Women: under 50
	Men: under 40
4. Blood pressure	Systolic: 130 or higher or
	Diastolic: 85 or higher
5. Fasting blood sugar	110 or higher(**)

(*) For some men, a 37- to 39-inch waist can be a risk factor.

(**) Recent recommendations classify a fasting blood sugar of 100 to 125 as "pre-diabetes."

Source: National Heart, Lung, and Blood Institute.

Researchers are trying to figure out why apples are at greater risk. Fat that's stored deep in the abdomen may hold the answer.

"On average, 80 to 90 percent of fat is subcutaneous, or just under the skin," says Klein. "The remaining 10 to 20 percent is the visceral fat that's deep inside the abdomen and the fat in nonadipose tissue like muscle, liver, and heart."

Researchers aren't sure why visceral fat is so much worse.

"It's very active," says Scherer. "And it releases free fatty acids that cause inflammation and insulin resistance." Visceral fat also secretes more inflammatory agents like interleukin-6 and tumor necrosis factor-alpha.

Another theory: "Visceral fat is close to the liver and pancreas, so when you move fat out of the fat cells, it goes directly to those organs," says Slentz.

Limits of Liposuction

When people lose weight, they lose both visceral and subcutaneous fat. And that lowers their risk of heart disease and diabetes. Not so when the fat is vacuumed out of them.

Klein and his co-workers recently used liposuction to remove roughly 20 pounds of subcutaneous fat from the bellies of 15 obese women.[1]

The result: "If you lose fat by liposuction, it improves only the cosmetic problem," says Klein.

Losing 20 pounds of fat had no impact on the women's metabolic health—their insulin resistance, adiponectin, or inflammatory proteins (C-reactive protein, interleukin-6, or tumor necrosis factor-alpha). Nor did the weight loss improve their blood pressure, blood sugar, cholesterol, or any other risk factors for heart disease. Zip.

In contrast, says Klein, "losing as little as five percent of your weight by eating less and increasing physical ac-

Diet Digest

Low-carb or low-fat? Researchers still don't know which diets are best for keeping weight off over the long term. Until more results are in, look for a healthy hybrid like the South Beach Diet. Our basic advice:

• **Less bad.** Cut back on calories from bad fats and bad carbs. (That includes french fries, burgers, pizza, movie-theater popcorn, nachos, sweets, etc.)

• **More good.** Build your diet around vegetables, seafood, poultry, low-fat dairy foods, beans, and whole grains, plus some oils, nuts, and other unsaturated fats.

• **Eat half out.** With most restaurant meals in the 1,000-calorie range, think about ordering one entree for even/two people (or taking half home).

tivity can lower insulin resistance, blood pressure, cholesterol, and the risk of diabetes."

Why so much metabolic bang for your buck? When people lose weight by diet and exercise, they run a calorie deficit—that is, they burn more calories than they take in.

"That causes fat to leave your fat cells, which makes them shrink," says Klein. "And you remove fat from your muscles and liver, which may also help. If you reduce fat by sucking it out, you change the number, but not the size, of fat cells."

The trick, says Klein, is keeping the weight off. "That's the Achilles' heel for most dieters."

Strategies

If liposuction doesn't lower your risk of disease, what does? Getting off your duff is first on the agenda.

"In our study, overweight men and women who averaged 30 minutes of vigorous exercise six days a week for six months lost eight percent of their visceral fat," says Slentz, describing research he conducted with Duke University's William Kraus and others.

"Vigorous" isn't as intimidating as it sounds. "No one actually ran," says Slentz. "They walked on a treadmill on an incline at a brisk pace or used an elliptical trainer," an exercise machine that's even less stressful than a treadmill.

The intensity was equivalent to jogging, he adds, "but we don't recommend jogging to people who are overweight."

What stunned the researchers wasn't the fat loss in the exercisers, but the fat gain in the sedentary "control" group.[2]

"The controls got much worse than we expected," says Slentz. Visceral fat jumped six percent in the men and 12 percent in the women, and they gained an average of about two pounds.

"People think inactivity is a holding pattern," he notes. "But if you gain two pounds in six months, think what you would look like in 10 years. We haven't figured out how to lose weight and keep it off, but if we can just prevent weight gain, that's half the battle."

Researchers see less of a weight gain looking at all adults, not just the obese, but it's still troubling. "Between the ages of 20 and 40, Americans gain about two pounds a year," says obesity researcher Xavier Pi-Sunyer of Columbia University. "That's 40 pounds over 20 years. It's incredible."

And it's not just a question of going up a dress size, says Slentz. "After six months, we saw an increase in the controls in insulin resistance and an increase in small, dense LDL particles," which are the most likely to clog arteries.

Surprisingly, Slentz didn't have to drag people kicking and screaming to the treadmill. "It's extremely easy to recruit overweight people for these studies," he says. "They desperately want to exercise, but they know they need help to get started."

Once they begin, most people keep with it because they feel and look better. "Even if people don't lose much weight, they like being trimmer and less flabby," says Slentz.

His participants might have lost more weight if they had also cut calories. Alice Ryan and co-workers at the University of Maryland School of Medicine put 37 overweight or obese women on a lower-calorie diet for six months.[3] The women also walked at moderate intensity on a treadmill for 45 minutes three times a week.

"This wasn't a crash diet," says Ryan. "They lost 10 percent of their body weight in six months—about half a pound to a pound a week—so it was certainly achievable." Along with the weight, the women walked off 17 percent of their visceral fat.

What's more, says Ryan, "their levels of pro-inflammatory proteins fell. That may explain why their insulin resistance dropped."

What You Eat

Clearly, how much you eat makes a difference to your fat cells. Could *what* you eat also matter? It's too early to say, but a few researchers have come up with intriguing results.

"Our study showed very significant weight loss over three months without restricting calories, just by changing people to a very-low-fat diet," says Scott Weigle of the University of Washington School of Medicine in Seattle.

"That's nothing new," he explains. "We know from studies on the Pritikin and Ornish diets that very-low-fat diets lead to weight loss."

What's new is the diet's impact on leptin.[4] "Leptin levels dropped, as expected with weight loss," says Weigle. "But the participants didn't complain of being hungry, so we infer that the brain's sensitivity to leptin increased."

What's more, his subjects showed no rise in ghrelin, a hormone released by the stomach that spurs hunger. "A rise in ghrelin occurs with weight loss if you achieve it by any other diet," says Weigle.

If his study is confirmed by others, it may mean that a very-low-fat diet somehow skirts the usual pitfalls—like a drop in leptin and a rise in ghrelin—that make it so hard for people to keep weight off.

Whether people can stick to a very-low-fat diet is another question. "To successfully implement it takes nothing short of remaking your life," says Weigle.

The Bottom Line

Though scientists know more than ever about fat, they have yet to find the magic bullet to keep us happily slender and shaped like movie stars, not fruit.

In fact, some researchers are even more convinced that, for some people, severe obesity is hard-wired.

"People who have a gastric bypass markedly reduce their intake to 700 calories a day," explains Rockefeller University's Jeffrey Friedman. "I'd be a rail if I ate only that much. These people lose weight but they're still obese because their metabolism slows so much."

It's fine to encourage people to lose weight, he adds. But we have to be much less judgmental about the fact that many people fail over the long term.

"The public needs to recognize that there is a real biological difficulty in maintaining substantial weight loss," says Friedman.

Fortunately, most people don't have to lose as much weight as someone who is severely obese. And when it comes to health, you don't need to lose every excess pound.

"Even a ten-pound weight loss can have important health benefits," says Friedman. "And that's achievable for most people."

The other take-home message: it's far better to not gain weight in the first place. "That's the real public health issue," says Columbia University's Xavier Pi-Sunyer. "Given our toxic food environment, we need to teach people to be restrained eaters."

And we need to change an environment where calorie-dense food is thrust under our noses 24/7. "Like any epidemic, we need to change the environment," says diabetes researcher Eric Ravussin of the Pennington Biomedical Research Center in Baton Rouge, Louisiana.

"If you have malaria, you drain the swamp. If you have death on the roads, you impose seatbelts. Maybe we need to tax junk foods to get people to subsidize healthy foods."

[1]*New Eng. J. Med. 350: 2549, 2004.*
[2]*Arch. Intern. Med. 164: 31, 2004.*
[3]*Diabetes Care 27:1699, 2004.*
[4]*J. Clin. Endocrinol. Metab. 88: 1577, 2003.*

UNIT 5
Health Claims

Unit Selections

Key Points to Consider

• How can consumers protect themselves from misinformation in the nutrition field?

• What is your opinion of assessing your own risk for degenerative disease and self- prescribing supplements?

• What should the role of the FDA be in monitoring and regulating use of supplements, herbs and functional foods?

DUSHKIN ONLINE **Links: www.dushkin.com/online/**
These sites are annotated in the World Wide Web pages.

Federal Trade Commission (FTC): Diet, Health & Fitness
http://www.ftc.gov/bcp/menu-health.htm

Food and Drug Administration (FDA)
http://www.fda.gov/default.htm

National Council Against Health Fraud (NCAHF)
http://www.ncahf.org

QuackWatch
http://www.quackwatch.com

Americans spend approximately $25 billion on alternative treatments. According to an American Dietetic Association (ADA) Survey, ninety percent of consumers polled get their nutrition information from television, magazines, and newspapers.

It is very discouraging that Americans are so confused and overwhelmed about the controversies surrounding food and health that they have stopped paying attention to the contradictory claims reported by news media. The media frequently misinterpret results, simplify them, and take them out of context. Additionally the media is too eager to publish sensational information and not solid science. A new source of information is the Internet, which allows distribution and promotion of just about anything. About 29 percent of Americans turn to the Internet for information. We need to be vigilant as to the type of information we get from different websites.

Functional foods are foods that may provide a health benefit beyond basic nutrition and are becoming one of the fastest growing segments of the food industry—especially among affluent baby boomers. The U.S. government has no regulatory category of functional foods. Despite their popularity, their efficacy and safety is questionable because they lack scientific evidence. So, we are far from declaring them "magic bullets" to improve health and prevent disease. The consumer should be advised to eat a variety of foods as part of an overall healthful diet. Moderate wine intake has been touted to be protective against heart disease and for having beneficial effects on the lungs and the nervous system. Caution needs to be exercised in balancing its health benefits versus the adverse effects as wine consumption has increased the last decade.

Herbal supplements have become very popular in the U.S. but what the consumer does not know is that manufacturers have problems with quality control. Activity of the herbal product components depends on many factors and what the label describes is not usually what is in the bottle. Safety of herbal supplements and their interactions with other herbs and medications are generally unknown. It is unsettling to discover the adverse health problems through cases of people who died due to interactions. The herb Ephedra has been touted as a diet pill. Yet Ephedra has taken lives due to the irresponsibility of product manufacturers whose primary goal is financial gain. Their audacity is illustrated in their suit against the federal government to keep their "poison" pills on the market.

Finally, to vitamin advocates who have thoroughly researched the literature and are guided by The Journal of Medical Association's statement that "all adults should take one multivitamin daily," vitamins help you optimize your health by customizing your vitamin supplement plan. But, keep in mind that there is no regulation for supplements by the government. The consumer cannot trust what the label claims including that the supplement does not contain contaminants. Laboratory tests reveal that labels often overstate the amount of the active ingredient in a pill.

Q & A on Functional Foods

Q. What are "functional foods"?

"Functional foods" is simply a convenient way to describe foods or their components which may provide a health benefit beyond basic nutrition. In other words, functional foods do more than meet your minimum daily requirements of nutrients—they also can play a role in reducing risk of disease and promoting good health. While all foods are functional in that they provide nutrients, "functional foods" tend to be those with health-promoting ingredients or natural components that have been found to have potential benefit in the body. They can include whole foods as well as fortified, enriched or enhanced foods and dietary supplements that have a beneficial effect on health.

The concept of functional foods is not entirely new, although it has evolved considerably over the years. In the early 1900s, food manufacturers in the United States began adding iodine to salt in an effort to prevent goiter, representing one of the first attempts at creating a functional component through fortification. Today, researchers have identified hundreds of compounds with functional qualities, and they continue to make new discoveries surrounding the complex benefits of phytochemicals in foods.

Q. How does a food become "functional"?

Since many of these foods are just natural, whole foods with new information about their potential health qualities, they do not become "functional" except for the way we perceive them. On the other hand, functional foods can result from agricultural breeding or added nutrients/ingredients.

Many—if not most—fruits, vegetables, grains, fish, and dairy and meat products contain several natural components that deliver benefits beyond basic nutrition, such as lycopene in tomatoes, omega-3 fatty acids in salmon or saponins in soy. Even tea and chocolate have been noted in some studies as possessing functional attributes.

Agricultural scientists are able to boost the nutritional content of certain crops through the same breeding techniques that are used to bring out other beneficial traits in plants and animals—everything from beta-carotene-rich rice to vitamin-enhanced broccoli and soybeans, just to name a couple of examples. And research is under way to improve the nutritional quality of dozens of other crops.

Below is a sampling of a few functional foods, their components and their potential benefits for human health.

Functional Component	Source	Potential Health Benefit
Lutein	Green vegetables	Contributes to maintenance of healthy vision
Insoluble fiber	Wheat bran	May reduce risk of breast and/or colon cancer
Lactobacillus	Yogurt, other dairy	May improve gastrointestinal health
Soy protein	Soy-based foods	May reduce risk of cardiovascular disease
Omega-3 fatty acids	Salmon, tuna, fish/marine oils	May reduce risk of cardiovascular disease and improve mental, visual functions
Xylitol	Nutritional bars, beverages	Improves oral health; Does not promote tooth decay

Other foods may be specially formulated with nutrients or other ingredients. This is true of products such as orange juice fortified with calcium, cereals with added vitamins or minerals, or flour with added folic acid. In fact, more and more foods are being fortified with nutrients and other physiologically active components (such as plant stanols and sterols) as researchers uncover more evidence about their role in health and even disease risk reduction.

Q. What are some of the health benefits associated with functional foods?

The scientific community has only just begun to understand the complex interactions between nutritional components and the human body. However, there is already a large body of scientific evidence showing that eating foods with functional benefits on a regular basis as part of a varied diet can help reduce the risk of, or manage a number of health concerns, including cancer, heart and cardiovascular disease, gastrointestinal health, menopausal symptoms, osteoporosis and eye health, to name a few.

Q. How can I get more functional foods in my diet?

The most effective way to reap the health benefits from foods is to eat a balanced and varied diet, including fruits and vegetables as well as foods with added beneficial components. Watch labels and read articles for information about foods and health. Before you decide to make any major dietary changes, however, take the time to evaluate your personal health, or speak to your health care provider on ways to help reduce your risk of certain diseases. It is also important to remember that there is no single "magic bullet" food that can cure or prevent most health concerns, even when eaten in abundance. The best advice is to choose foods wisely from each level of the food guide pyramid in order to incorporate many potentially beneficial components into the diet.

Q. Where can I learn about scientific research related to the functional benefits of foods?

There are several universities and research institutions conducting scientific studies on various food components. You can find out more about current research by visiting the home page of the Functional Foods for Health program administered by the University of Illinois at Urbana-Champaign and Chicago. Information on functional foods research is also available from the U.S. Department of Agriculture's Agricultural Research Service, the Institute of Food Technologists, the American Dietetic Association, and the food science programs at Rutgers University and the University of California, Davis.

Q. Are functional foods regulated by the federal government?

Yes. "Functional foods" has no official meaning and do not constitute a distinctly separate category of foods. Most often they are simply natural whole foods we have been eating for thousands of years. Therefore, the Food and Drug Administration (FDA) regulates them in the same way they regulate all foods—safety of ingredients must be assured in advance, and all claims must be substantiated, truthful, and non-misleading.

A significant amount of credible scientific data is needed to confirm any "health claims"—messages pertaining to a relationship between dietary components and a disease or health condition, for example soy protein and heart disease. Foods also can bear another type of claim to convey their potential benefits, and those are called "structure/function claims." These statements describe or imply a relationship between the product itself, or its components, and normal bodily functions (for example, "may help support digestion"). All such claims must be adequately substantiated.

A 1994 law stipulates that dietary supplements-for example an herb, vitamin, mineral or other substance added to one's total diet—shall continue to be treated as foods for regulatory purposes, but with just a few differences in approach. Regardless of any differences in approach, like all other foods, supplements are regulated by FDA to assure safety and accuracy of label claims.

There has been some criticism of certain foods containing herbal ingredients—whether or not such ingredients are allowed in food and whether their label claims are substantiated. The FDA is looking into these allegations. While herb-containing foods may be considered "functional", it is important to keep in mind that they represent only a small number of the broad spectrum of foods that are thought of as "functional foods".

Consumers need to remember that functional foods represent an important breakthrough in understanding the connection between diet, health, and even disease risk reduction. With regard to all claims pertaining to diseases and health conditions, consumers may be reassured to know that they must be pre-approved by FDA and substantiated by a large body of credible scientific evidence. And, although structure/function claims do not require FDA pre-approval, they too must be adequately substantiated by the producers of the food.

Q. What health claims have been approved so far by FDA?

Since 1993, FDA has approved 14 health claims, eight of which are related to the functional benefits of food:

- Potassium and reduced risk of high blood pressure and stroke
- Plant sterol and plant stanol esters and coronary heart disease
- Soy protein and coronary heart disease
- Calcium and reduced risk of osteoporosis
- Fiber-containing grain products, fruits and vegetables and cancer

- Fruits, vegetables and grain products that contain fiber, particularly soluble fiber, and risk of coronary heart disease
- Fruits and vegetables and cancer
- Folate and neural tube birth defects
- Dietary soluble fiber, such as that found in whole oats and psyllium seed husk, and coronary heart disease
- Dietary sugar alcohol and dental caries (cavaties)

The remaining three are based on diets low in "negative" nutrients in food, such as sodium:

- Dietary fat and cancer
- Dietary saturated fat and cholesterol and risk of coronary heart disease
- Sodium and high blood pressure

Q. What is the relationship between biotechnology and functional foods?

While many of the nutritional compounds in functional foods are either naturally present or added during processing, some may be the result of agricultural breeding techniques, including conventional crossbreeding and biotechnology.

Crossbreeding a plant for a specific genetic trait, such as higher vitamin A content, can take as long as a decade or more. Modern biotechnology, however, makes it possible to select a specific genetic trait from any plant and move it into the genetic code of another plant in a much shorter time span, and with more precision than crossbreeding allows.

Researchers are working with farmers around the world to develop dozens of functional foods through the use of this promising technology.

From *International Food Information Council Foundation*, November 2002. © 2002 by International Food Information Council Foundation.

HERBAL LOTTERY

What's on a dietary supplement's label may not be what's in the bottle

JANET RALOFF

Echinacea is a commercial success. The dietary supplement—made from the flowers, stems, and leaves of the purple coneflower—has become a popular and lucrative over-the-counter cold remedy. It's also one of the few nutraceuticals—natural products with medicinal reputations—that have substantial scientific evidence to support its purported functions: Various studies suggest that echinacea supplements can boost immunity or shorten the duration of colds.

Several years ago, however, Christine M. Gilroy of the University of Colorado Health Sciences Center in Denver was unsure whether to trust data from those experiments because few reports included biochemical proof of which species of purple coneflower had been used. That's important, she notes, because three species—*Echinacea pallida, Echinacea purpurea*, and *Echinacea angustifolia*—turn up in supplements "and only the first two have data indicating they might make colds better."

Not Twins—*Echinacea pallida* and *Echinacea purpurea* look different, but manufacturers sometimes swap one for the other in dietary supplements—even though the plants contain different chemicals and may perform differently.

Curious about *E. pallida's* reputed power against colds, Gilroy designed a study and then ordered dried samples from three suppliers. She sent some of each delivery out for analysis of chemicals that were known to distinguish the species and that might even have therapeutic activity.

The data that came back put her study on hold. They showed no batch containing pure *E. pallida*. The one from a bulk wholesaler that supplies herbal-products companies contained almost no *Echinacea* from any species, and what little there was consisted solely of *E. purpurea*. The other batches, acquired directly from coneflower growers, did contain *E. pallida*—but also contaminating plants, including *E. angustifolia*.

Gilroy then turned to 59 commercial echinacea products from local stores. Her team's analyses, reported in the March 24 *Archives of Internal Medicine*, show that none offered con-

sumers what had been promised by its label. Six contained no evidence of any echinacea, and 28 failed to contain the specific species that was listed on the box. Some offered echinacea in quantities exceeding or, more often, falling below the quantity on the label, sometimes substantially.

These findings call into question the conclusions of the many earlier studies of echinacea's purported cure for the common cold, says Gilroy. At the least, they suggest that health effects seen with one sample of supplement might not hold for others.

This is just the latest in a string of studies revealing variability in the ingredients of dietary supplements on the market today. Uniform products require consistent ingredients and processes throughout every stage of manufacturing. The troubling findings suggest that many herbal-product makers aren't maintaining adequate quality control.

Several weeks ago, the Food and Drug Administration proposed rules designed to stem quality-control problems in dietary supplements, including nutraceuticals. The agency would mandate so-called good manufacturing practices, or GMPs, in the industry. Under GMPs like those now governing pharmaceuticals, all manufacturers of dietary supplements would have to chemically validate their ingredients and keep stringent records. These would include temperature readings from each batch as it's made and notes about any breakdowns of factory equipment.

However, representatives of the nutraceutical industry say they plan to call for amendments to the proposed FDA rules. They're currently analyzing the hundreds of pages of details before requesting changes. Moreover, any set of standard practices may be severely challenged by the complex makeup of herbal products, several scientists told *Science News*.

"For the most part, with [herbal] supplements, we still don't know what all the active ingredients are," so nobody knows the ideal formulation of most supplements, observes Bill J. Gurley of the University of Arkansas for Medical Sciences in Little Rock.

Says David J. Newman of the National Cancer Institute in Frederick, Md., "The bottom line remains *caveat emptor*," or let the buyer beware.

Beyond Echinacea

There's evidence for poor quality control in the making of many dietary supplements, says Chien M. Wai of the University of Idaho in Moscow. His work focuses on those made from leaves of the maidenhair tree (*Ginkgo biloba L.*). Ginkgo supplements fight memory loss and reinvigorate blood flow in the brain, according to users of the herb.

Scientists have identified five purported active ingredients in ginkgo. In most cases, Wai finds, a product's label describes only how much bulk ginkgo tissue a tablet, powder, or tincture contains without quantifying the active agents. Concentrations of those agents can vary widely in plant tissue.

In 2001, Wai's group reported data showing that, for instance, supposedly equally potent ginkgo supplements could contain anywhere from 0 to almost 4 milligrams of active compounds. Brands varied in which active chemicals dominated them, and some brands exhibited large batch-to-batch variation.

His subsequent studies, Wai says, indicate "the situation is not getting better."

Consumers can't use his team's reports to avoid supplements with weak or erratic ingredients because the researchers haven't published any brand names. Companies challenge any implied criticism of their products, Wai explains, and "we can't afford the time to fight lawsuits."

Gurley has named brands in his published analyses of supplements containing the weight-loss stimulant ephedra and indeed "stirred up a hornet's nest," he notes. It started 3 years ago, when his team first surveyed 20 over-the-counter ephedra products. As Gilroy found with echinacea, the ingredients often didn't match label claims.

Tissues from the *Ephedra sinica* plant, like ginkgo, contain at least five purported active ingredients, which are in the chemical family named alkaloids. Each alkaloid has a different effectiveness as a stimulant, and its concentration varies among individual plants. Most supplements that are labeled with ingredient information claim only to have some specified quantity of mixed ephedra alkaloids—information too general to offer much gauge of potency, says Gurley.

Although one brand that his team tested contained none of the five stimulant alkaloids, most had several, but the amounts varied among brands. When the researchers tested several batches of a brand, some differed in concentration by up to tenfold. Only 13 of the 20 products listed a total quantity of alkaloids on the label; others just listed quantities of the raw source plant. In many cases, Gurley says, those values bore no relation to what was present. His group published its findings in 2000. Since then, the researchers' tests of 130 additional ephedra products found far fewer discrepancies between labels and contents, "although they do still occur," says Gurley.

His team has lately turned to St. John's wort (*Hypericum perforatum*), a possible antidepressant. The researchers are finding a wide range of concentrations of St. John's wort's purported active ingredient, which is called hyperforin. Batch-to-batch hyperforin differences in one supplement brand varied 15-fold.

Gurley acknowledges that some herbal-supplement companies reliably produce what their labels promise. The trick is identifying them, Gurley says, a task beyond the capability of most consumers.

Many Explanations

Quality-control problems in herbal supplements often start with the hundreds of chemicals that plants contain. The type and quantity of these compounds vary in response to the environment in which a plant grew: its soil type and nutrition, water availability, excessive heat or cold, exposure to toxic minerals, degree of shading, and any hybridization.

One team is studying horticulturally triggered variations in several citrus compounds that are regarded as potential nutraceuticals because they've inhibited cancers in laboratory animals. Data collected by Bhimanagouda S. Patil and his colleagues at Texas A&M University in Weslaco show that concentrations of one such chemical—limonin glycoside—peaks midway through the crop's harvest season. So, when it comes to this agent, Patil says, "you must eat two grapefruit in May to get what one picked around Christmas will give you."

He's also been quantifying lycopene, a potential anticancer carotenoid that turns plants red. When his group planted Florida-derived rootstock of Star Ruby grapefruit in Texas, the fruit produced some 50 percent more of this carotenoid than it had in Florida.

Researchers at the University of Newcastle in Ourimbah, Australia, are studying effects of manufacturing techniques on nutraceutical quality. For instance, Douglas L. Stuart and Ron B.H. Wills report that high temperatures reduce concentrations of one of the potential therapeutic agents derived from *E. purpurea*. The scientists report in the March 15 *Journal of Agricultural and Food Chemistry* that drying the plant at 40°C results in one-third more cichoric acid than drying it at 70°C does.

Moreover, Wai's team has shown that whether oil, alcohol, or water is used can effect which chemicals are extracted from a plant. These products can have different potencies.

Even if purported active ingredients make it into a supplement, poor manufacturing techniques can yield tablets that don't effectively release those chemicals, notes Larry L. Augsburger of the University of Maryland in Baltimore.

Working with a synthetic version of melatonin, a hormone that promotes sleep, seems to fight jet lag (*SN: 5/13/95, p. 300*), and maybe even battles cancer (*SN: 10/17/98, p. 252*: http://www.sciencenews.org/sn_arc98/10_17_98/19981017fob.asp), his team showed that tablets don't always release their contents in a timely fashion. Although industry standards for the breakdown of conventional drugs is generally 30 minutes or less, his test-tube studies showed that some commercial melatonin supplements didn't disintegrate or release their contents for periods of 4 hours to more than 20 hours, by which time an ingested tablet may well have been excreted.

Help on the Way?

In the early 1990s, nutraceutical manufacturers feared that FDA would challenge their label claims. Then, the 1994 Dietary Supplement Health and Education Act was passed, permitting the sale of nutraceuticals and other supplements that are nontoxic and make no curative claims.

Immediately following the act's passage, sales of herbal supplements skyrocketed, with many companies regularly reporting up to 11 percent annual growth. But by 2000, U.S. sales started flagging, observes Clare M. Hasler of the University of Illinois at Urbana-Champaign. Reports were emerging of health risks associated with some products, such as ephedra; uncertain efficacy of others; and quality-control problems in the industry.

Because that last item appears to be the easiest for manufacturers to fix, some nutraceutical makers have been voluntarily adopting GMPs of their own design, says Nancy Childs of St. Joseph's University in Philadelphia. These companies tend to be the large prescription-drug manufacturers that have entered the nutraceuticals market in the past half-decade, she adds.

Most nutraceutical makers are far smaller than those companies, notes Kim Smith, an attorney with the National Nutritional Food Association (NNFA) of Newport Beach, Calif. Since 1999, her trade group—which represents many nutraceutical makers with 20 to 500 employees—has provided guidance for developing voluntary GMPs. NNFA also officially supports FDA's March 28 proposal for mandatory GMPs. "It will go a long way toward improving credibility in the industry," Smith says.

However, she adds, small firms could have a hard time paying for stringent FDA-required monitoring and record keeping. The agency estimates that first-year costs for small firms will run about $100,000, with annual costs of $60,000 or so thereafter. In fact, Smith says, her group suspects FDA is substantially underestimating those costs.

Success in complying with mandatory GMPs, Hasler suspects, "is going to sort out the [nutraceutical industry's] major players from the fly-by-night companies and probably put some small players out of business." She adds, " I'm not sure that's a bad thing."

Allen Montgomery, executive director of the American Nutraceuticals Association in Birmingham, Ala., which represents pharmacists and other health professionals, agrees. He says, "I don't know of any other billion-dollar industry that makes ingested products for which [mandatory] GMPs are not in place."

Within the nutraceutical industry generally, Gurley charges, "there are so many bad actors right now, that it's giving the whole industry a bad name."

Fortunately, Montgomery notes, several independent groups—such as the U.S. Pharmacopoeia (USP) of Rockville, Md.—have already begun validating voluntary GMPs for several products. USP is the official standards-setting body for all U.S. medicines and dietary supplements.

Companies that want to carry the USP logo must submit products for a series of stringent tests of such features as a product's purity, potency, and consistency. Also, USP inspectors visit factories to confirm that GMPs are in place, notes Sherrie L. Borden, the organization's spokesperson. "Then we do postmarket surveillance [of a supplement] once a product is on the shelf. It's very rigorous," she notes, "because this mark carries a lot of credibility."

All this sounds comforting, Gurley says, except that pharmaceutical-grade uniformity in herbal products may be amazingly difficult to achieve, and FDA's new rules don't address the complexity of a plant's make-up. Synthetic drugs and vitamins tend to have only one or two well-characterized active ingredients, he explains, while herbal supplements "are a veritable pharmacological Pandora's box."

Indeed, the 48 nutraceuticals that USP recently vetted—all produced under the Nature Made or Kirkland Signature labels—contain only vitamins, minerals, or fish oil—not complex herbal products.

Since plant tissue may contain hundreds of compounds with perhaps dozens of active ingredients, Gurley asks, who knows which of these should be standardized in each product? This "truly daunting" problem would challenge the best pharmaceutical manufacturer, he says, let alone a 30-employee herbal-products company.

Wai and Newman say that they'd like to see the herbal-supplements market develop into a natural-products offshoot of the over-the-counter drug industry. They argue that the best route for making safe and effective nutraceuticals would be to identify each plant's active agents, isolate them for testing in the same kind of trials that conventional pharmaceuticals go through, and then package the proven chemicals in carefully measured doses.

An advantage to this approach for manufacturers, Newman argues, is that unlike an herb, the recipe for a cocktail of natural chemicals is patentable. Thus, it might be market forces after all that bring consistency to the nutraceutical marketplace.

The Latest Scoop on Soy

Twenty-eight percent of Americans consume soyfoods or soy beverages once a week or more, according to the United Soybean Board's 2003–04 annual study, "Consumer Attitudes about Nutrition." According to the survey, soymilk, tofu, and soy veggie burgers are the top soy products regularly consumed (see table).

The USB study found that significantly more consumers are aware of soymilk, soy ice cream or cheese, miso, and tempeh compared to 2002. In addition to becoming more aware of soy products, consumers are also learning more about soy's health benefits. The study found that 74% of U.S. consumers perceive soy as healthy. Heart health is the main benefit that consumers associate with soy. Other areas of awareness include menopause relief, obesity prevention/ weight loss, cancer prevention, and protein source.

As awareness grows and as research accumulates, so do the soy ingredients that companies offer. Ingredients such as soy protein isolates, soy protein concentrates, soy isoflavones, soy flour, and soy nuggets have evolved through the years to become more functional for manufacturers' needs. Solubility and flavor of soy ingredients are two areas that have vastly improved.

Here's a brief update on some of the latest soy news related to health and ingredient offerings.

The Healthy Side of Soy

Soy is most commonly known for its cardiovascular benefits, particularly soy protein. This is evident in the Food and Drug Administration's approved soy protein health claim linking it to a reduced risk for heart disease. The health claim is based on clinical trials showing that consumption of soy protein can lower total and low-density-lipoprotein (LDL) cholesterol levels.

> Soy is most commonly known for its cardiovascular benefits [but] bone health, prostate cancer, and menopause are three main areas where consumers may soon be learning more about soy's benefits.

Additional research and clinical trials are pointing to other potential health benefits of soy protein and soy isoflavones. Bone health, prostate cancer, and menopause are three main areas where consumers may soon be learning more about soy's benefits.

Bone Health

"In my view, there is probably the most support for the skeletal benefits of soy protein and isoflavones," said Mark Messina, Adjunct Associate Professor at California's Loma Linda University and co-owner of Nutrition Matters Inc. "When soy protein is substituted for milk protein, several studies have found that urinary calcium excretion is decreased. The metabolism of the sulfur amino acids in protein leads to the production of acid, which requires buffering. The skeletal system is the largest source of buffering agent in the body. In response to acid, the bones are broken down, which leads to an increase in urinary calcium. Since soy protein contains lower amounts of sulfur amino acids than milk protein, it causes less calcium excretion."

In addition to soy protein, isoflavones may have possible skeletal benefits. Messina discussed two studies that have drawn attention to this. "A recent one-year trial found that genistein, the main isoflavone in soybeans, was even more effective than conventional hormone replacement therapy (HRT) at reducing bone loss at the hip in postmenopausal women and was only slightly less effective than HRT at the spine," he said. "Another recently presented two-year trial found that isoflavone-rich soymilk reduced bone loss at the hip and spine in comparison to soymilk low in isoflavones."

He added that long-term studies are currently underway to firmly conclude that isoflavones have the same effect as HRT in reducing fracture risk. "Nevertheless, because soy protein is high quality, the current data justify recommending that isoflavone-rich soyfoods be part of an overall bone-healthy diet. When using soy in place of dairy products, calcium-fortified soy products should be used."

Breast and Prostate Cancer

"There is a large body of literature on the cancer prevention actions of a diet that includes soy. These data support a beneficial effect especially on breast cancer and prostate cancer risk," stated Debra Miller, Director, Nutrition Science Communications, The Solae Co., St. Louis, Mo.

For example, a recent Japanese study suggested that eating foods rich in isoflavones reduced the risk of breast cancer, especially in postmenopausal women. Frequent consumption of soy-rich miso soup was found to be particularly effective (Yamamoto et al., 2003).

Researchers from the National Cancer Center Research Institute in Japan evaluated the relationship between isoflavone consumption and breast cancer risk among women as part of the Ja-

What consumers say about soy foods, according to the United Soybean Board's 2003–04 annual study	
Soy products used regularly	**Soy products tried at least once during the year**
1. Soymilk (17%)	1. Tofu (48%)
2. Tofu (12%)	2. Soy veggie burgers (44%)
3. Soy veggie burgers (12%)	3. Soymilk (39%)
4. Soy protein bars (5%)	4. Soy nuts (26%)
5. Soy nuts (4%)	5. Soy protein bars (22%)

pan Public Health Center-based prospective study on cancer and cardiovascular diseases.

The JPHC study began in 1990, when nearly 22,000 Japanese female residents age 40–59 years from four public health center areas completed a questionnaire which included items about the frequency of soy consumption. Ten years later, 179 of these women had been diagnosed with breast cancer.

Researchers found that while soyfoods alone did not have a significant effect, both consumption of miso soup and overall isoflavone intake reduced the risk of breast cancer. In addition, the researchers reported that the association was found to be stronger in postmenopausal women.

Because of increasing evidence of the benefits of isoflavones, a European Union-funded project, called the Isoheart project, has recently been established to explore the physiological effects from eating foods with added soy-derived isoflavones. One of the project's aims is to establish the presumed health benefits of phytoestrogens in reducing the risk of heart disease in postmenopausal women, as well as to study the consumer acceptability of foods enriched with isoflavones.

In men, soy isoflavones are believed to help in preventing prostate cancer. "Personally, I am most excited about the role that soy may have in preventing and even treating prostate cancer," said Messina. "One key to preventing prostate cancer mortality is preventing the latent (small, clinically irrelevant) tumors from progressing to the larger tumors that can metastasize and which are life threatening," he said. "The International Prostate Health Council concluded that isoflavones stop this progression. Animal

studies are very supportive of this hypothesis, and a recent pilot study found that isoflavones were of benefit to prostate cancer patients resistant to conventional medical treatment. Still, all this remains speculative, although I strongly recommend that men consume soy."

Research presented at a recent American Urological Association meeting in Chicago showed that genistein reduced prostate-specific antigen (PSA) levels in men with untreated cancer, in some cases by almost two thirds.

PSA is a protein produced by the cells of the prostate gland. PSA levels tend to rise if the prostate gland is enlarged due to cancer. The researchers from the University of California Davis Cancer Center said their study suggested that genistein could help men at risk of developing prostate cancer.

The researchers studied 62 men known to have prostate cancer and elevated PSA levels. The men were given 5 g of a dietary supplement containing genistein every day for six months. Sixteen of the men had untreated prostate cancer—they were in the "watchful waiting" group, where the cancer is slow-growing and causing no symptoms. In this group, three had to stop the therapy because they suffered from diarrhea, but eight saw their PSA level fall between 3 and 61%. The remaining five (38%) saw their PSA levels rise, but the researchers say this is a far smaller proportion than in the remaining 46 men who had been treated for prostate cancer, 98% of whom saw a rise.

Ralph de Vere White, Director of the UC-Davis Cancer Center, said, "It must be interpreted cautiously because the numbers of men enrolled are small. He added, however, that "patients on watchful waiting may do better due to grade of

disease or distribution and concentration of genistein within the prostate."

Menopausal Symptoms

A number of studies have shown that consuming both soy protein and soy isoflavone extracts can help reduce the severity and frequency of hot flashes, said Miller. "It should be noted, however, that consuming soyfoods or supplements will not result in the powerful and quick results that HRT provides. However HRT has recently been associated with a number of long-term health risks such as heart attack, stroke, breast cancer, and Alzheimer's disease. In light of these risks, many women find consuming soyfoods a healthy option."

In an article in the *Journal of Medicinal Food*, Messina and Hughes (2003) reviewed the evidence to date on the impact of soyfoods and soy isoflavones on hot flush symptoms in women. They found a statistically significant relationship between initial hot flush frequency and treatment efficacy.

"Initial hot flush frequency explained about 46 percent of the treatment effects, and hot flush frequency decreased by about 5 percent (above placebo or control effects) for every additional initial hot flush per day in women whose initial hot flush frequency was five or more per day," the authors reported.

Soy has received attention as an alternative to HRT largely because it is a unique dietary source of isoflavones. However, there have been conflicting results from trials measuring the ability of isoflavones to reduce menopausal symptoms. In their review, Messina and Hughes eliminated trials on breast cancer patients. They also eliminated nonblinded trials.

Out of 11 studies on soyfoods, only one found that women showed a significant decrease in hot flush frequency. The researchers noted, however, that "the large placebo effect makes most of these trials underpowered to detect modest effects." In four out of six studies on isoflavone supplements, there was a positive link to reduced menopausal symptoms. But the baseline level of hot flush frequency was higher on average among participants in the supplement trials. This led the authors to the theory that efficacy increased with hot flush frequency, so that those women having around 10 hot flushes each day saw this frequency halved, while those experiencing only seven daily only saw a reduction of around three flushes, after taking isoflavones.

The researchers wrote that although conclusions based on the analysis should be considered tentative, "the available data justify the recommendation that patients with frequent hot flushes consider trying soyfoods or isoflavone supplements for the alleviation of their symptoms."

They added that future trials involving soyfoods and isoflavone supplements are warranted, "but should focus on women who have frequent hot flushes." The correlation between initial hot flush frequency and the extent of reduction of symptoms should also be studied, they said.

Weight Management/Diabetes Control

"Given the enormous problem with obesity and its secondary effects, such as type 2 diabetes in the Western world, many people are looking at alterations in diet. Many have opted for high protein/lower carbohydrate diets and found success with such diets," said Miller. "However, health professionals are concerned with long-term high animal protein consumption. Eating large amounts of meat, cheese, and eggs can cause calcium loss from bones and cause the kidneys to work harder than usual (a big risk factor for those who have type 2 diabetes already). Interestingly, soy protein, as a vegetable protein, does not cause calcium loss and is actually the protein recommended to many patients on dialysis to prevent protein malnutrition because

even patients with impaired renal function can tolerate soy protein."

Soy protein and its constituents have also been linked to enhancements in glucose tolerance and reductions in insulin resistance, added Miller. "This research is encouraging. Certainly adding soy protein to food in place of carbohydrates can help reduce the glycemic index of foods."

Soy proteins and isoflavones are becoming more versatile and functional for various products.

Cognitive Ability

"One of the most exciting areas of research regarding soy foods is the association with better recognition and recall ability in memory testing when people eat a diet high in soy compared to those on a low-soy diet," said Miller. Research is ongoing in this area.

Improvements in Soy Ingredients

"Who thought that soy protein would be used in cold cereal four or five years ago?" said Mian Riaz, Head of the Extrusion Technology Program and Research Scientist at the Food Protein Research and Development Center at Texas A&M University, College Station. "With improved ingredients, we will see more soy-cultured products with improved flavor and taste, real soy cheese and ice cream, which taste just like traditional cheese and ice cream products, soy water, soy tea, and soy candy."

He added that there is a lot of research going on to process a soy meat analog that is very close to real meat. "This meat texture will resemble fresh meat and have the same composition as real meat you buy from the butcher (with 70% moisture content)."

Novel soy products such as these would not have been possible if not for the continuous improvement of soy ingredients. From the following information from three soy suppliers, we can see that the ingredients are becoming more refined and tailored for specific food product applications. Both soy proteins and isofla-

vones are becoming more versatile and functional for various products.

New Soy Ingredient Developments

"What's happened overall with soy ingredients is that companies have figured out how to create better-tasting ingredients for different applications. That now has allowed us to put together food systems with better taste and texture," said Tony DeLio, Vice President, Marketing and External Affairs, Archer Daniels Midland Co., Natural Health and Nutrition Division, Decatur, Ill.

The company offers a range of soy products, from flours, to soy protein concentrates and isolates, to soy isoflavones. "It all depends on what your end product is. Our soy flours enable us to work in bread applications, for example. Utilizing our baking expertise, we can easily get 6.25 g of soy protein into two slices of sandwich bread without compromising texture and flavor," said DeLio.

A new addition to the company's *NutriSoy* line is *Wholebean Soy Powder*, an organic ingredient for soymilk and other dairy-like products. It offers the superior nutrition of whole soybeans—fiber and isoflavones—in a form that can be easily incorporated into virtually any dairy or dairy analog product, he said.

"We can also incorporate soy into chocolate coating systems and have worked with a number of companies to create soy rice crispies for nutrition bars," DeLio added. "On the meat analog side, we tend to use soy concentrates and isolates to get a higher level of protein. We are currently developing technology to simulate whole-muscle meat products. We hope to have this revolutionary new product on the market within the next six months."

Regarding isoflavones, approximately 125 different retail product labels carry the *NovaSoy* brand name. "Isoflavones have gone from being primarily in dietary supplements to functional foods such as beverages and snack bars," he said. "We provide all different concentration levels of isoflavones. We have recently licensed technology that allows the time release of isoflavones. For example, you could have a time-released steady stream of isoflavones in a product."

DeLio concluded that with the innovation in soy ingredients, there is no reason why the food industry can't have a line of branded soy products that cut across all food segments. This would be similar to the line of *Healthy Choice* products that cater to low salt and low fat demand. "The consumer interest is there and the time is right for somebody."

Concept Beverage with Soy Isoflavones.

A ready-to-drink raspberry tea that supports bone health was unveiled by Cargill Health & Food Technologies, Minneapolis, Minn., at the Institute of Food Technologists' Annual Meeting + Food Expo® last month. The prototype beverage, named *Bone Appetit*, contains Cargill's *AdvantaSoy™* Clear isoflavones, *Oliggo-Fiber™* inulin, and calcium. Proprietary processing technology results in beverages that retain their traditional flavor, color, and consistency. "*AdvantaSoy Clear* isoflavones allow us to meet the challenge of creating new functional beverages that promote health and retain the delicious flavor and aroma which made them popular in the first place," said Steve Snyder, Cargill's Director of Sales and Marketing, Nutraceuticals.

"What we try to do is look at the retail market and create a product solution based on consumer input," said Lee Knudson, *Advantasoy* Product Manager. "This will help our customers be more successful in key product launches. The ready-to-drink tea is one example."

The *AdvantaSoy line* is available in three different forms depending on the application, he explained. Produced using proprietary technology and available in isoflavone concentrations of up to 50%, *AdvantaSoy Clear* has improved solubility, a whiter appearance, and reduced undesirable taste and odor, ideal for beverages and more-attractive food product applications. The product is GRAS for beverages, nutrition bars, yogurt, meal replacement, and confections. *AdvantaSoy Complete Isoflavones* are created using a natural, solvent-free processing technique. The ingredient is a combination of soy protein and isoflavones, ideal for breads, cereals, and meal replacements. *AdvantaSoy Compress*, available in isoflavone concentrations of up to 50%, is formulated for dietary supplements.

"Our soy isoflavones are really next-generation ingredients in the sense that we concentrate ours in a proprietary process from the soy germ," said Snyder. "The first generation of isoflavones was concentrated from the soy protein isolate manufacturing process."

In the future, said Snyder, we'll see soy ingredients that are easier to formulate, with better taste attributes. "Ingredients will be tailored to individual food products."

Improved Flavor and Functional Performance

New soy developments center on improving the flavor and functional performance and developing new ingredient forms to allow use in a wider array of food products. "We have also focused on innovations that contribute unique textures in food products," said Jim Holbrook, Vice President, Food Science Research and Development, The Solae Co. For example, the company's *Supro® XT* proteins, based on soy isolate technology, provide flavor and functional improvements in beverages. The *Alpha®* proteins, based on a revolutionary new manufacturing process, provide improved flavor performance in beverages and a range of dairy alternative products.

Other new offerings include extruded soy nuggets, now delivering protein contents up to 80% protein and providing unique texture and crunch in nutritional food bars and other grain-based foods. "For meat alternatives, we have introduced a range of high-moisture extruded ingredients for use in this application, which provide consumers a more meat-like eating experience," Holbrook said. "We have also introduced a number of products that offer enhanced nutritional attributes, such as soy proteins co-processed with other ingredients, such as calcium phosphate, carbohydrates, and fibers to enhance the nutritional value and functional performance of our ingredients in various food products. We also offer products with guaranteed levels of isoflavones, important health-promoting components found in soy."

Applications that will benefit from Solae's innovations include beverages, nutrition bars, and meat alternatives. "We have recently introduced new technology that makes soy protein more functional in acidic beverages, a big growth area for soy protein today," Holbrook said. "We are looking at both powdered isolate and extruded soy nuggets as technologies we can employ to positively affect shelf life in bars. We are also continuing to innovate with new extruded products and forms for meat alternatives. Additionally, we are very excited about our new *Alpha* technology, based on an innovative new process that delivers very bland-flavored soy proteins. We believe this technology has tremendous potential for future development across a spectrum of new applications."

Better Soy Ingredients

So, in the future, we can expect soy ingredients with improved flavor, texture, color, and mouthfeel. "The food industry will be able to find soy ingredients with very specific functionality, like foaming, whipping, emulsification, solubility, and texturization for specific food applications," said Riaz. "Improved soy ingredients will be available for soy beverages without the chalky flavor. There will be improvement in soybean oil for taste, flavor, and overall quality without the hydrogenation. The food industry will also find soy flour with higher protein levels, through breeding and improved processing techniques."

Expect more great things to come from soy!

REFERENCES

1. Messina, M. and Hughes, C. 2003. Efficacy of soyfoods and soybean isoflavone supplements for alleviating menopausal symptoms is positively related to initial hot flush frequency. J. Medicinal Food 6(1): 1–11.
2. Yamamoto, S., Sobue, T., Kobayashi, M., Sasaki, S., and Tsugane, S. 2003. Soy, isoflavones, and breast cancer risk in Japan. J. Natl. Cancer Inst. 95: 906–913.

How Low Can You *Go?*

Cutting Calories to Extend Life

**Some sing the praises of calorie restriction.
Animal research supports the claim.
Does the science hold up in the human equation?**

By Kate Jackson

It may seem paradoxical to those who associate sustenance with abundance, but research has demonstrated that members of a number of species—including mice, worms, dogs, monkeys, and fruit flies—live longer when fed less. For these and other animals, reducing calories by one-third increases the lifespan by as much as 50% while it decreases disease and minimizes the signs of aging.

A number of theories have been proposed to explain this reaction in animals. Digestion of food and metabolism results in the production of free radicals, which are harmful to the genetic material of cells. With less fuel for the metabolic process, fewer free radicals are produced, so less damage is done to the cells. Another possibility is that calorie restriction slows cell division in some tissues, while still another is that it essentially conserves energy.

What Science Says

Scientists at the National Institutes of Health and other research centers are eager to find out if slashing calories will allow humans, like animals, to live significantly longer, but the results of their studies may be some time in coming. "Scientists don't have time to follow their subjects for a life-time," says Katherine Tallmadge, MA, RD, LD, president of Personalized Nutrition, author of *Diet Simple* (LifeLine Press, 2004), and national spokesperson for the American Dietetic Association. "So to shorten the process, they're looking for things like biomarkers, which research has told them are important biological signs that aging may be slowing." It's known, for example, that people who live longer usually have lower sex hormone levels, lower body temperatures, and lower plasma insulin levels, she explains. Still, researchers have not amassed evidence that will tempt great numbers of Americans to eat like monks.

Nevertheless, intrigued by the promise of this research, a calorie restriction movement has arisen, its ranks swelled by those who aren't waiting for the scientific verdict. The Calorie Restriction (CR) Society, in Gardena, Calif. (www.calorierestriction.org), for example, boasts nearly 1,200 members, all of whom believe reducing normal caloric intake by as much as 40% will greatly slow the aging process and lengthen life. "The purpose of the CR Society," says its public relations representative, Warren Taylor, "is to retard aging and disease by advancing the science, instruction, and application of calorie restriction principles. The society,

which grew from an Internet-based Usenet discussion group created by Brian M. Delaney, helps people to live longer, with those extra years in superior health." The calorie restriction diet, says Taylor, "increases average lifespan, maximum lifespan, and total health span." Its members, known as CRONies (Calorie Restriction with Optimal Nutrition), he adds, "eat to live rather than live to eat."

While these believers may sound overzealous, their beliefs stem from a considerable amount of solid scientific evidence that calorie restriction produces these effects in animals. For more than six decades, researchers have extended the lives of laboratory rats and other creatures by reducing their calorie intake. Roy L. Walford, MD, a University of California, Los Angeles School of Medicine professor of pathology, is credited with publicizing the research and promise of the low-calorie path to longevity. His books, including *Maximum Life Span, Beyond the 120 Year Diet,* and *The Anti-Aging Plan*, and his dietary trials in the Biosphere experiment of the 1990s garnered enormous attention and are often credited with catalyzing the calorie restriction movement.

Numerous studies bolster the movement's suppositions. In early 2003, for example, a study by investigators at the National

Institute on Aging (NIA) Intramural Research program found that reducing caloric intake "protects nerve cells from genetically induced damage, delays the onset of Huntington's disease-like symptoms in mice, and prolongs the lives of affected rodents." Studies further have indicated that calorie-restricted diets have retarded age-related disease and changes—including diabetes, certain cancers, kidney disease, and immune system dysfunction—in a variety of animals.

The Human Equation

The question at the core of the controversy surrounding calorie restriction is: Will it work in humans? The CR Society, of course, believes it will—and its members live by that belief. "We place our bets on the laboratory research that shows the robustness and universality of the calorie restriction effect in all animal species. And human lab measurements show the same remarkable physiological benefits as seen in animals," explains Taylor. And many researchers tentatively suggest this belief may not be far off the mark. In a press release announcing the NIA's study of calorie restriction and Huntington's disease-like symptoms in mice, Mark P. Mattson, PhD, chief of the NIA's laboratory of neurosciences, said, "If reducing food intake has the same effects in humans as it does in mice, then it may be theoretically possible to delay the onset of the disease and extend the lives of Huntington's patients by prescribing low-caloric diets or diets with reduced meal frequency."

But even some who devote a considerable amount of their professional undertakings to its study not only discourage individuals from participating in a severely calorie-restricted lifestyle but also doubt the application of animal research to humans. Without question, says Charles V. Mobbs, PhD, associate professor in neurobiology and geriatrics, Mt. Sinai School of Medicine, "calorie restriction is robustly effective across the species under standard laboratory conditions." While this type of dietetic restriction is not necessarily healthy even for animals, he observes, it effectively increases their lifespan in what he describes as the relatively benign conditions under which they live, but he speculates that if you put calorie-restricted animals out in the wild, they probably wouldn't live longer.

Mobbs isn't convinced that the lifestyle can be practiced in a healthy way by humans or, more to the point, that it will extend human life. His reasoning is simple:

"Throughout history, there have been so many kinds of people that have basically functioned under calorie restriction, and yet there's no evidence that anyone ever lived beyond maximum lifespan." One would think, he speculates, that some monks or nuns, for example, who have lived the caloric restriction lifestyle for whatever reason, would have been documented to have lived longer than 120 years, but no such documentation exists. "This is how millions of Buddhist monks lived their lives," he notes, "not to mention peasants throughout history—99% of the human population—who never had more than 1,200 calories a day." Such an ample diet, he says, is an absolutely modern invention, yet those earlier populations never lived beyond 120 years, although many did live to a ripe old age.

If he's so convinced that calorie restriction won't lengthen human life, why is he committed to researching the proposition? Animal research indicates that there's a mechanism for extending lifespan, and in experimental models with mice, calorie restriction appears to trigger that mechanism. Although he doesn't think calorie restriction will work similarly in humans, Mobbs does believe a molecular mechanism to extend life does exist in humans and can likely be activated by some means other than caloric restriction.

How Low Should You Go?

Experts agree that those who are overweight or consume an excess of calories should significantly cut back on calories while maintaining adequate nutrition. "Obviously people would be better off generally if they ate fewer calories," says Mobbs. "If they're overweight, absolutely they should cut back from 2,400 calories a day to 1,800 calories," he suggests, adding, "it's not going to increase their maximum lifespan, and it's not even going to increase their average lifespan by much, but they'll certainly be healthier." In such cases, cutting back by 20% or 10% of calories will reverse obesity or overweightness and decrease the risk of weight-related diseases, but going to extremes of reducing calories by 30% merely puts people at risk. Moreover, he observes, "Most of us don't have the discipline or motivation to do this very difficult thing."

Despite his belief in the potential of research leading to longer-lasting life, Mobbs is opposed to severe caloric restriction in humans not only because there's little evidence that it will extend life but also

because it's tough on the body and a rather unpleasant way to live. "People claim that they get used to it—maybe it's true, I don't know." Beyond the difficulty, among the more serious risks of calorie restriction, he observes, is the likelihood of developing osteoporosis. Additional negative side effects of severe calorie restriction, as described by the CR Society, include hunger, anemia, negative appearance changes, cold sensitivity, physical discomfort due to reduced padding that protects body tissues, depression, reduced energy reserves, loss of libido, menstrual irregularities, infertility, risks in pregnancy, loss of stamina, slower wound healing, and an inability to combat long-term illness.

Mobbs is concerned as well about the potential for developing eating disorders as a result of severe calorie restrictions. "It can be a fine line between calorie restriction and anorexia, and obviously anorexia can kill you." Tallmadge is equally concerned with the potential for the development of eating disorders. "I wouldn't feel comfortable advocating calorie restriction with clients," she explains. "I've seen the negative consequences of rigid dieting: eating disorders and weight fluctuation." Furthermore, she says, "It basically advocates lowering metabolism to create less oxidative stress. But you counter this oxidative stress by eating more fruits and vegetables and foods with antioxidants."

Those who desire longevity beyond current reasonable expectation may be drawn to a calorie restriction lifestyle, despite the lack of evidence of a life-extending effect in humans and despite the risks and challenges. While many experts might suggest that it's too soon to say whether or not there's a truly healthful way to severely curtail calories, they'd advise those who wish to attempt this lifestyle to do so only under the care of a physician and dietitian. "They must be very careful about having an otherwise balanced diet and possibly changing the composition of their diet," says Mobbs, who adds that he's most concerned that those who restrict calories will not get adequate protein.

The question at the core of the controversy surrounding calorie restriction is: Will it work in humans? The CR Society, of course, believes it will.

Older adults are particularly vulnerable to both the lure and potential negative consequences of caloric restriction. "During aging, muscles begin to atrophy," says Mobbs, a condition that he speculates could worsen with inadequate calories. "It's very possible that calorie restriction will worsen many age-related changes—glucocorticoids, for example, become elevated during aging and are also elevated by caloric restriction." Older adults, agrees Tallmadge, have increased nutrient requirements and are at high risk for not getting enough protein. "They're not the population that should be exploring this," she insists. Not only can calorie restriction be more dangerous for older people, Mobbs explains, it's even less likely to extend life in that population. Even if he were inclined to believe it will work in humans, "certainly the older you are when you start caloric restriction, the less effective it would be. So it's very likely that if you start it after midlife, it probably wouldn't do much good."

The Real Message

Like Mobbs, Tallmadge comes down against calorie restriction because the benefits are uncertain and some of the disadvantages are clear. "I'd feel comfortable telling people to avoid severe calorie restriction at this time," she says. Instead, she advises clients to achieve an ideal weight through healthful eating and activity. "It sounds simple, but those are the things that science has proven will improve your quality of life and longevity."

The take-home message of calorie restriction studies, suggests Tallmadge, is not that we have to abnormally restrict calories to 25% or 30% below normal but rather that we should not overeat. "These studies underline the importance of eating the right amount of calories from a high-quality diet full of antioxidants and adding exercise to give you some of the same benefits of calorie restriction." She suggests focusing on the most promising aspects of the research: "There are certain aspects of aging that we can change. Exercising and weight loss bring many of the benefits you would receive by restricting calories. It reduces plasma insulin levels, keeps you from eating too many calories, and you can eat foods high in antioxidants to prevent oxidative damage."

More active people, she adds, expend more calories than those who are inactive, which would be physiologically similar to being on a restricted energy intake diet, and, she's quick to point out, they tend to live longer.

While the benefits of calorie restriction may be demonstrated by science in the future and its promise of longevity may one day be realized, few scientists or healthcare providers will go out on a limb to support it at this time. "There's a danger in jumping on the bandwagon too soon," concludes Tallmadge. "There's just too much that we don't know."

—Kate Jackson is a staff writer for *Today's Dietitian*

MULTIPLE CHOICES

THE RIGHT VITAMINS FOR YOU

Two unabashed vitamin advocates offer tailor-made solutions

By Nancy Bruning and Shari Lieberman, Ph.D.

WE BELIEVE IN SUPPLEMENTS. We've delved into the research, seen the strengths and weaknesses of the studies, understood the depth of the debate. And in the past few years, we've heard the "You can get everything you need from food" refrain start to fade: In 2002 *The Journal of the American Medical Association* published a groundbreaking article that concluded, "All adults [should] take one multivitamin daily."

We couldn't agree more. There's a difference, though, between filling your nutritional holes and optimizing your health, and we're going to show you how you can do better than one size fits all. But first things first.

What do vitamins and minerals do for you? Nearly everything. Without them, you could not lift a baby, kiss a lover, eat a peach, or fight a cold. Vitamins and minerals act as coenzymes, which are at the heart of every bodily and neural function, from breathing to memory. Many nutrients also function as antioxidants, controlling the free-radical activity that wears our bodies down and, eventually, out. And recent studies show that vitamins and minerals help control chronic inflammation, now believed to be at the root of aging, degeneration, and dozens of diseases.

A balanced, healthy diet is the most critical source of all nutrients, but it's not enough. For one thing, we live busy lives, and most of us find it difficult to eat a perfect diet every day, including the recommended 5–9 servings of fruits and vegetables; whole grains and healthy fats; and minimal sugar. Moreover, much of our food has had the life sucked out of it: It is grown in nutritionally depleted soil, shipped long distances, stored a long time, and then, often, heavily processed—and that's before we deplete more nutrients through cutting and cooking. And even as our food becomes less nutritious, the pace and strain of our modern lives further depletes us; stress, pollution, and nutrient-sapping medications all increase our need for vitamins and minerals.

But which ones? And how much of each? It depends on a host of variables, from lifestyle choices (exercise, smoking) to genetics. For optimal health, most people can benefit from taking higher amounts of certain nutrients than are found in a typical multivitamin. What's more, we now know that it's possible to custom design a supplement plan to help ward off many of the diseases of our day.

In this article, we help you cut through supplement-buying guesswork. You'll find out whether our basic optimal-health regimen is right for you, or whether you need a plan that targets cardiovascular disease, cancer, immune problems, osteoporosis, or aging skin. As in our book, *The Real Vitamin & Mineral Book* (Avery, 2003, 3d ed.), the recommendations we make here are based on a multitude of scientific studies and the clinical experience of knowledgeable health practitioners.

True or False. I spent a lot of time in the sun as a child.

Design Your Own Supplement Plan

Since people are individuals, with different health risks and nutritional needs, we've created six customized vitamin regimens: the basic Optimal Health plan, and then five variations designed to slow down skin aging, boost immunity, and help prevent osteoporosis, heart disease, and cancer. To help gauge your risk for each condition, take the following series of quizzes. Answer "True" ("T") or "False" ("F") for each statement, and refer to "6 Customized Plans of Action," below, for your personalized vitamin plan.

When it comes to buying vitamins, we recommend finding a full-spectrum multi-vitamin-and-mineral formula that comes close to the Optimal Health plan. Start with that as a foundation, and buy nutrients you need higher amounts of individually. (For tips on getting the most out of your supplements, see "Absorption Is Everything" on next page.)

Remember that eating well, exercising regularly, minimizing stress, and limiting your exposure to toxins are the bedrock of prevention. Note that our quizzes aren't a substitute for a medical assessment—see your doctor if you're concerned about any of the conditions discussed here.

Feed Your Mind

In the 1950s, progressive physicians began treating schizophrenics with high doses of vitamin B3 (niacin) along with standard treatment; the success rate increased.

This was the first scientific evidence that nutrition was a factor in psychiatric diseases. Today we're using nutritional therapy, primarily the B vitamins, to help prevent and manage a slew of mind-related conditions. Stress, depression, insomnia, anxiety, mental fatigue and burn-out, nervousness, mood swings, and poor memory and cognition–you name it, B vitamins (25–300 mg a day) can help.

As is the case with heart disease, folic acid (a B vitamin) is in the spotlight as a memory and cognitive-function enhancer for the aging brain; this B vitamin may help because of its ability to reduce levels of homocysteine, which is linked to declining brain function. Vitamins C and E have also been linked with a lowered risk and slowed progression of Alzheimer's disease.

OPTIMAL HEALTH

1. Health and longevity run in my family . . . . T | F

2. I eat a diet plentiful in fruits, vegetables, and whole grains and moderate in healthy fats and protein foods. . . . T | F

3. I rarely eat foods containing sugar or foods that have been cooked at high temperatures. . . . . T | F

4. I don't smoke or drink alcohol. T | F

5. I live where there is clean, unpolluted air and water. . . . . T | F

6. I get an hour of moderate, aerobic exercise (such as walking, running, or biking) at least five times a week. T | F

7. I get at least some exercise every day. . . . . T | F

8. I am not on a weight-reducing diet now and have seldom been in the past . . . . T | F

9. I do not take prescription drugs, including birth-control pills, regularly. T | F

10. I am under a minimum amount of emotional stress, and when stress comes along I manage it well. . . . . T | F

If you circled "False" for five or more of these statements, you are at average risk for serious chronic diseases. You're in good company: While a lucky few among us don't need to take anything beyond a multivitamin, even the average "healthy" person has enough nutritional holes and lifestyle stressors to merit some extra protection from chronic illness. Our Optimal Health plan will cover many people's needs for coenzymes, antioxidants, and anti-inflammatory vitamins and minerals.

SKIN-AGING PREVENTION

1. The people in my family generally look young for their age. . . . . T | F

2. I limit my sun exposure and wear sun protection when in the sun. . . . . . T | F

3. I have naturally dark skin with no or few freckles . . . . T | F

4. I spent little time in the sun as a child . . . . T | F

5. I have never smoked cigarettes (or cigars) . . . . T | F

6. I drink at least eight glasses of water, mineral water, or herbal teas a day . . . . T | F

If you circled "False" for five or more statements in the Optimal Health section and for four or more of the above statements, you may be at higher-than-average risk for prematurely aging skin. Since this condition is primarily due to cumulative free-radical damage, the prevention plan contains protective antioxidants. Vitamin A and carotenes, vitamin C, and vitamin E can help protect your skin from damage. In addition to taking supplements, you may want to use skin products rich in antioxidants. It's not just hype; a growing body of studies show that if you apply these nutrients directly to your skin, they penetrate skin layers and help stimulate collagen, slow the progress of wrinkles and fine lines, and reduce discoloration and inflammation.

Absorption is Everything

If you swallowed a nail, you would be ingesting a lot of iron, but how much would your body actually be able to absorb and use? Very little, if any, since the iron in a nail is not in a form your body can use. Fortunately, there are ways to maximize your supplements' effectiveness.

¶ **Take a full-spectrum supplement.** Vitamins and minerals work synergistically in the body, so don't just load up on one or two nutrients.

¶ **Buy natural and mixed.** There's evidence that several nutrients are better absorbed and used in their natural form, particularly vitamin E and beta-carotene. Studies show that synthetic forms of fat-soluble vitamins such as vitamin E and beta-carotene may actually interfere with the absorption of the natural forms. Also, vitamin E supplements should contain a mixture of tocopherols and tocotrienols, not just alphatocopherol, and mixed carotenes are preferable to just beta-carotene.

¶ **Time it right.** Take supplements immediately before or after a balanced meal. Nature intended us to get our nutrients from food, so don't take supplements on an empty stomach, and be sure to include some fat so that fat-soluble vitamins get absorbed.

¶ **Divide your doses.** Your body can absorb only so much at one time. Divide your total daily supplement amount by three, and take this amount with breakfast, lunch, and dinner.

¶ **Exercise.** Studies show that regular exercise—at a minimum, a half hour of moderate aerobic exercise three times a week—helps your body use nutrients more efficiently.

CARDIOVASCULAR-DISEASE PREVENTION

1. Cardiovascular disease does not run in my family . . . . T | F

2. I get an hour of moderate, aerobic exercise (such as walking, running, or biking) at least five times a week. . . . T | F

3. I have low overall cholesterol; favorable ratios and amounts of LDL, HDL, and triglycerides; and low levels of

6 Customized Plans of Action

These dosages have been found to be safe in clinical studies, but keep your physician informed about any supplements you're taking. If you have a medical condition or may be pregnant, consult your doctor *before* taking supplements. Each column represents a daily regimen; if you're at risk for multiple conditions, use the higher dosage—do not add the dosages together.

NUTRIENT	OPTIMAL HEALTH	SKIN *AGING PREVENTION	HEART-DISEASE PREVENTION	IMMUNE-SYSTEM BOOSTING	OSTEOPOROSIS PREVENTION	CANCER PREVENTION
Vitamin A	5,000 IU	10,000–25,000 IU*	5,000–10,000 IU	10,000–25,000 IU*	5,000 IU	10,000–50,000 IU*
Carotenoids	11,000 IU	25,000–100,000 IU	11,000–25,000 IU	25,000–50,000 IU	11,000 IU	25,000–100,000 IU
B complex	25 mg	25 mg	50–100 mg	50 mg	25 mg	50–150 mg
Vitamin C	500 mg	3,000–5,000 mg	500–3,000 mg	1,000–5,000 mg	500 mg	5,000–10,000 mg
Vitamin D	400 IU	400 IU	400 IU	400 IU	400–800 IU	400–800 IU
Vitamin E	400 IU	400 IU	400–800 IU	400 IU	400 IU	400–800 IU
Vitamin K	80 mg	80 mg	80 mg	80 mg	80 mg	80 mg
Boron	3 mg	3 mg	3 mg	3 mg	3–6 mg	3 mg
Calcium	1,000 mg	1,000 mg	1,000 mg	1,000 mg	1,500–2,000 mg	1,000 mg
Chromium	200 mcg	200 mcg	400 mcg	200 mcg	200 mcg	400 mcg
Copper	0.5 mg	0.5 mg	0.5 mg	0.5 mg	0.5 mg	0.5 mg
Iodine	150 mcg	150 mcg	150 mcg	150 mcg	150 mcg	150 mcg
Iron	15 mg	15 mg	15 mg	15 mg	15 mg	15 mg
Magnesium	500 mg	500 mg	500 mg	500 mg	500–1,000 mg	500 mg
Manganese	15 mg	15 mg	15 mg	15 mg	15–50 mg	15–50 mg
Phosphorous	Obtained from food	Obtained from food	Obtained from food	Obtained from food	200–400 mg	Obtained from food
Potassium	Obtained from food	Obtained from food	Obtained from food	Obtained from food	Obtained from food	Obtained from food
Selenium	100 mcg	200–400 mcg	100–400 mcg	100–200 mcg	100 mcg	100–400 mcg
Zinc	22.5 mg	22.5–50 mg	22.5 mg	30–50 mg	22.5 mg	22.5 mg

*NOTE: Vitamin A may be toxic when consumed in very high doses. If you are taking more than 25,000 mg, work with a knowledgeable health-care provider.

homocysteine and C-reactive protein in my blood. . . . . T | F
4. I have low or average blood pressure. T | F
5. I am of a healthy weight. . . . . . T | F
6. I have not had a heart attack, stroke, or other type of heart disease. . . . . . . T | F

If you circled "False" for five or more statements in the Optimal Health section and for four or more of the statements above, you may be at higher-than-average risk for cardiovascular disease. Antioxidant nutrients are at the heart of the Cardiovascular-Disease Prevention plan. Studies show that vitamin C helps prevent hypertension and atherosclerosis, as well as reducing cholesterol and increasing HDL, or "good," cholesterol. Studies on vitamin E are mixed but tantalizing; results from two large stud-

ies suggested an impressive reduction in risk (about 40 percent) of heart disease in both women and men who had high intakes of vitamin E (mostly from supplements). The B vitamins may also lower your risk, especially B6, B12, and folic acid, all of which reduce excess homocysteine in the blood. Calcium, chromium, and selenium may help lower your risk of heart disease, too.

True or False: I have high blood pressure.

IMMUNE-SYSTEM BOOSTING

1. The people in my family are very healthy and rarely get sick. . . . . . . T | F
2. I generally get enough sleep so I wake up refreshed. . . . . T | F

3. I rarely catch colds, the flu, or other infections. . . . . T | F
4. I am rarely around young children. T | F
5. I rarely let myself get run down. . . . . T | F
6. I have not taken antibiotics frequently for infections or acne . . . . T | F

If you circled "False" for five or more statements in the Optimal Health section and for four or more of the statements above, you may be at higher-than-average risk for having a compromised immune system. The Immune-System Boosting plan contains a number of nutrients essential for building a strong immune system. Vitamin A, for instance, strengthens the immune system by enhancing white-blood-cell function and antibody activity. Vitamin C, which stimulates and supports many components of the immune system, may help reduce the duration and intensity of cold symptoms. Studies also support the use of B complex, selenium, and zinc as immune boosters.

<u>True</u> or False. Osteoporosis runs in my family.

OSTEOPOROSIS PREVENTION

1. Osteoporosis does not run in my family .T | F
2. I do weight-bearing exercise or weight training three to five times a week. . . . . T | F
3. I ate plenty of green leafy vegetables and other calcium-rich foods such as milk and dairy products every day as a child, teen, and young adult, and still do today. . . . . T | F
4. I don't smoke or drink caffeinated beverages or sodas to excess. . . . . T | F
5. I have not crash-dieted.. . . . . . . T | F
6. I'm not thin, white, or small-boned. . . . . T | F

If you circled "False" for five or more statements in the Optimal Health section and for four or more of these statements, you may be at higher-than-average risk for osteoporosis. Calcium is considered to be the crucial component of bone; hundreds of studies support its use as a supplement. The Osteoporosis Prevention plan also contains plentiful amounts of the minerals magnesium, manganese, boron, and phosphorus as well as vitamin D, crucial minerals for calcium to work most effectively. Bone loss can begin by age 30, so start supplementation early to help create a foundation of strong, mineral-rich bones.

CANCER PREVENTION

1. Cancer does not run in my family . . . . .T | F
2. I have not been exposed to excess radiation, such as dental X-rays, chest X-rays, or more than three mammograms . . . . .T | F
3. I regularly eat organic food and drink bottled or filtered water . . . . .T | F

4. I live in an area where there is little or no air pollution. . . . . T | F
5. I have not taken any medicines for a year or longer that increase the risk of cancer. . . . . T | F
6. I am neither overweight nor underweight. . . . . T | F

If you circled "False" for five or more statements in the Optimal Health section and for four or more of the statements above, you may be at higher-than-average risk for cancer. Antioxidants, again, are key to the Cancer Prevention plan. Higher blood levels of the carotenoids are associated with a lower incidence of many types of cancer. Most recently, the carotenoid lycopene has been in the news; it may help prevent prostate cancer. Vitamin C, vitamin E, and selenium (the "anticancer mineral") are all potent antioxidants and work together synergistically to reduce free-radical damage; vitamin C's added benefit is its ability to disarm carcinogens in the liver. Vitamin D has been in the spotlight because of its association with a reduced risk of colon cancer.

Food-Friendly Bugs Do the Body Good

Trillions of bacteria naturally occur in your gut, but don't be alarmed! Many of the bacteria are good and may help protect the body from certain diseases. A number of factors can upset the balance between the levels of good and bad bacteria. However, there is evidence that consuming foods that have "good" bacteria, called probiotics, and food that aid the function of probiotics, called prebiotics, may help maintain a healthy balance of bacteria in the body and help improve certain disease conditions.

"Food-Friendly Bugs"

Our bodies have four lines of defense against infection: skin, mucosal lining, immune system, and gut microflora, sometimes referred to as gut microbiota. Research has shown that adding "friendly" bacteria to your diet will improve the health of your gut microflora, and may help protect both the lining of your intestinal tract and your immune system. An article written by Negendra Shah, associate professor of food science at the School of Life Sciences and Technology, Victoria University of Technology, Australia, in the November 2001 issue of *Food Technology,* highlights the common practice of adding probiotics, similar to bacteria already present in your body, to fermented foods such as yogurt. Probiotics are defined as live microbial food ingredients that have a beneficial effect on human health, when ingested live and in sufficient numbers.

Knowledge of the health benefits of probiotics can be traced back many years when a Nobel Prize winning scientist and director of the Pasteur Institute, Elie Metchnikoff, hypothesized that Bulgarian peasants owed their health and longevity to the consumption of fermented milk products containing lactobacillus, a probiotic bacterium. By 1997, the use of probiotics was becoming well established in Europe, with fermented dairy products accounting for 65 percent of the European "functional food" market. According to an article by Catherine Stanton and colleagues in the *American Journal of Clinical Nutrition* in 2001, health-conscious Americans are realizing the potential health benefits of supplementing their diets with good bacteria and are the fastest growing segment of consumers of probiotic foods.

Different Types of Probiotics

The two most common bacteria added in the production of probiotic foods are lactobacilli and bifidobacteria. According to an article by Fooks and Gibson, published in a supplement of the *British Journal of Nutrition* in 2002, there are numerous species of lactobacilli and bifidobacteria; the main species thought to have probiotic characteristics are *L. casei, B. lactis, L. johnsonii, B. breve, L. bulgaricus, B. animalis, L. rhamnosus, B. infantis, L. reuteri, B. longum,* and *L. acidophilus.*

Today there are more than 70 lactic acid bacteria-containing products worldwide, including sour cream, buttermilk, yogurt, powdered milk, and frozen desserts. According to Shah, more than 53 different types of probiotic milk products are marketed in Japan alone. In an article published in the *American Journal of Clinical Nutrition* in 2000, Belgian expert Marcel Roberfroid states that probiotics have traditionally been consumed as fermented dairy products such as yogurt but have also recently been incorporated into drinks, and in the future may be found in fermented vegetables and meats. They are also being marketed as dietary supplements in tablet, capsule, and freeze-dried preparations.

Health Effects of Probiotics

The health of the gut largely relies on the balance between good and bad bacteria, and probiotics may help the gut prevent an imbalance in which there are too many harmful bacteria. Most of the research on probiotics has been conducted through small clinical studies or epidemiological (observational) studies. This research has shown that probiotics may be promising as treatments for a number of diseases and conditions including: lactose intolerance, diarrhea secondary to antibiotic use or *E. coli* infections, other gastrointestinal infections, vaginal candida (yeast) infections, and lactose malabsorption due to chemotherapy. Research has reasonably well established that probiotics improve the body's ability to resist intestinal infection and improve digestion. Only limited evidence, however, suggests that probiotics have cholesterol-lowering benefits, reduce the risk of cancer, produce vitamins, and reduce the risk of urogenital infections other than candida. Although there is relatively little harm in taking probiotics, more research is necessary to establish a firm basis for using probiotics for specific health benefits.

Prebiotics, The Companion Nutrient

Gut microflora need an environment in which to thrive. Dennis T. Gordon, Ph.D., professor and chair of the department of cereal science at North Dakota State University, explains, "Fermentable dietary fiber is a source of prebiotics and the necessary energy source for our intestinal microbiota." According to an article by Christopher Duggan of Children's Hospital in Boston, Mass., published in the *American Journal of Clinical Nutrition* in 2002, inulin and oligofructose are the two most commonly studied prebiotics. Both inulin and oligofructose are found naturally in many fruits and vegetables as well as in whole-grain foods. They are also widely used commercially to add fiber to foods without adding bulk.

Health Effects of Prebiotics

Most of the research on the potential health benefits of prebiotics has been done in studies with animals or *in vitro* (in a test tube). Studies of inulin have shown that it may have a promising role to play in providing relief from constipation and suppressing diarrhea. Some studies also suggest a possible benefit for reduced risk of osteoporosis through increased calcium absorption, reduced risk of atherosclerosis through decreased cholesterol and triglycerides and improved insulin response, obesity and possibly type 2 diabetes (Roberfroid, *American Journal of Clinical Nutrition*, 2000).

The Lowdown on Consuming Probiotics and Prebiotics

Probiotics and prebiotics are safe to eat and have many positive health

---

Food Sources of Probiotics

- Yogurt
- Buttermilk
- Kefir
- Tempeh
- Miso
- Kim Chi
- Sauerkraut
- Other "fermented" foods

(source:**www.cancer.med.umich.edu/ news/pro09spr02.htm**)

---

benefits. Eating a combination of pre- and probiotic foods, or symbiotic foods, those that contain both pre- and probiotics, may provide the most health benefits. Probiotic and prebiotic products are now widely available. Manufacturers formulate their products with different types and amounts of probiotic bacteria. Most work best when refrigerated or vacuum-packed to preserve the freshness of the bacteria.

Currently, there are no established recommended consumption levels of pre- and probiotics for beneficial effects. More research is needed to determine who will benefit most from consumption of those foods, and who should potentially avoid them. For example, as stated by Sanders in an article published in the November 1999 issue of *Food Technology*, immuno-compromised individuals (e.g., young, elderly, patients with AIDS, Crohn's Disease or enteric infection, etc.) should check with their doctor before consuming probiotics and prebiotics. As always, it is important that individuals not self-diagnose any health condition and speak to their healthcare professionals for advice on the nutritional component of any treatment plan

---

Food Sources of Prebiotics

- Oatmeal
- Flax
- Barley
- Other whole grains
- Onions
- Greens (especially dandelion greens, but also spinach, collard greens, chard, kale, and mustard greens)
- Berries, bananas, and other fruit
- Legumes (lentils, kidney beans, chickpeas, navy beans, white beans, black beans, etc.)

(source: **www.cancer.med.umich.edu/ news/pro09spr02.htm**)

The Future of Probiotics and Prebiotics

Pre- and probiotics are exciting areas of food and nutrition research; however, more studies are needed to substantiate some of the links between these nutrients and health.

Dr. Gordon sums up the current state of the science by saying, "Probiotics are helping us to not only understand but also improve intestinal health. Emerging research is also revealing an important supporting role for prebiotics." The determination of specific strains of beneficial bacteria may help address various gastrointestinal diseases including Crohn's disease and ulcerative colitis, irritable bowel syndrome, and infections in the stomach and small intestine. Research may also find ways for probiotics to improve tube feedings and infant formula as well as improve the nutritional health of the elderly.

ARE YOUR SUPPLEMENTS SAFE?

**Which supplements are safe? Which aren't? Which should you avoid if
you're taking blood-thinners or antidepressants?**

**Don't bother asking the manufacturers...or the government, for that matter. When it comes
to herbs and other over-the-counter supplements, you're pretty much on your own.**

Seven out of every ten adults in the U.S take vitamins, minerals, herbs, or other supplements, according to a 2002 Harris Poll. Some—calcium, folic acid, glucosamine, and saw palmetto, for example—are beneficial. Others—soy isoflavones, ginseng, ginkgo—may or may not be. And still others—ephedra, usnic acid, kava—can be dangerous.

And *any* supplement can do damage if you take too much or take it in the wrong combinations.

"How many supplement takers suffer adverse reactions, no one really knows," says Christine Haller, a medical toxicologist at the University of California at San Francisco who has analyzed reports on the toxicity of ephedra for the Food and Drug Administration (FDA). (Ephedra, which has been called an "herbal fat burner," was linked to the death of Baltimore Orioles pitcher Steve Bechler last spring.)

"We really can't tell how serious the safety questions are for dietary supplements until we look at these products more carefully," says Mary Palmer, an emergency room physician and toxicologist in Alexandria, Virginia.

Palmer, Haller, and their colleagues recently analyzed nearly 500 calls about bad reactions to supplements that had been phoned in to 11 poison control centers in the U.S. in 1998.[1]

"When I started the study I thought that maybe the safety problems with supplements really were mild and that my worries were unfounded," says Palmer. "I was very surprised to see how serious the adverse reactions really were." A third of them included heart attacks, liver failure, bleeding, seizures, and death.

Prescription medications cause an estimated 100,000 deaths and 2.2 million adverse reactions each year. While the toll from supplements is nowhere near as great, it's far from trivial. For example, more than 20,000 complaints about weight-loss products containing ephedra, including scores of deaths, have been registered during the past decade.

Supplements are regulated so much more loosely than drugs that it's impossible to know how much harm they cause.

"Drugs can be sold only if companies have enough evidence to convince the FDA and panels of independent experts that they're safe and effective and that their benefits justify their risks," says Bruce Silverglade, director of legal affairs at the Center for Science in the Public Interest (publisher of *Nutrition Action Healthletter*).

In contrast, "The dietary supplement market is the Wild West," says Congressman Henry Waxman, a California Democrat and longtime champion of measures to protect consumers' health.

"There are no requirements that a company prove anything about either the safety or the effectiveness of its products before they go to market."

Most people don't realize that.

"About 60 percent of U.S. consumers believe that dietary supplements must be approved by a government agency like the Food and Drug Administration before they can be sold to the public," says Nancy Wong of the Harris Poll.

Not so. Congress made sure of that when it passed the Dietary Supplement Health and Education Act (DSHEA) in 1994. "DSHEA put manufacturers in the driver's seat when it comes to which supplements are sold and what claims can be made for them," notes Palmer.

Before DSHEA, if the FDA questioned a supplement's safety, the manufacturer had to prove that it was safe. "DSHEA shifted the burden of proof," says Silverglade. "With drugs, food additives, and pesticides, it's always up to the manufacturer to prove safety. But thanks to DSHEA, the FDA has to prove that supplements are dangerous."

"Because of DSHEA," says Silverglade, "the FDA has been reduced to regulating by press release."

When the agency considers a supplement unsafe, it typically issues a consumer advisory and then discourages—but doesn't prohibit—companies from continuing to sell the product. How many consumers hear about these FDA advisories? "We don't know," concedes FDA spokesperson Sebastian Cianci. "To find that out would require research we don't have the resources to do."

Bottom line: The FDA can only bark, not bite.

In late 2001, for example, the agency received reports of young adults who developed liver damage or failure soon after starting to use a weight-loss product called Li-poKinetix. (It contained usnic acid, the same substance thought to have destroyed Jennifer Rosenthal's liver a year later.) In response, the agency put out a press release advising consumers to "immediately stop use of LipoKinetix."

But the FDA didn't ban or suspend its sale. "Given the serious hazard presented by the use of your product," the agency wrote in a letter to the manufacturer, "we strongly recommend that you take prompt action to remove Lipo-Kinetix from the market." (As it happened, the company had already suspended production because it couldn't get a steady supply of one ingredient.) Two years later, anyone can still purchase supplements that contain usnic acid on the Internet.

Consumers are protected from unsafe *drugs* by at least three lines of defense: The law requires manufacturers to test drugs for safety before they're sold, the FDA removes drugs from the marketplace when serious problems become evident, and manufacturers must track and disclose adverse effects, drug interactions, and other safety problems.

But against potentially unsafe *dietary supplements*, consumers are left to fend for themselves. Among the obstacles they face:

No Safety Testing

Pharmaceutical companies have to test their drugs to make sure they don't cause cancer, interfere with reproduction, damage organs, or cause other problems greater than they solve. In contrast, "Supplement companies have no obligation to test their products for safety before they market them," points out Christine Haller of the University of California at San Francisco.

"Some companies do small studies, but certainly not of the magnitude you would need to detect adverse effects," adds toxicologist Mary Palmer. "In many cases, there will be no information at all about a product's safety. But that doesn't mean it's safe."

"The dietary supplement market is the Wild West."

"Supplement manufacturers like to say that their products are safe because they've been used for centuries in other cultures," says Haller. "But traditional use didn't mean taking capsules of herbs day after day, so it was really different from the way we use them now." Continual exposure to concentrated extracts "probably changes the body's response to the herbs," notes Haller. "So these products might become ineffective or even have a detrimental effect."

How can an herb that has been used for centuries still be dangerous? If it causes cancer in, say, one out of every 100 people 20 years after they take it, the increased risk would never be noticed. Yet the government calls some food additives pesticides, and drugs carcinogens if they cause cancer in one out of every *million* people. That's the level that animal studies on those substances are designed to detect.

Supplement manufacturers, on the other hand, don't even have to understand how the body metabolizes their products. If they did, physicians would have learned long ago that St. John's wort can be life-threatening. (It can interfere with HIV drugs and immunosuppressants for transplant patients.)

And if companies had been required to thoroughly research the safety of hydroxycitrate before putting it in weight-loss supplements, they would have learned that the pharmaceutical giant Hoffman-La Roche abandoned the compound in the 1980s because of toxicity problems.

"We dropped hydroxycitrate when we saw that it seemed to cause testicular atrophy and other toxicities in animals," said a Hoffmann-La Roche spokesperson. "We never got as far as testing it in humans."

When told about the potential problems, a spokesperson for the firm that produces one of the two most popular hydroxycitrate formulations sold in the U.S. said, "I'm really, really surprised."

"There's no incentive for supplement companies to study the safety of their products," says Palmer. "It would be nothing but trouble for them, because they have a good deal right now." If anything's going to hurt their sales, "it's going to be safety issues. So why would they go looking for trouble?"

Take usnic acid. It's produced by lichen plants, so it falls within the loose definition of a dietary supplement. You can buy it on the Internet in the form of Usnea Lichen liquid herbal extracts. (We found one company that sells bottles of usnic acid capsules "for experimental research use only and not for human consumption" to anyone who claims to be at least 18 years old.)

Yet usnic acid may have destroyed the livers of at least half a dozen people in the U.S. over the past few years. Apparently that's not enough to motivate the companies that sell it—or the FDA—to investigate its toxicity.

"I don't know anyone else who's working on the toxicity of usnic acid besides me," says Neil Kaplowitz, director of the University of Southern California Research Center for Liver Diseases in Los Angeles.

Underreported Reactions

"Mild symptoms are definitely underreported to physicians and health agencies, and, as a result, there are probably many problems with supplements that are not being described," says toxicologist Christine Haller. A 2001 report by the U.S. Department of Health and Human Services estimated that only about one out of every 100 adverse reactions is reported to the FDA.[2]

EIGHT TO AVOID

Despite evidence that these eight products can cause serious problems, most are still available, either over the counter or via the Internet.

- **Aristolochic acid.** The ingredient in some traditional Chinese medicines is toxic to the kidneys.
- **Chaparral.** In 1992, the FDA advised consumers to "stop taking chaparral immediately" because it can cause hepatitis.
- **Comfrey.** It can cause chronic liver disease.
- **Ephedra.** It has been linked to high blood pressure, strokes, and heart attacks and is 200 times more likely to cause an adverse reaction than all other herbs combined.
- **Kava.** It's a suspect in liver damage that has resulted in 11 liver transplants over the last several years.

- **PC SPES and SPES.** These supplements, which held promise as prostate-cancer fighters, turned out to be frauds. They worked like hormones only because they were spiked with hormones, a blood thinner, an anti-inflammatory, and several other drugs.
- **Tiratricol.** In 2000, the FDA warned consumers not to use weight-loss supplements containing this thyroid hormone, which can cause strokes and heart attacks.
- **Usnic acid.** This "natural" compound (it's found in lichen), which is used in some herbal mixtures, appears to be toxic to the liver.

Sources: Food and Drug Administration (*www.cfsan.fda.gov/%7Edms/ds-warn.html*) and CSPI.

"People are somewhat embarrassed when they have a problem with a supplement that they think maybe they shouldn't have been taking, like one of the weight-loss products," says Haller. "Why tell your doctor if your doctor didn't know you were taking it?"

What's more, people may not make the connection between a bad reaction and a "natural" supplement. And even if people call the consumer complaint number that's on the product label, "manufacturers sometimes don't do anything with those complaints," says Haller.

Troublesome Interactions

"There's competition in the marketplace now to give consumers the most for their dollar by offering combinations of herbs and other ingredients," says Haller. "But combining ingredients, especially herbs, isn't a good idea, because we really don't understand a lot about how they interact."

In their analysis of calls to poison control centers in the U.S., Haller and her colleagues found that multiple-ingredient supplements were more likely than single-ingredient ones to produce severe adverse effects.

No Required Warnings

"About two-thirds of the U.S. public believes that the government requires the labels of dietary supplements to include warnings about potential side effects or dangers," says Nancy Wong of the Harris Poll.

Not so. Unlike drug labels, supplement labels don't have to disclose who shouldn't take the product, what drugs it shouldn't be taken with, or other warnings.

So, for example, beta-carotene supplements labels don't have to disclose who shouldn't take the product, what drugs it shouldn't be taken with, or other warnings.

So, for example, beta-carotene supplements are unlikely to warn smokers that high doses (at least 25 mg, or 42,000 IU) may increase their risk of lung cancer. And zinc supplement labels are unlikely to disclose that too much zinc can compromise the immune system.

Unreported Problems

"The FDA maintains surveillance of prescription drugs by requiring prompt reports from manufacturers of all adverse events brought to their attention," says Arthur Grollman, chair of pharmacology at the State University of New York at Stony Brook.

"But there is no mandatory requirement for manufacturers of supplements to record, investigate, or forward to the FDA reports of adverse effects they might receive," he adds. "Under current regulations, there is no penalty for withholding these reports." Grollman wants Congress to require companies to report safety problems.

For years, Metabolife, the leading manufacturer of weight-loss pills that contain ephedra, denied that it knew of any serious complaints about its products. Then last year, lawyers who were suing the company on behalf of injured consumers learned that Metabolife had, in fact, received more than 13,000 complaints from users.

The Top Ten Supplements: How Safe?

How safe are the 10 most popular herbal supplements? Here's what you need to know. Just keep in mind that most reactions are rare; in some cases they're based on just one or two reports from physicians. Until more research is done, it's probably wise for children and pregnant or nursing women not to take any of these supplements.

Supplement	What Consumers Expect	Reported Reactions	Who Should be Especially Careful	May Interact With
Black Cohosh	To relieve symptoms of menopause.	Mild gastrointestinal distress.	Women who have had breast cancer (in an animal study, black cohosh caused cancer to spread).	No drug interactions known.
Cranberry	To prevent or treat urinary tract infections.	Regular use of cranberry concentrate tablets might increase the risk of kidney stones.	People susceptible to kidney stones.	Antidepressants and prescription painkillers.
Echinacea	To prevent or treat colds or other infections.	Minor gastrointestinal symptoms. Increased urination. Allergic reactions.	People with autoimmune diseases (like multiple sclerosis, lupus, and rheumatoid arthritis). May also trigger episodes of erythema nodosum, an inflammation that produces tender nodules under the skin.	No drug interactions known.
Garlic	To lower cholesterol levels.	Unpleasant breath odor. Heartburn and flatulence.	People who are about to have—or have just had—surgery (garlic thins the blood). Women just before or after labor or delivery.	Blood-thinning drugs like Coumadin (warfarin), heparin, or aspirin. Blood-thinning supplements like ginko or high doses of vitamin E. Chloroxazone, which is used to treat painful muscle conditions. HIV drugs.
Ginkgo Biloba	To improve memory.	Mild headache. Upset stomach. Seizures (possibly caused by contamination with ginkgo seeds, which are toxic).	People with bleeding disorders like hemophilia. People who are about to have—or have just had—surgery. Women just before or after labor or delivery. People with diabetes.	Blood-thinning drugs like Coumadin (warfarin), heparin, or aspirin. Blood-thinning supplements like high doses of vitamin E. The antidepressant trazodone. Anti-diabetes drugs. Thiazide diuretics.
Ginseng	To increase energy and relieve stress.	Insomnia. Menstrual abnormalities and breast tenderness with long-term use.	Women who had had breast cancer (ginseng stimulated the growth of breast cancer cells in test tubes). People with high blood pressure who aren't taking medication to lower it.	Any drug metabolized by the enzyme CYP 3A4 (ask your physician). MAO inhibitor drugs or digitalis. May increase the activity of insulin and oral hypoglycemics and decrease the activity of Coumadin (warfarin) and ticlopidine.
Saw Palmetto	To prevent or relieve the symptoms of an enlarged prostate.	Mild gastrointestinal distress.	People with bleeding disorders like hemophilia. People who are about to have—or have just had—surgery.	Blood-thinning drugs like Coumadin (warfarin), heparin, or aspirin. Blood-thinning supplements like ginkgo or high doses of vitamin E.
Soy Isoflavones	To relieve menopausal symptoms, prevent breast or prostate cancer, and strengthen bones.	None reported.	Women who have had—or are at high risk for—breast cancer (soy isoflavones may increase cell proliferation). Pregnant women. People with impaired thyroid function.	No drug interactions known.
St. John's Wort	To alleviate depression.	Mild gastrointestinal distress. Rash. Tiredness. Restlessness.	People with skin that's sensitive to sunlight. People taking UV treatment. People with bipolar disorder.	Ritalin, ephedrine (found in ephedra), and caffeine. May increase the activity of protease inhibitors (for HIV), digitalis (for high cholesterol), warfarin (blood-thinner), chemotherapy drugs, oral contraceptives, tricyclic antidepressants, olanzapine and clozapine (for schizophrenia), and theophylline (for asthma). May increase sensitivity to sunlight if combined with sulfa drugs, Feldene (anti-inflammatory), or Prilosec or Prevacid (for acid reflux).
Valerian	To induce sleep or relaxation.	May impair attention for a few hours.	People about to operate heavy machinery or drive.	May increase the activity of central-nervous-system depressants like barbiturates (such as Seconal) and benzodiazepines (such as Valium or Halcion).

Source: The Natural Pharmacist, Healthnotes, and CSPI.

Among them were more than 1,000 reports of significant adverse reactions, including 18 heart attacks, 26 strokes, 43 seizures, and five deaths.[3]

An angry FDA has asked the Department of Justice to pursue filing criminal charges against Metabolife officials for lying to the agency.

Unavailable Adverse Reaction Reports

For years, the Food and Drug Administration has been collecting reports of adverse reactions to dietary supplements. But last year the agency pulled the database from its Web site, saying that the information was confusing.

Last June, the FDA installed a new system (the Center for Food Safety and Applied Nutrition Adverse Events Reporting System, or CAERS) to track complaints by consumers and physicians to its MedWatch hotline (800-FDA-1088 or *fda.gov/medwatch/report/consumer/consumer.htm*).

But health professionals and the public can't view the complaints that have been submitted to CAERS.

"We're working on a way to give the public access to this information, but that's at least a year away," says FDA spokesperson Sebastian Cianci. "Until then, you need to file a Freedom of Information Act [FOIA] request to see the information."

That can take months, which is far too long to help people track down what's causing a reaction. And it certainly would have been too long for people like Jennifer Rosenthal, the California mother who paid a steep price for her lesson in supplement safety.

Notes

1. *Lancet 361*: 101, 2003.
2. Department of Health and Human Services, Office of the Inspector General: *Adverse Event Reporting for Dietary Supplements, An Inadequate Safety Valve.* OEI-01-00180, April 2001.
3. Government Accounting Office: *Dietary Supplements Containing Ephedra.* GAO-03-1042T, July 2003.

UNIT 6
Food Safety/Technology

Unit Selections

Key Points to Consider

- What are some of the main factors that compromise food safety?

- What action should you take to avoid or minimize your risk from exposure to environmental contaminants in the food chain?

- What should your role be as a consumer in ensuring food safety from production to sale?

- Survey your neighborhood supermarkets about the origin of the salmon sold.

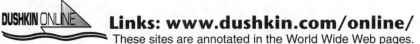 **Links: www.dushkin.com/online/**
These sites are annotated in the World Wide Web pages.

American Council on Science and Health (ACSH)
http://www.acsh.org/food/

Centers for Disease Control and Prevention (CDC)
http://www.cdc.gov

FDA Center for Food Safety and Applied Nutrition
http://vm.cfsan.fda.gov

Food Safety Project (FSP)
http://www.extension.iastate.edu/foodsafety/

National Food Safety Programs
http://vm.cfsan.fda.gov/~dms/fs-toc.html

USDA Food Safety and Inspection Service (FSIS)
http://www.fsis.usda.gov

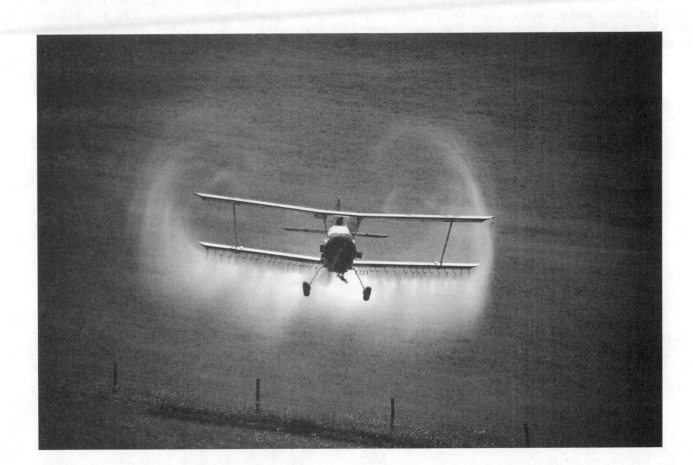

Food-borne disease constitutes an important public health problem in the United States. The U.S. Centers for Disease Control has reported 76 million cases of food-borne illness each year—5,000 that end in death. The annual cost of losses in productivity ranges from 20 to 40 billion dollars. Food-borne disease results primarily from microbial contamination and from naturally occurring toxicants, environmental contaminants, pesticide residues, and food additives.

The first Food and Drug Act was passed in 1906 and was followed by tighter control on the use of additives that might be carcinogenic. In 1958, the Delaney Clause was passed and a list of additives that were considered as safe for human consumption (GRAS list) was developed. The Food and Drug Administration (FDA) controls and regulates procedures dealing with food safety, food service, and production. The FDA has established rules (Hazard Analysis and Critical Control Points) to improve safety control and to monitor the production of seafood, meat, and poultry. Even though there have been outbreaks of food poisoning traced to errors at the commercial processing stage, the culprit is usually mishandling of food. Surveys show that over 95 percent of the time people do not follow proper sanitation methods when working with food. Therefore, the U.S. government, launched the Food Safety Initiative program to minimize foodborne disease and to educate the public about safe food handling practice.

Consumer concerns have shifted to include concerns about consuming food that may contain antibiotics, hormones, pesticides, mercury, dioxin, and PCBs and about the cloning of animals. Crowding living conditions of animals necessitate the use of germ-fighting antibiotics that eventually become part of the food chain. These antibiotics increase risk of exposure to consumers and may result in the development of antibiotic resistance. Growth hormones injected into cattle may also disrupt human hormone systems. Toxic pesticides in trace amounts are found in vegetables, fruits, meats, milk and trans fat found in fast foods, bakery products, margarines, and shortenings raise our risk of chronic disease. More recently the safety issue of consuming farmed salmon is under question since mercury, PCBs,— and dioxin contamination is making the public and scientists uneasy about dietary recommendations. Dioxin is a potent carcinogen, found in incinerator emissions and spills from electrical transformers. It may end up in our cheeseburgers, chicken, and pizza—to name a few. Dioxin accumulates in our bodies and may trigger cancers such as lung, especially in people who consume a diet high in animal fat. It may also decrease learning ability, affect reproduction, decrease sperm production, cause birth defects and impair the immune system. Topping off the list of consumer food concerns are food irradiation to combat food borne illness and reduce food spoilage and questions about genetically modified food and its labeling.

The recent scare in Europe about "mad cow" disease that killed over 100 people during the last few years, has increased awareness of the disease in the U.S. These events have forced the government to look at the gaps in its system and ensure that the disease will be prevented here. The most recent newcomer is the possibility that meat from cloned animals may be coming to a market near you. The FDA's Veterinary Committee has concluded that animal clones "appear to be safe" and there is no reason for product labeling. Buying organic is a safety valve for consumers who are concerned and would like to know what they are eating. The U.S.D.A. has set the criteria to be met by foods before they are given the stamp of "certified organic." The National Organic Rule, defines "organic" as foods that are produced without insecticides, herbicides, chemical fertilizers, radiation, genetic modification, hormones, or antibiotics. This is a breakthrough for consumers since it informs them of what is organic and what is not.

tainted food

Is there anything that's really safe to eat? That depends on what lurks in your fridge

DANYLO HAWALESHKA with BRIAN BETHUNE and SUE FERGUSON

FROZEN ORGANIC beef hamburger patties, $9.78/kg. Grade No. 1 organic onions, $2.26. On-the-vine, hothouse organic tomatoes, $11/kg. Eating a hamburger that doesn't load you down with chemicals, priceless. Well, maybe. Some shoppers would just say pricey. Those organic ingredients—when compared to the common ones regrettably seasoned with traces of antibiotics, growth hormones and pesticides—can cost anywhere from 15 to 170 per cent more. But it's come to this, hasn't it? Most Canadians would never accept a two-tiered health-care system, yet that's the direction in which we seem to be heading with our food. Consumers who are at least reasonably well-off can afford the good stuff, while those who are financially strapped make do. As shown by the scares with mad cow disease and tainted farmed salmon, our increasingly industrialized food chain may turn out to be the pitfall that keeps us from what could otherwise be a long, healthy life.

In the early 1900s, socialist author Upton Sinclair's *The Jungle* brought to light the horrifically unsanitary conditions in Chicago slaughterhouses and packing plants. He described the steam-filled tank rooms with their open vats. Because some of the vat openings were almost level with the shop floor, workers sometimes slipped and fell in. Occasionally, before anyone noticed, the unfortunate soul's remains would re-emerge

Anxiety in the icebox

Common food items may contain harmful and/or controversial substances (all amounts are within federally regulated limits):

1. Beef rib roast
antibiotics, hormones, pesticides
2. Milk
pesticides
3. Chicken
antibiotics, dioxins
4. Ham
nitrates
Bell peppers
pesticides
6. Grapes
pesticides
7. Cantaloupe
pesticides
8. Cucumbers
pesticides
9. Farmed salmon
dioxins, PCBs
10. Muffins baked with margarine
trans fat
11. Bacon
nitrates and nitrites
12. Eggs
dioxins
13. Black Forest cake with maraschino cherries
trans fats, red synthetic dye
14. Stuffed olives
red synthetic dye

days later—packaged as Durham's Pure Leaf Lard. In writing his book, Sinclair wanted to draw attention to the inhumane work conditions under which immigrants toiled. Instead, the U.S. public and its legislators were so shocked that Congress passed the federal Pure Food and Drug and Meat Inspection Act in 1906. Later, Sinclair famously remarked: "I aimed at the public's heart and by accident I hit it in the stomach."

What we're seeing in the news lately amounts to a similar blow to the gut. While we've dealt with those century-old problems in our abattoirs, we now have new ones to contend with, and they go well beyond two North American mad cow cases in the past year. The recent study on farmed Atlantic salmon published in the journal *Science* found high levels of PCBs, dioxins, DDT and other toxins linked to increased risks of cancer and birth defects. Yet this is only one element of a larger problem with food production. Industrialized farming and widespread pollution, critics argue, are the real culprits today. We must rethink how we put food on our tables.

Giant agribusinesses pack together cattle, pigs, chickens and fish by the hundreds and thousands, necessitating the use of germ-fighting antibiotics that we end up swallowing. Studies suggest these ingested drugs can increase the risk of harmful bacteria in humans developing antibiotic resistance. Growth hormones

The dirty dozen

According to the Sierra Club of Canada, if you can afford to buy only some organic produce, you should focus on the following fruits and vegetables—especially if you're serving them to children. Typically, these items are heavily sprayed with pesticides.

apricots	grapes
bananas	green beans
bell peppers	lettuce
cantaloupe	potatoes
cherries	spinach
cucumbers	tomatoes

pumped into cattle raise concerns over disruption of our own hormone systems. Our fruit, vegetables, meat and milk are found to contain toxic pesticides in trace amounts. Processed meats are preserved with nitrite and nitrate salts that guard against the bacterial growth that causes botulism, but have been linked to cancer. Trans fatty acids in margarines, shortenings, fast foods and common bakery products increase the risk of heart disease. There are worries about genetically modified food and the incessant push by business to irradiate meat to sterilize it.

It used to be that if you wanted to eat healthy, you'd eat fish. Now, we have to consider whether seafood might not be better considered a potential biohazard. Consider that the U.S. Food and Drug Administration warns pregnant women, nursing mothers and small children against eating tuna and shellfish on a regular basis. There's too much mercury in them. Health Canada says it sets strict limits on the toxins allowed in the fish we eat, and in conjunction with the Canadian Food Inspection Agency, contends that "consuming farmed salmon does not pose a health risk to consumers." Others aren't so sure. "The Canadian government says that arguably we have the safest and best food in the world," notes Herb Barbolet, founder of the FarmFolk/CityFolk Society, a non-profit organization in Vancouver concerned with food, farming, health and the environment. "I think on the whole that's probably correct, but the problems in the food system, nonetheless, are enormous."

Even the water we drink can be tainted in countless ways. Pesticides, industrial chemicals and micro-organisms constantly have to be monitored and kept at bay. Scientists worry about excreted pharmaceutical drugs in the water we drink. Bottled water—the guidelines are outdated—is often no more than filtered tap water. (Health Canada has undertaken a review and expects to toughen rules on, for example, arsenic levels.)

Karen Dodds, director general of Health Canada's health products and food branch, stands by the quality of our food safety systems. She disputes the need to restrict consumption of farmed salmon, as the *Science* paper recommends. "Levels found in the study were well below our guidelines," notes Dodds. "There is no reason for concern."

What can the consumer do? Andrea Peart, the Ottawa-based director of the health and environment program for the Sierra Club of Canada, says buying organic foods is a start, but not the ultimate answer. "Above all else," counsels Peart, "buy local, whether it's a pig or a tomato." That supports often hard-pressed farmers and helps decentralize food production, she adds. The fruits and vegetables tend to have less pesticide residue, too. "A lot of additional chemicals are applied just in shipments to stop moulding," she notes. "Immediately, by buying from farmers close to home, that's cut out of the equation." Other food-safety options: buy meat products that are raised without antibiotics and growth hormones, and contain no dyes.

Cooking a meal from scratch once in a while, if not regularly, is another not-so-revolutionary activity that many families have strayed from. The food's better than, say, packaged lasagna, whose meat could be the very last and worst scraps taken off the bone. The tomato sauce may be oozing with trans fats, and the cheese is perhaps from factory-farmed animals and thus could contain growth hormones.

Janet Nicol, a high-school teacher in Toronto, has been buying organic products for a decade. When stories about suspect food make the news, Nicol is content in knowing she's on top of the situation and that she and her three children—Emmet, 5, and 18-week-old twins Austin and Myles—are safe. At the same time, the salmon report caused some concern. Because the cost of wild fish is so high, her family eats farm-raised salmon about once a month. Still, Nicol, 38, has taken a wait-and-see approach. "I don't tend to immediately stop just because there's been one report. It's something to follow." She encourages friends to opt for organics whenever possible, but wonders if her own family can maintain its current degree of commitment. "Prices are going down," observes Nicol, "but frankly, I'm going to have three growing boys. We're going to have to cut back on our consumption because it's so much more expensive."

In general, North Americans aren't exactly eager to reach for their wallets at the checkout counter. "We spend less than 10 per cent of our disposable income on food," notes Barbolet. "That's the least that any place in the world spends on food. Because of this, we're getting, basically, fat, salt and sugar—the things that are cheap." If, for example, overweight people needed any more convincing, yet another study earlier this month pointed to obesity as a killer. Published in the *Canadian Journal of Public Health*, the study shows that one in 10 deaths in people aged 20 to 64 years can be blamed on excess weight. Unfortunately, good food costs money, but it at least holds out the lure of better health.

After decades of urban sprawl and loss of farmland, can we revive the family farm? Tom Manley, chairman of the Canadian Organic Growers' Ottawa chapter, thinks we can. Instead of independent farmers selling their grain to distant, industrialized livestock operations as they do today, Manley says farmers could raise and feed their own cattle. "The increase in production in the last 40 years," says Manley, "has largely been done with genetics, breeding and selecting plants and animals to produce more per unit of space or time." Currently, drug- and pesticide-free production lags behind factory farming, Manley adds, because most organic farmers are still learning their craft. "But if you compare experienced, skilful organic farmers to conventional farmers in a similar environment," Manley says, "you'll get very comparable results, if not better."

Austin, Tex.-based Whole Foods Market Inc. bills itself as the world's largest retailer of natural and organic foods. It has 149 stores in North America, including a single Canadian outlet that opened in Toronto in 2002. Another in the area is in the final stages of planning, and a third is set to open in Vancouver by next September. The success of Whole Foods—a single store with 19 employees started it all in 1980—shows just how popular eating well has become, at least in a significant subset of the population. "Everything in the store is at least 'natural,' and then we try to offer an organic option wherever possible," says Stefanie Artis, the chain's Toronto-based spokeswoman. By natural, Artis means free of any artificial colours, flavours, preservatives and sweeteners. The company is selective about the salmon it offers. "First of all,

there's PCBs in everything," says Artis, "which the average person doesn't necessarily know." The store's farmed salmon, she adds, was tested by a private laboratory and showed 340 times less dioxin and over 1,000 times less PCBs than wild salmon.

A BRAVE NEW WORLD of food production awaits us. In 2000, Kraft Foods helped create a heavy-hitting research consortium called NanoteK, a play on the word nanotechnology, the science of manipulating atoms and molecules to do our bidding. For instance, Kraft wants to learn how nanoparticles can improve fla-

vour. Some of the thinking is way out there—we're talking food that changes colour, flavour and nutrient value to suit a person's health or palate. We're talking filters to remove toxins. We're even talking packaging that can detect whether food has gone bad. But are we talking madness, or progress? Who can say with certainty? Eating well has always been about ensuring a balanced diet. Increasingly, however, it also means balancing commerce and nutrition, and finding ways to produce food without polluting it.

With Brian Bethune and Sue Ferguson

CERTIFIED ORGANIC

STAMP OF APPROVAL: New government rules will define 'organic.' The sale of these fruits, veggies and snack foods has soared, but we still aren't sure what good they do. Here's a guide to how purer products affect the health of our families and the planet.

BY GEOFFREY COWLEY

OTTO KRAMM USED TO COME home from work at night and warn his toddlers to keep their distance until he'd bathed and changed his clothes. He wasn't just trying to keep them clean. As a vegetable farmer in California's Salinas Valley, Kramm spent his days covered in pesticides, herbicides and fungicides, and he worried about their effects on young children. "I didn't know what was on my clothes," he says, "or how it might affect the kids 15 years down the road." The more he thought about it, the less he liked the feeling. So in 1996, Kramm did something radical. He bought into a farm that was being cultivated organically. "It was scary," he says. "I couldn't fall back on the tools I'd always used to fight the pests and the weeds." But he worked out a new relationship with the soil and ended up not only cleaner but more prosperous. Today Kramm has 6,000 acres on three farms. The nation's largest organic-produce distributor, Earthbound Farm, is buying up everything he can grow. And he's never off-limits to his kids.

Organic farms are still sprouts in a forest of industrial giants. They provide less than 2 percent of the nation's food supply and take up less than 1 percent of its cropland. But they're flourishing as never before. Over the past decade the market for organic food has grown by 15 to 20 percent every year—five times faster than food sales in general. Nearly 40 percent of U.S. consumers now reach occasionally for something labeled organic, and sales are expected to top $11 billion this year. Could dusty neighborhood co-ops sell that many wormy little apples? Well, no. That was the old organic. The new organic is all about bigger farms, heartier crops, better distribution and slicker packaging and promotion. Conglomerates as big as Heinz and General Mills are now launching or buying organic lines—and selling them in mainstream supermarkets.

What exactly are consumers getting out of the deal? Until now, the definition of "organic" has varied from one state to the next, leaving shoppers to assume it means something like "way more expensive but probably better for you." Not anymore. As of Oct. 21, any food sold as organic will have to meet criteria set by the United States Department of Agriculture. The National Organic Rule—the product of 10 years' deliberation by growers, scientists and consumers—reserves the terms "100 percent organic" and "organic" (at least 95 percent) for foods produced without hormones, antibiotics, herbicides, insecticides, chemical fertilizers, genetic modification or germ-killing radiation. Food makers who document their compliance will qualify for a new USDA seal declaring their products "certified organic." "This really signifies the start of a new era," says Margaret Wittenberg of the Whole Foods supermarket chain. "From now on, consumers will get a very solid idea of what is organic and what is not."

Yet for all the clarity they provide, the standards say nothing about what's worth putting in your shopping cart. "This is not a food-safety program," says Barbara Robinson, the USDA official overseeing the effort. "We're not saying that organic food is safer or better than other kinds of food." How, then, should we read the new label?

Does "certified organic" tell us anything worth knowing about a chicken breast or a candy bar? Are organically grown grapes more nutritious than conventional ones? And is organic agriculture a viable alternative to modern factory farming? These are complicated, politically charged questions, but they're questions worth asking ourselves—both as consumers and citizens.

When the counterculture embraced organic food and farming in the early '70s, the motivation was more philosophical than practical. Maria Rodale, whose family runs the pro-organic Rodale Institute in Kutztown, Pa., sees the current boom as evidence that people are still "expressing their values about the environment and even spirituality and politics through the food choices they make." Market research suggests she's about 26 percent right. When the Hartman Group of Bellevue, Wash., surveyed consumers two years ago, only one in four cited concern about the environment as a "top motivator" for buying organic food. Flavor was a bigger concern, cited by 38 percent as reason enough to pay a premium of 15 percent or more. Sophisticated chefs have responded in droves, many now serving only fresh, seasonal food from small local growers. "The difference is huge," says Peter Hoffman, owner of New York's Restaurant Savoy and chairman of the Chefs' Collaborative. "When people taste asparagus or string beans grown in richly composted soil, they can't get over the depth and vibrancy of the flavor."

To most consumers, though, organic means healthier. Fully 66 percent of the Hartman Group's respondents cited health as a "top motivator"—as will almost any shopper on the street. "Buying an apple that has poison on it, even if you wash it you don't know how much has come off," says Wendy Abrams, a suburban Chicago mother with four kids at home. Abrams buys organic milk and stocks her pantry with Newman's Own pretzels and raisins on the theory that anything organic is less likely to harbor cancer-causing chemicals. "There have been six cases of cancer on my street," she says. "It's just weird."

All of these folks—market analysts refer to them as "true naturals," "connoisseurs" and "health seekers"—seem happy with their purchases. But are they getting what they're seeking? It's hard to argue with the connoisseurs, and not just because they know what they like. A tomato grown on a vast commercial plot is bred less for taste than for durability, notes Bob Scowcroft of the nonprofit Organic Farming Research Foundation. It has to resist disease and ship well. Organic growers, with their smaller harvests and their reliance on nearby markets, can plant delicate heirloom strains and give the fruit more time on the vine. "They pick it when it's ripe," says Marion Cunningham, author of "The Fannie Farmer Cookbook." "No one goes around picking organic fruits when they're as hard as little rocks."

Managed property, organic farms can match conventional ones for productivity, and beat them during drought conditions.

The health seekers may have common sense on their side, but no one has found a way to determine whether people eating well-balanced organic diets are healthier than those eating well-balanced conventional ones. No one denies that nonorganic produce contains pesticide residues that would be toxic at high doses. Nor is there any question that children (because of their size) consume those residues in higher concentrations than adults. But there is still no evidence that pesticides cause ill health at the doses found in food, or that people who eschew them come out ahead. Technological optimists find it ludicrous that anyone would fret over pesticide residues when the hazards of foodborne bacteria are

so much clearer. *E. coli* is "perhaps the deadliest risk in our modern food supply," says Dennis Avery of the Hudson Institute—"and its primary hiding place is the cattle manure with which organic farmers fertilize food crops." So wash your produce, but don't let it scare you. Organic or conventional, fruits and vegetables are the best fuel you can put in your body.

Dangerous bacteria are even more common in animal products, but the organic program is not a germ-control initiative. Under the new guidelines, meat and dairy labeled organic must come from creatures that are raised on organic grains or grasses, given access to the outdoors and spared treatment with growth hormones and antibiotics. Experts agree that by spiking animal feed with antibiotics, conventional farmers are speeding the emergence of drug-resistant bacteria. Buying organic is one way to vote against that practice. But in terms of your own health, you'll profit more from holding back on animal products than by eating organic ones. In one study, Danish research found that organic chickens were actually more likely than conventional ones to carry campylobacter, a pathogen that can cause severe diarrhea.

So organic food is tastier and more appealing, but not demonstrably better for you. If you're shopping with only yourself in mind, maybe you'll save your money. But if you pause to think about what you're buying into with every food purchase, organic goods start to look like a bargain. Our current agricultural system took off in the years following World War II, when farmers discovered that chemical fertilizers could force higher yields out of tired soil—and that pesticides could clear croplands of competing species. As farmers saw what the new chemicals made possible, American agriculture was transformed from a rural art into a heavy industry dominated by large corporations growing single crops on vast stretches of poisoned soil.

As any ecologist might have predicted, the new approach was hard to sustain. A small, varied farm can renew itself endlessly when managed with care. Last year's bean stocks help nourish next year's cantaloupes, and a bad year for tomatoes may be a good year for eggplant. As they lost sight of those lessons, the factory farmers grew ever more dependent on chemicals. Insects died off conveniently at

first. But each application of insecticide left a few heart survivors, and within a few generations whole populations were resistant. Today, says Scowcroft, "we're applying three times as much chemical as we were 40 years ago to kill the same pests." It's not just insects. Conventional farmers now use herbicides to kill weeds, fungicides to kill fungi, rodenticides to kill field mice and gophers, avicides to kill fruit-eating birds and molluscicides to kill snails. Strawberry growers now favor all-purpose fumigants such as methyl bromide. "You inject it into the soil and put a tarp over it," says Monica Moore of the Pesticide Action Network of North America. "It kills everything from mammals to microbes. It's a complete biocide."

These practices may not be poisoning our food, but there is no question they're killing off wildlife, endangering farmworkers and degrading the soil and water that life itself depends on. Pesticides now kill 67 million American birds each year. The Mississippi River dumps enough synthetic fertilizer into the Gulf of Mexico to maintain a 60-mile-wide "dead zone" too choked with algae to support fish. And soil erosion threatens to turn much of the world's arable land into desert. "Conventional agriculture still delivers cheap, abundant food," says Fred Kirschenmann of the Leopold Center for Sustainable Agriculture in Ames, Iowa. "But when you factor in the government subsidies and the environmental costs, it gets very expensive. We're drawing down our ecological capital. At some point, the systems will start to break down."

Can organic agriculture save the day? Not if it's just a boutique alternative. But as demand grows, more and more farmers are taking a leap backward—and landing on their feet. They're discovering they can enrich the soil and manage some pests simply by rotating their crops. They're learning that they can often control insects with other insects—or lure them away from cash crops by planting things they prefer. Well-run organic farms often match conventional ones for productivity, even beat them when water is scarce. Creating a sustainable food supply may well require advanced technology as well as ecological awareness. But an organic ethic could be the very key to our survival.

With ANNE UNDERWOOD
and KAREN SPRINGEN

Send in the Clones

Will the FDA allow food products derived from animal clones to be sold without any labeling requirements?

By Kate Jackson

Could food from cloned animals be coming soon to a market near you? Will you dine on roasted rack of cloned lamb, feast on ribs from a cloned pig, or down a glass of cold milk from a cloned cow? The answer is likely to be yes, but the real question is: Will you know it if you do?

A recent announcement by the FDA—based on ongoing assessments indicating that consumption of food from animal clones "appears to be safe"—suggests that it won't be long until these products are approved to enter the U.S. food supply and find their way into stores and restaurants. If that prospect makes you squeamish, this might make you downright queasy: The FDA currently sees no reason for labels that would let consumers know that they're purchasing food from animal clones.

The Ongoing Review

Somatic cell nuclear transfer is the name of the process by which animals are cloned. Through this fusion of a cell's nucleus from the body of the parent animal to an unfertilized egg cell, an identical genetic copy of the parent animal is created. The process has been used for the purpose of improving quality and increasing productivity at a cost of as much as $20,000 to clone a single

goat, pig, or cow. At this cost, it's unlikely that these animal clones will themselves enter the food supply, but their progeny are likely to reach American tables once they are approved by the government.

Before that can happen, the government must conclude its ongoing process of reviewing the scientific research concerning the safety of human consumption of cloned animal products. The FDA's risk analysis began nearly two years ago when it asked the National Academy of Sciences (NAS) to investigate the evidence. On October 31, 2003, the FDA issued a draft executive summary of its risk assessment, which it says builds upon the NAS findings. The academy determined that although animal clones "posed only a low level of food safety concern, it would be prudent to have more data in order to minimize further safety concerns." Before it could make policy decisions concerning animal clones, the FDA concluded that a risk assessment was necessary, to be followed by a review of risk management options. Information has and will continue to be communicated at public meetings and all future information will be publicly available through the FDA's Web site.

With the release of the draft executive summary, the FDA also an-

nounced that a voluntary moratorium on releasing animal clones remains in effect until further data are evaluated. The summary reveals that an advisory panel has reached the tentative opinion that food from "animal clones and their offspring is likely to be as safe to eat as food from their nonclone counterparts, based on all the evidence available." A public meeting was held November 4, 2003, at the Center for Veterinary Medicine in Rockville, Md., during which some panel members insisted on the need for further data to support the FDA's presumption of safety while others urged the agency to pay greater attention to the ethical issues surrounding animal cloning, including the suffering of cloned animals. The transcripts of this meeting explaining the review process are available online at www.fda.gov/cvm/index/vmac/VMACFall2003.htm.

The FDA is continuing to review the issues and inviting comments from the public before making a final decision. While the biotechnology industry pushes for FDA approval and suggests that cloned animals will provide a reproducible, healthful, cost-effective alternative to natural animal products, others are voicing concerns that cloning animals for food is not only potentially unsafe and perhaps un-ethical but also unnecessary and just plain distasteful.

Safety

The FDA's presumption of safety is based on the fact that its Veterinary Medicine Advisory Committee—like an NAS study released the previous year—could discern no difference between mature cloned animals and their counterparts in nature. Its con-clusions were based on studies of cattle but extended to pigs and goats. This conclusion supports the FDA's suggestion that labels on food con-taining the products of animal clones would be unnecessary. If there's no difference in the products, the agency indicates, there would be no need for special labels.

> **The FDA currently sees no reason for labels that would let consumers know that they're purchasing food from animal clones.**

In a swift response to the FDA's announcement of its tentative sup-port of cloning, George Siemon, CEO of Organic Valley, told the press, "American families should not be guinea pigs for corporate greed. Contrary to what the FDA says, there is no level of 'acceptable risk' when it comes to putting unproven science on the table for dinner."

When the FDA comments that consumption of cloned products ap-pears to be safe, adds Michael Le-vine, president, Organic Meat Company, a wholly owned subsid-iary of Organic Valley, it's taking a leap of faith that hurdles a chasm of uncertainty. The agency indicates that it has no reason to believe cloned products are unsafe. That, suggests Levine, isn't evidence that they are safe. "What makes me par-ticularly uncomfortable," he says, "is that there's a lack of knowledge, so consequently we can't find the risks

because we don't understand it well enough."

The notion that since science can't distinguish a difference between natural and cloned animals there must not be a difference "borders on ignorance and egotism," says Le-vine. "We know what we know, and beyond that, we'll find out." Rather than cater to business interest, he in-sists, we should err on the side of caution.

Ethics and the Unknown

According to Levine, "There is an enormous amount of uncertainty as to where this will lead." Once cloned products are released, there's no re-turning, he suggests. "You can't call it back," he says. "Once it's out and the genetic material is allowed to blend with regular genetic material, then it essentially infects."

"Whether it's genetically engi-neered crops, cross-pollinating with wild weeds, genetically modified salmon breeding with wild fish, or future concerns with clone mam-mals, the risks to the balance in eco-systems worldwide are great," said Siemon. Ethical concerns have been raised as well about the welfare of the animals themselves, many of which are born with deformities or disease as a result of the cloning technology.

The Yuck Factor

Levine believes the prospect of eating the products of cloned ani-mals makes people uncomfortable enough that there will be a strong consumer outcry regarding the need for labeling. "It's one thing when it's a tomato, but when it's a living, breathing animal—a created, processed creature—that's some-thing else," he says. Once a need for labeling is established and people see the labels, he speculates, people won't want the products. Much like irradiated foods, says Levine, "there's enough uncertainty and discomfort at the consumer level that it will prevent it from wide-spread distribution."

Wahida Karmally, DrPH, RD, CDE, director of nutrition, Irving Center for Clinical Research at Co-lumbia University, took an informal survey of colleagues, asking whether or not they'd eat cloned animals or products from cloned animals. Most, she says, were not so inclined. How-ever, among her sampling were three doctors, each of whom had no qualms about it. The scientists among the group claimed they could see no difference, while those op-posed to eating cloned animal prod-ucts cited concerns about safety and the unknowns. Some, in addition, merely question the need for clon-ing, asking, "Why not leave animal reproduction to nature?"

Karmally, herself not a big meat eater, says she finds the idea dis-tasteful. Although she has no reason to believe these products are hazard-ous to human health, she's con-cerned that the government's assessment discusses the appearance rather than the certainty of safety. Why, she wonders, do they just ap-pear to be safe, and what's prevent-ing the government from using more conclusive language? "I'm not to-tally convinced that it's without haz-ards, but I really don't know," says Karmally.

"Ultimately what will happen if the business interests push through ... somehow they'll be able to dis-guise it and then it's out there and there's nothing we'll be able to do because the market, in face of igno-rance, will accept it," she continues. "Knowledge, though, is a remark-ably powerful tool, and if consumers have the knowledge that it's out there, I believe they will opt not to participate."

Necessity

Like her colleagues, Karmally questions the necessity for cloning in the first place, asking, "Don't we have enough production?" Katherine Tall-madge, American Dietetic Associa-tion spokesperson, agrees. "We have plenty of food. Why do we need to clone?"

"Obviously from my perspective, the organic protocol and the organic system is the right way to raise animals," says Levine. "But even conventionally speaking, the quality level of animals is high enough. There's no need."

Labeling

Even many who believe there's no harm to human health and/or for concern about eating the products of animal clones believe the public has a right to know where their food comes from. "I think we should let people decide whether they want to eat [food from cloned] animals," says Karmally, "People need to make informed decisions." Echoes Tallmadge, "The more educated the consumer is, the better, so the more labeling, the better." One reason labels may be important, says Karmally, is to assure consumers that the cloned animal has the equivalent nutrient content. They may want to know that the cloned product offers the same amount of protein, for example.

Even though Levine clearly believes that if animal clone products are released into the food supply they should be labeled, he's uncomfortable with the statement. "I'd rather say it should never get to that."

Making Choices

If products from animal clones are permitted to enter the food supply and the FDA determines that labeling is necessary, consumers will be able to recognize cloned products and make their own choices. If these products are permitted without labeling, only consumers who purchase organic meat products will be certain that their food is not from animal clones. "Buying organic is a safety valve across so many different levels," says Levine. "The organic protocol is about raising animals and crops in harmony with nature, as nature intended. So you don't have any of these issues because they're not within the organic system."

Staying Tuned

The FDA risk assessment will continue and its findings will be published on the agency's Web site, possibly by early this year, after the public has had an opportunity to comment. The FDA will then look at risk management and regulatory options. To stay current, follow the risk assessment process or offer comment on the FDA's Web site at www.fda.gov/cvm.

— Kate Jackson is a staff writer for *Today's Dietitian.*

Hooked on fish? There might be some catches

Health-conscious people eat it three, even four times a week. But farm-raised fish and worries about mercury contamination are churning the waters.

The advantage of eating fish has become one of those health-advice truisms, ranking right up there with getting exercise and eating fruits and vegetables. "Studies show that fish consumption lowers your risk of... "—you can fill in the blank, although the evidence remains strongest for heart disease.

The topic has spawned plenty of research. We recently did a quick computer search of the medical literature for fish-consumption studies. Within minutes we found research papers on stroke in American women, prostate cancer in Swedish men, Alzheimer's disease in French seniors, and leptin

(an appetite hormone) levels in Tanzania. Not surprisingly, all came out swimmingly for the fish eaters.

Farm vs. Wild

The glowing health reports have whet the American appetite for fish, and the millions of pounds of farm-raised fish produced each year help meet that demand. In addition to farm-raised catfish, salmon, and trout, we now have tilapia, striped bass, sturgeon, and walleye on the menu and at the store. In Australia, they've started tuna "ranching"—catching the fish in large nets and

herding them into pens for several months of feeding.

Dilemmas abound. Farming fish makes a healthy food less expensive for consumers. The added supply almost certainly eases overfishing of dwindling stocks of some species. But some environmental groups are critical, especially of salmon operations on the West Coast, and want consumers to boycott farm-raised salmon. They say the "floating feedlots" harm fragile marine environments. There's also an argument that raising carnivorous fish like salmon is wasteful of natural resources because it takes several pounds of wild

---

What is it about fish?

When you eat carbohydrates (sugar or starch) or protein, your body shows little respect for the artistry of those molecules. It tears them apart and reassembles them to suit its own purposes. Carbohydrates and protein—they're just fodder.

But it's different with fat. Some gets roughed up during digestion and metabolism. But some gets through more or less intact, becomes part of our cell membranes, and thus has considerable say-so over how cells behave. We are the fat that we eat.

Fish is a special food because it contains two important varieties of *long-chain omega-3* fats that you won't find anywhere else in a conven-

tional diet. *Long-chain* refers to the number of carbon atoms, *omega-3* to a position of a certain chemical bond that puts a 45-degree kink in that chain. Both attributes determine how a fat molecule is going to fit into cell membranes and what it's going to do once it gets there.

As it turns out, long-chain omega-3 fats in fish are just the sort of fat molecules that any healthy cell should gladly welcome into its membranes. One of them, *eicosapentaenoic acid,* manages to displace molecules that could otherwise give rise to active prostaglandins, leukotrienes, and other inflammatory compounds. And inflammation seems to be a root cause of many diseases. *Eicosapentaenoic acid* also seems to be the

omega-3 with the most pronounced cardiac benefits.

The other main omega-3 in fish is *docosahexaenoic acid* (DHA). It's important to brain and vision development in infants and is added to infant formulas.

Sometimes there's some confusion about where the *alpha-linolenic acid* in walnuts, flaxseed oil, and soy products fits in. It's also an omega-3 fat, but has fewer carbon atoms and therefore isn't a long-chain omega-3. Being short-changed those few carbon atoms makes a difference because alpha-linolenic acid doesn't have as many health benefits as the more carbon-blessed omega-3s in fish.

fish like herring or anchovy to produce a pound of salmon. The industry says it has responded by cutting back on antibiotics, switching to low-phosphorous feeds that make fish waste less polluting, and experimenting with soy and other vegetable-based feeds.

Nutritional Issues

Coddled and cooped up, farm fish tend to be anywhere from two to five times fattier overall than wild fish, although the fat content of wild fish varies tremendously depending on the season and where the creature is in its reproductive cycle. That extra fat means more calories. But fattier (oilier) fish also tend to have more of the omega-3 fats that are the main reason fish is such a health food. (*See sidebar.*) A meal of an oily fish like bluefish will give you twice as many omega-3s as a like-sized serving of halibut, and four times as many as farmed catfish.

So farm-raised fish—simply because they're fattier—tend to have more omega-3s than wild fish. But actual comparisons become complicated. Both the amount and type of fat in farmed fish depend on their feed, particularly the type of oil (fat) it contains.

When we looked up the omega-3 content of farmed and wild Atlantic salmon in a nutritional database compiled by the United States Department of Agriculture (USDA), they were the same. But wild Atlantic salmon is scarce and not commercially available very often. A more realistic comparison is farmed Atlantic with other wild salmon species. And according to the USDA database, wild coho salmon, for example, contains half the amount of omega-3s as farmed Atlantic salmon.

Researchers at Oregon Health & Science University have made their own comparisons. So far, their tests haven't shown any difference in the omega-3 content of farmed and wild salmon, according to Dr. William E. Connor, one of the researchers. But when they tested catfish, the omega-3 content of the wild fish was much higher than the farmed.

Fish Feed

Fish feeds vary tremendously with the species. There is also continual ex-perimentation with, for example, different sorts of enzymes to make the fish metabolize feed more efficiently and thus grow faster. British scientists announced last year that they had successfully added *pheromones* to feed to make it more appetizing. Red coloring in the form of synthetic carotenoids is added to salmon feed to give the flesh that rosy color that consumers have come to expect.

For consumers, the oil content of the feed is a key issue because it influences omega-3 levels. Currently, most of the oil used for fish feed comes from small fish like herring and menhaden—and it's rich in omega-3s. But the industry is worried about dwindling supplies and rising costs and thus interested in plant-based alternatives. Researchers at the University of Stirling in Scotland have published several studies showing that replacing fish oil with plant-derived substitutes is feasible, but, not surprisingly, a high proportion of plant oil significantly reduces the omega-3 content of salmon.

Omega-3 and mercury content of select fish			
Omega-3 fats (grams in 3-oz. serving)*		**Mercury (parts per million)****	
Atlantic salmon, farmed	1.8	Tilefish	1.45
Anchovy	1.7	Swordfish	1.00
Sardines	1.4	Shark	0.96
Rainbow trout, farmed	1.0	King mackerel	0.73
Coho salmon, wild	0.9	Tuna (fresh and frozen)	0.32
Bluefish	0.8	Halibut	0.23
Striped bass	0.8	Mahi mahi	0.19
Swordfish	0.7	Tuna (canned)	0.17
Tuna, white, canned	0.7	Catfish	0.07
Halibut	0.4	Salmon	Not detectable
Catfish, channel, farmed	0.2	Tilapia	Not detectable

*SOURCE: USDA NUTRIENT DATABASE

**SOURCE: FDA

Some experts we talked to said feed makers are more likely to switch from fish to vegetable (soy) sources of protein, not fat. For one thing, some species—notably salmon, trout, and steelhead—need omega-3 oil to flourish. The industry also has an interest in preserving the reputation of fish as a healthy food, which means keeping the omega-3 levels as high as possible.

As for farm vs. wild taste, we defer to the palate of Roger Berkowitz, CEO of Legal Sea Foods, a chain of seafood restaurants based in Boston. He says that wild fish, especially salmon, has a gamier, more intense flavor. It's also more expensive. Berkowitz says farm-raised flounder has foundered because of poor taste and texture.

Mercury Contamination

But an even bigger worry these days is that the fish we're urged to eat for health may contain some very unhealthy contaminants, particularly mercury. Most research suggests that if the mercury in fish causes harm, the danger is primarily to the developing nervous systems of children, although studies have suggested a link between mercury and the atherosclerosis that underlies heart disease. Last spring, the FDA advised pregnant women and all women of childbearing age not to eat any shark, swordfish, king mackerel, and tilefish because of their high mercury content, and to limit consumption of all fish to 12 ounces (about two servings) per week. Harvard researchers recently published a study in the *New England Journal of Medicine* showing that Americans who eat more fish have higher levels of the metal in their bodies (more specifically, in their toenails), although they don't believe the levels cause harm. No one is recommending routine mercury testing. But the contaminant does seem to pose a damned-if-you-do, damned-if-you-don't problem for people who want to eat a lot of fish for health reasons. Mercury tends to accumulate in the food chain: the higher on the chain, the greater the concentration of mercury. But species rich in omega-3 fats also tend to be the food chain's higher-ups, including swordfish, mackerel, and tuna.

The FDA is correct to take a better-safe-than-sorry approach to mercury in fish. But consider the risks and benefits. The amount of mercury you're exposed to by occasionally eating swordfish and mackerel is very small. Besides, you have other choices. Salmon, for example, is high in omega-3s and so far has tested very low for mercury. Smaller tuna are used for canning, so apart from all that mayonnaise, eating a tunafish sandwich, a couple times per week isn't a major hazard.

In November 2002, the American Heart Association re-emphasized its recommendation that all adults should eat at least two servings of fish per week because of the cardiovascular benefits. The association takes the position that for adult men and older women not having children, any risk from mercury is offset by the advantages.

So you can have your fish and enjoy it, too. Eating fish remains one of the better health bets out there.

Excerpted from the January 2003 issue of the *Harvard Health Letter* Copyright © 2003, President and Fellows of Harvard College. www.health.harvard.edu

Ensuring the Safety of Dietary Supplements

Michelle Meadows

When taken appropriately, some dietary supplements have clear benefits. Folic acid lowers the risk of some birth defects. Calcium supplements can strengthen bones and help prevent osteoporosis. But some dietary supplements pose health risks. They may be improperly manufactured or handled, or their ingredients may cause harmful effects on the body.

Under the Dietary Supplement Health and Education Act of 1994 (DSHEA), dietary supplements are regulated like foods. Unlike new drugs, dietary supplements don't generally have to go through review by the Food and Drug Administration for safety and effectiveness or be "approved" before they can be marketed. But manufacturers must provide premarket notice and evidence of safety for any supplements they plan to sell that contain dietary ingredients that were not on the market before DSHEA was passed.

The FDA evaluates the safety of dietary supplements after they are on the market primarily through research and adverse event monitoring. Those who market and make dietary supplements are responsible for ensuring that any claims are substantiated with adequate evidence, and they cannot claim that the dietary supplements will treat or cure any disease.

Monitoring Industry

The dietary supplement industry has changed a lot in the last decade. When DSHEA was passed, there were about 4,000 dietary supplements on the market. Now there are about 29,000 on the market, with another 1,000 new products introduced each year, according to a recent Institute of Medicine report that was sponsored by the FDA. "We have seen a huge growth in the industry over the last 10 years, including the introduction of products that seem far removed from the vitamins and minerals of the pre-DSHEA days," says Dr. Lester M. Crawford, Acting FDA Commissioner. "Unlike most foods, some dietary supplements are pharmacologically active." When a substance is pharmacologically active, it can cause changes in the body. Such a substance could be toxic on its own or cause dangerous interactions with over-the-counter or prescription drugs.

The FDA is developing regulations on the standards for manufacturing and handling dietary supplements.

Ephedra, which was often marketed for weight control and improved energy, was linked to cardiovascular problems, such as increased blood pressure and irregular heart rhythm. In the first formal action to stop the sale of a dietary supplement since DSHEA was passed, the FDA banned ephedra last year. "This is an example of how we can get a dietary supplement off the market if we have solid scientific proof that it does more harm than good," Crawford says.

The dietary supplement industry has changed a lot in the last decade.

Manufacturers and retailers can make claims about the impact of dietary supplements on the structure or function of the body, but these claims must be truthful. An example of such a claim is "calcium builds strong bones." The FDA plans to issue guidance for what data substantiates these types of claims. The agency has worked closely with the Federal Trade Commission to aggressively enforce the law against dietary supplements that are labeled with fraudulent health claims. In April 2004, the FDA sent warning letters to 16 firms, asking them to stop making false claims for weight loss.

From November 2003 to April 2004, the FDA inspected 180 domestic dietary supplement manufacturers, sent 119 warning letters to dietary supplement distributors, refused entry to 1,171 foreign shipments of dietary supplements, and seized or supervised the voluntary destruction of almost $18 million worth of mislabeled or adulterated dietary supplement products.

In March 2004, the FDA requested that 23 companies stop distributing dietary supplements containing androstenedione, also known as "andro." Widely marketed to athletes and body builders, androstenedione has been touted as a way to increase muscle growth and reduce fat. However, it acts like a steroid in the body and increases the risk of serious diseases. For example, women who use these products may be at increased risk for breast cancer and endometrial cancer. Children who use these products are at risk of early onset of puberty and of premature cessation of bone growth.

Additionally, the FDA is developing regulations for industry on good manufacturing practices (GMPs) for dietary supplements. When finalized, the rule will set standards for the manufacturing and handling of dietary supplements to ensure that consumers are provided with high-quality dietary supplements.

"The GMP regulation is the linchpin for properly regulating dietary supplements," Crawford says. "It gives FDA benchmarks for regulating dietary supplements and it gives clear instructions to the industry on how to manufacture products that meet rigorous quality standards."

Continuing Research

Crawford says that these initiatives are an important part of the agency's science-based approach to regulating dietary supplements. He also notes that the FDA was pleased to welcome Barbara O. Schneeman, Ph.D., as the new director of the Office of Nutritional Products, Labeling, and Dietary Supplements, part of the FDA's Center for Food Safety and Applied Nutrition. Schneeman has an extensive background in nutrition science and has served on the faculty of the University of California, Davis, since 1976.

The FDA continues to collaborate with federal research partners at the National Institutes of Health and other organizations to gather evidence about the safety and effectiveness of dietary supplements. "In evaluating dietary supplements, we look at scientific infor-

mation from a range of sources," Crawford says, "including published research, evidence-based reports, and data about the pharmacology or toxicology of a compound." Crawford notes that the agency has particular interest in gathering safety data about certain dietary supplements suspected to pose human health risks, including:

- an ephedra substitute called *Citrus aurantium*, also known as bitter orange, which may present health risks similar to ephedra

- usnic acid, marketed for weight loss and linked to liver damage

- kava, a botanical ingredient that has caused liver failure

- pyrrolizidine alkaloids, which are found in some plants and have been shown to have toxic effects that can cause liver damage.

The FDA recommends that consumers talk with a health care provider before using a dietary supplement. People who think they have been harmed by a dietary supplement should contact their health providers, and also report it to the FDA's MedWatch program by calling (800) FDA-1088 (332-1088), or visiting *www.fda.gov/medwatch/*.

From *FDA Consumer*, July/August 2004. Published by U.S. Food and Drug Administration.

UNIT 7

World Hunger and Malnutrition

Unit Selections

Key Points to Consider

- How extensive is global hunger and malnutrition?

- What is the role of global food companies to world hunger and malnutrition?

- Offer several solutions to decreasing or eliminating food insecurity and malnutrition.

- What sort of role will genetically modified food have in feeding people in developing countries?

DUSHKIN ONLINE **Links: www.dushkin.com/online/**
These sites are annotated in the World Wide Web pages.

Population Reference Bureau
http://www.prb.org
World Health Organization (WHO)
http://www.who.int/en/
WWW Virtual Library: Demography & Population Studies
http://demography.anu.edu.au/VirtualLibrary/

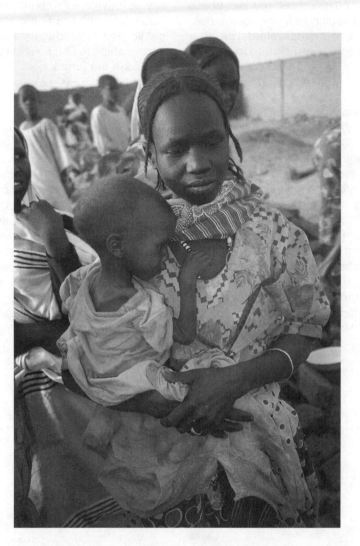

The cause of malnutrition worldwide is poverty. The United Nations Food and Agriculture Organization (FAO) determined that a body mass index (BMI) (body weight divided by the square root of height) of 18.5 is indicative of chronic energy deficit in adults. Approximately 840 million people are malnourished in the developing world; Asia has the largest number and children under 5 years of age that are the most susceptible. Infectious disease kills approximately 10 million children each year. Thus, in 1994 the director general of FAO launched, a special Programme for Food Security (SPFS) for low-income, food-deficit countries (LIFDCs), which was endorsed by the World Food Summit held in Rome in 1996. They pledged to increase food production and access to food in LIFDCs so that the number of malnourished people would be reduced by half. They set goals to increase sustainable agricultural production within the cultural, political, and economic millieu of the country to improve access to food, increase the role of trade, and to deal effectively with food emergencies.

Malnutrition is also the main culprit for lowered resistance to disease, infection, and death—especially in children. The malnutrition-infection combination results in stunted growth, lowered mental development in children, lowered productivity, and higher incidence of degenerative disease in adulthood. This directly affects the economies of developing countries. Globally, over one billion people suffer from micronutrient malnutrition frequently called "hidden hunger." Additionally, partnerships between the public and private sectors may prove valuable in combating malnutrition. Solutions to these problems may combat hunger and nutrient deficiencies. Some solutions include building sustainability through Indigenous knowledge and practices—that are community based and environmentally friendly such as biofortification and dietary diversification.

Nutrient deficiencies magnify the effect of disease and result in more severe symptoms and greater complications of the disease. For example, vitamin A deficiency leads to blindness in about 250,000-300,000 children annually—and exacerbates the symptoms of measles. Iron deficiency, which is widespread among pregnant women and those in the child-bearing years in developing countries, increases the risk of death from hemorrhage in their offspring and reduces physical productivity and learning capacity. Finally, iodine deficiency causes brain damage and mental retardation. It is estimated that 1.5 billion people are at risk for iodine deficiency disorders.

Malnutrition affects children and adults in developing countries and in this country. Thirty million Americans (11 million are children), experience food insecurity and hunger. In a country where one-fifth of the food is wasted and 130 pounds of food per person is disposed of, it is unacceptable that Americans go hungry. The primary nutrient deficiencies in this country, as in developing countries, are iron deficiency anemia, (common in infants, young children, and teens), and lead poisoning. Undernourished pregnant women give birth to low-weight babies who suffer developmental delays and increases in mortality rate. Another group in the United States that experiences health problems due to hunger is the elderly. Many charities and relief funds are working together to alleviate hunger in America.

A recent paradox some of the poorest countries are facing along with food insecurity and malnutrition—is obesity and malnutrition. The World Health Organization in their recent report on "Diet, Nutrition and the Prevention of Chronic Disease" questions the role and contribution of global food companies on the increasing incidence of obesity in developing countries. The creation of the Mega Country Health Promotion Network by the WHO, to identify public health strategies that involve public and private partnerships to find solutions to the obesity problem, is expected in the future.

Biotechnologists believe that genetically modified (GM) foods such as rice that is fortified with beta-carotene and iron may help feed the world, and eradicate nutritional deficiencies. Additionally, GM foods may decrease damage to crops from pests, viruses, bacteria, and drought. Yet it seems too good to be true. If farmers cannot afford to grow GM crops or afford to buy the food, if the infrastructure for transport and distribution is not available, the products may never reach the consumers. Since the safety of humans and the efficacy for the environment of GM crops has not been adequately studied, many scientists and consumers believe that genetic engineering is by no means the panacea for hunger. The potential of GM foods to cause allergies is real. It is so real, that the E.P.A. gathered scientists from universities and government laboratories in workshops to discuss strategies in assessing the allergenic potential of GM foods. The debate of the health risks of GM foods and the need for labeling will rage for years to come.

Undernourishment around the world

Hunger and mortality

MILLIONS OF PEOPLE, including 6 million children under the age of five, die each year as a result of hunger. Of these millions, relatively few are the victims of famines that attract headlines, video crews and emergency aid. Far more die unnoticed, killed by the effects of chronic hunger and malnutrition, a "covert famine" that stunts their development, saps their strength and cripples their immune systems.

Where prevalence of hunger is high, mortality rates for infants and children under five are also high, and life expectancy is low (see map and graphs). In the worst affected countries, a newborn child can look forward to an average of barely 38 years of healthy life (compared to over 70 years of life in "full health" in 24 wealthy nations). One in seven children born in the countries where hunger is most common will die before reaching the age of five.

Not all of these shortened lives can be attributed to the effects of hunger, of course. Many other factors combine with hunger and malnutrition to sentence tens of millions of people to an early death. The HIV/AIDS pandemic, which is ravaging many of the same countries where hunger is most widespread, has reduced average life expectancy across all of sub-Saharan Africa by nearly five years for women and 2.5 years for men.

Even after compensating for the impact of HIV/AIDS and other factors, however, the correlation between chronic hunger and higher mortality rates remains striking. Numerous studies suggest that it is far from coincidental. Since the early 1990s, a series of analyses have confirmed that between 50 and 60 percent of all childhood deaths in the developing world are caused either directly or indirectly by hunger and malnutrition.

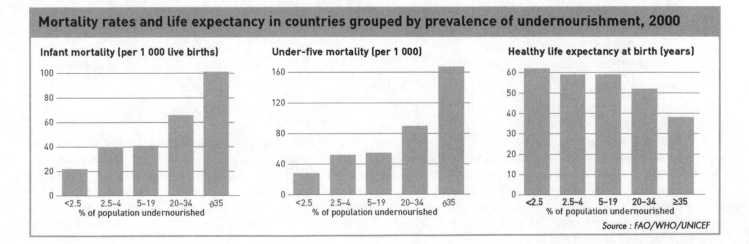

Mortality rates and life expectancy in countries grouped by prevalence of undernourishment, 2000

Infant mortality (per 1 000 live births) | Under-five mortality (per 1 000) | Healthy life expectancy at birth (years)

Source : FAO/WHO/UNICEF

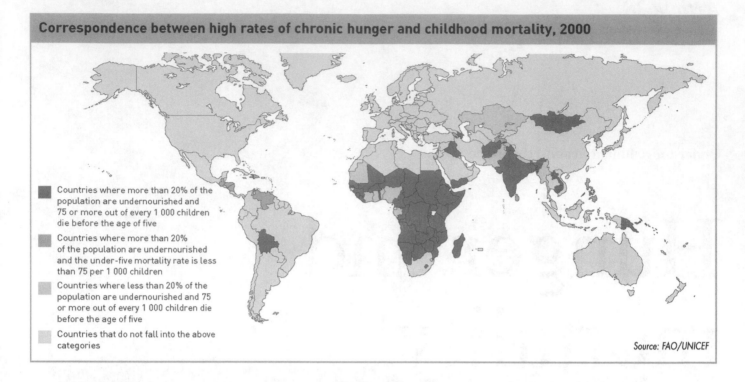

Correspondence between high rates of chronic hunger and childhood mortality, 2000

Countries where more than 20% of the population are undernourished and 75 or more out of every 1 000 children die before the age of five

Countries where more than 20% of the population are undernourished and the under-five mortality rate is less than 75 per 1 000 children

Countries where less than 20% of the population are undernourished and 75 or more out of every 1 000 children die before the age of five

Countries that do not fall into the above categories

Source: FAO/UNICEF

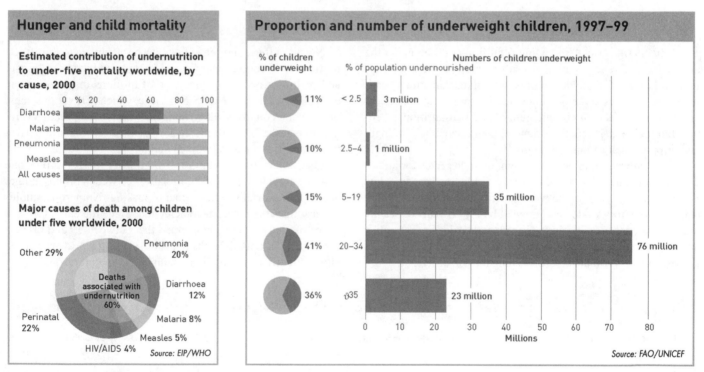

Hunger and child mortality

Estimated contribution of undernutrition to under-five mortality worldwide, by cause, 2000

Diarrhoea
Malaria
Pneumonia
Measles
All causes

Major causes of death among children under five worldwide, 2000

Other 29%
Pneumonia 20%

Deaths associated with undernutrition 60%

Diarrhoea 12%

Perinatal 22%

Malaria 8%

Measles 5%

HIV/AIDS 4%   *Source: EIP/WHO*

Proportion and number of underweight children, 1997–99

% of children underweight

Numbers of children underweight

% of population undernourished

11%   < 2.5   3 million

10%   2.5–4   1 million

15%   5–19   35 million

41%   20–34   76 million

36%   ⩾35   23 million

Millions

Source: FAO/UNICEF

Relatively few of those deaths are the result of starvation. Most are caused by a persistent lack of adequate food intake and essential nutrients that leaves children weak, underweight and vulnerable.

As might be expected, the vast majority of the 153 million underweight children under five in the developing world are concentrated in countries where the prevalence of undernourishment is high (see graph above).

Even mild-to-moderate malnutrition greatly increases the risk of children dying from common childhood diseases. Overall, analysis shows that the risk of death is 2.5 times higher for children with only mild malnutrition than it is for children who are adequately nourished. And the risk increases sharply along with the severity of malnutrition (as measured by their weight-to-age ratio). The risk of death is 4.6 times higher for children suffering from moderate malnutrition and 8.4 times higher for the severely malnourished.

Common diseases often fatal for malnourished children

Infectious diseases are the immediate cause of death for most of the 11 million children under the age of five who die each year in the developing world. But the risk of dying from those diseases is far greater for children who are hungry and malnourished.

The four biggest killers of children are diarrhoea, acute respiratory illness, malaria and measles. Taken together, these four diseases account for almost half of all deaths among children under the age of five. Analysis of data from hospitals and villages shows that all four of these diseases are far more deadly to children who are stunted or underweight.

In the case of diarrhoea, numerous studies show that the risk of death is as much as nine times higher for children who are significantly underweight, the most common indicator of chronic undernutrition. Similarly, underweight children are two to three times more likely to die of malaria and acute respiratory infections, including pneumonia, than well-nourished children.

Lack of dietary diversity and essential minerals and vitamins also contributes to increased child and adult mortality. Iron deficiency anaemia greatly increases the risk of death from malaria, and vitamin A deficiency impairs the immune system, increasing the annual death toll from measles and other diseases by an estimated 1.3–2.5 million children.

Improving nutrition to save lives

The weight of evidence clearly argues that eliminating hunger and malnutrition could save millions of lives each year. That conclusion has been confirmed by a study that examined factors that had helped reduce child mortality during the 1990s. Topping the list were the decline in the proportion of children who were malnourished and lacking access to adequate water, sanitation and housing.

The Scourge of "Hidden Hunger": Global Dimensions of Micronutrient Deficiencies

G. KENNEDY, G. NANTEL AND P. SHETTY

The most recent estimates from FAO indicate that 840 million people do not receive enough energy from their diets to meet their needs. The overwhelming majority of these people—799 million—live in developing countries. The global toll of people affected by micronutrient deficiency is estimated to be even higher and probably exceeds two billion. Micronutrient deficiencies can exist in populations even where the food supply is adequate in terms of meeting energy requirements. In these situations, people are not considered "hungry" in the classical sense, but their diets may be grossly deficient in one or more micronutrients. Blindness and goitre are two of the most visible external manifestations of micronutrient deficiency, and have helped to bring it into the limelight. However, they represent only a fraction of the problem, and subclinical deficiencies afflict a much larger proportion of the population. Today, the consequences of subclinical deficiency are becoming better understood and monitored, but they often go unnoticed within the community in spite of their insidious effects on immune system functioning, growth and cognitive development. It is for these reasons that micronutrient deficiencies have been referred to as "hidden hunger".

Micronutrient deficiencies are most prevalent in areas where the diet lacks variety, as is the case for many individuals in developing countries. When people cannot afford to diversify their diets with adequate amounts of fruits, vegetables or animal-source foods that contain large amounts of micronutrients, deficiencies are inevitable. In addition, a minimum amount of fat or vegetable oil is required in the diet for adequate absorption of the fat-soluble vitamins A, D, E and K.

Grave consequences, including continued and sustained loss of productivity, permanent mental disability, blindness, depressed immune system function and increased infant and maternal mortality can result from micronutrient deficiencies. The heaviest toll from these dietary deficiencies is borne disproportionately by women and children. Death and the disabilities caused by micronutrient deficiencies need not occur, because there are several short- and long-term strategies that can be employed to prevent the development of these deficiencies. Many actions can be undertaken by the communities them selves, once they recognize and understand the problem. This article provides an overview of the global prevalence of micronutrient malnutrition and discusses approaches that may be used to address the situation while emphasizing the role of food-based strategies favoured by FAO.

Global prevalence of hidden hunger

Micronutrients are the essential vitamins and minerals required by human beings to stimulate cellular growth and metabolism. Nineteen vitamins and minerals are considered essential for physical and mental development, immune system functioning and various metabolic processes.[1] Deficiencies of iron, iodine and vitamin A are the most widespread forms of micronutrient malnutrition with public health consequences. Other micronutrients have been shown to play a role in preventing specific disease conditions (e.g. folic acid and calcium) or in promoting growth (e.g. zinc). The global prevalence of zinc and folate deficiency has not yet been established, but it is predicted to be significant, as micronutrient deficiencies rarely occur in isolation. One reason is that deficiencies usually occur when the habitual diet lacks diversity or is overly dependent on a single staple food, as is the case with monotonous cereal- or tuber-based diets (FAO/WHO, 2002). Situations of food insecurity, where populations do not have enough to eat, will also inevitably result in micronutrient deficiency.

Iron, vitamin A and iodine deficiencies are the three micronutrient deficiencies of greatest public health significance in the developing world.

IRON

Iron deficiency anaemia

Anaemia is defined as a reduction in the oxygen-carrying capacity of red blood cells, which occurs as a result either of decreased haemoglobin or of a reduction in the total number of red blood cells (i.e. a decline in red blood cell mass). Iron deficiency is the most common cause of anaemia, although anaemia can also occur as a result of vitamin B_{12} or folate deficiencies, con genital hereditary defects in red cells, reproductive blood losses, or from infection by malarial parasites or infestations of the gut by parasites such as hookworm. The level of haemoglobin in the blood is the most commonly used indicator to screen for iron deficiency anaemia (IDA), and is thus the indicator for which there is the most data worldwide. The true prevalence of iron deficiency in a population, however, will be larger than the level of clinically detectable iron deficiency anaemia (WHO, 2001a), because most individuals are likely to be iron deficient long before there is a detectable drop in blood haemoglobin levels.

When people cannot afford to diversify their diets with adequate amounts of fruits, vegetables or animal-source foods that contain large amounts of micronutrients, deficiencies are inevitable

Nutritional iron deficiency, or habitual iron intake that is insufficient to cover requirements, is the most common cause of iron deficiency (FAO/WHO 2002). Dietary sources of iron are present in two forms, haem and non-haem iron. Haem iron, found in animal-source foods such as meat, poultry and fish, has greater bioavailability than does non-haem iron, found in cereals, pulses, fruits and vegetables. There are many dietary factors that can either inhibit or enhance absorption of non-haem iron. Iron absorption is inhibited by phytate, found in whole grains, seeds, nuts and legumes, and by the phenolic compounds (tannins) present in tea, coffee and red wine. By contrast, iron absorption is enhanced when consumed with ascorbic acid, present in many fruits and vegetables. Iron deficiency becomes more common when an individual's iron requirements are increased owing to physiological demands such as pregnancy, menstrual loss or periods of growth, or when iron is lost because of parasitic infections (hookworm or malaria). As a consequence of these compounding factors, people living in environments prone to infection from malaria and hookworm, and whose habitual diet is high in phytate with few animal-source foods are more likely to become iron deficient.

IDA is considered as a micronutrient deficiency of public health significance not only because it is widespread, with an estimated two billion persons affected worldwide, but also because of its serious consequences in both adults and children. IDA is more prevalent in women than in men, and is also prevalent among children and the elderly. IDA during pregnancy can result in serious consequences for both mother and baby. Iron-deficient women have a higher mortality risk during childbirth and an increased incidence of low-birth-weight babies (WHO, 2002). Figure 1 illustrates the prevalence of IDA in pregnant women. Southeast Asia shows the highest prevalence of anaemia in women, with over 50 percent of pregnant women affected (Mason *et al.*, 2001). In addition to the effects of anaemia during pregnancy, much more is now known of the deleterious effects of anaemia on the cognitive performance, behaviour and physical growth of infants and children of preschool and school age (WHO, 2001a). IDA in adults diminishes their stamina and work capacity by as much as 10-15 percent, and it has been estimated that this deficiency provokes losses in gross domestic product of up to 1.5 percent (FAO, 2002).

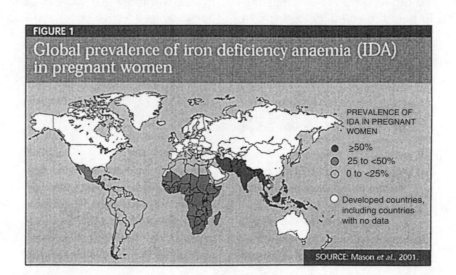

FIGURE 1

Global prevalence of iron deficiency anaemia (IDA) in pregnant women

PREVALENCE OF IDA IN PREGNANT WOMEN

● ≥50%

● 25 to <50%

○ 0 to <25%

○ Developed countries, including countries with no data

SOURCE: Mason *et al.*, 2001.

IODINE

Iodine deficiency

Iodine is an essential mineral required by the body to synthesize thyroid hormones, the most important of which is thyroxine, a metabolism-regulating substance. The iodine content of plant foods is heavily influenced by the presence of iodine in the soil or environment. Seaweed concentrates iodine from seawater and therefore constitutes a rich source of this nutrient. Seaweed and seafood, in general, are good dietary sources of iodine. Eggs, meat, milk and cereals also contain small amounts of iodine. Populations with little access to ocean fish or other marine products, for example persons living in mountainous areas, are the most likely to show iodine deficiencies resulting from a lack of natural dietary sources of iodine.

Clinical iodine deficiency is detected by the presence of goitre (swelling of the thyroid gland). Subclinical iodine deficiency can be detected by measuring urinary iodine or assessing thyroid function. Figure 2 shows the global prevalence of goitre. The latest estimates indicate that 741 million people, or 13 percent of the world's population, are affected by goitre (WHO, 2001b). As with IDA, the true prevalence of iodine deficiency is even more widespread than the numbers of those affected with goitre would seem to indicate; however, there are no global estimates for prevalence of low urinary iodine, which is the best subclinical indicator.

The most devastating consequence of iodine deficiency is reduced mental capacity. Fifty million people worldwide are mentally handicapped as a result of iodine deficiency (WHO, 2002). According to one source, it has been estimated that 100 000 children are born each year with irreversible brain damage because their mothers lacked iodine prior to and during pregnancy (ICCIDD, 2002). Maternal iodine deficiency can also lead to spontaneous abortions, stillbirth and impaired foetal development. In infancy and childhood, this deficiency is manifested by poor mental development and growth defects. Persons living in communities with endemic iodine deficiency may show an intelligence quotient 13.5 points lower than persons from similar communities with adequate iodine supplies (WHO, 2001b). Iodine deficiency is the most preventable cause of brain damage and one of the easiest disorders to prevent: it suffices to add small amounts of iodine to frequently consumed foods such as common table salt.

VITAMIN A

Vitamin A deficiency

Vitamin A is required by all body tissues for normal growth and tissue repair. The visual and immune systems are particularly dependent upon this vitamin for normal functioning. Vitamin A in the form of retinol is present in a variety of foods including eggs, milk and fish, or in its precursor form as carotene in yellow fruits and vegetables, green leafy vegetables and red palm oil. Retinol forms of vitamin A are more readily absorbed by the body than carotene, although the bioavailability of carotene can be enhanced by consuming dietary sources of fat at the same time. The efficiency in converting carotene (and other carotenoids) into the active form of the vitamin is now thought to be considerably poorer than previously assumed; this topic is currently an active area of investigation.

Blindness resulting from vitamin A deficiency (VAD) has been largely responsible for sensitizing communities and raising international awareness of the devastating consequences of this deficiency. VAD is still the leading cause of preventable blindness in children. However, clinical forms of the deficiency are now becoming less frequent, and detection of subclinical deficiency is gaining

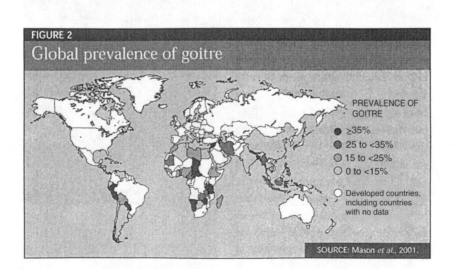

FIGURE 2
Global prevalence of goitre

PREVALENCE OF GOITRE

● ≥35%
● 25 to <35%
○ 15 to <25%
○ 0 to <15%
○ Developed countries, including countries with no data

SOURCE: Mason *et al.*, 2001.

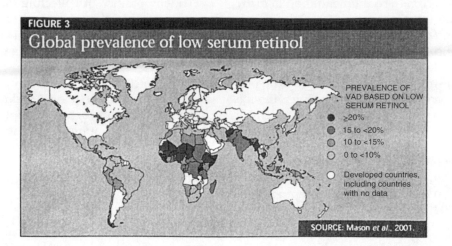

FIGURE 3

Global prevalence of low serum retinol

PREVALENCE OF VAD BASED ON LOW SERUM RETINOL

● ≥20%
● 15 to <20%
○ 10 to <15%
○ 0 to <10%

○ Developed countries, including countries with no data

SOURCE: Mason *et al.*, 2001.

more importance (Mason *et al.*, 2001). Optimal vitamin A status is necessary for the immune system to function normally. Subclinical deficiency has been linked to increased childhood illness and death. It is estimated that improving the vitamin A status of children would decrease overall child mortality rates by 25 percent, measles death rates by 50 percent and death caused by diarrhoea by 40 percent (UNICEF, 2002).

Previously, the most common indicators used to assess VAD were clinical signs affecting the eye. Collectively known as xerophthalmia, these range from relatively mild, reversible conditions to permanent blindness as a result of keratomalacia (irreversible corneal damage). Subclinical deficiency can be detected through measurement of serum retinol. This indicator can be used to identify populations at risk from increased morbidity and mortality and can also be used to classify the severity of the problem. The World Health Organization (WHO) recommends that VAD be regarded as a severe public health problem in populations where more than 20 percent of the children have serum retinol levels equal to or lower than 0.7 mmol/l (WHO, 1996). Figure 3 shows the global prevalence of low serum retinol.

Other micronutrients

Deficiencies of the micronutrients vitamin A, iron and iodine are those considered to be of the greatest public health significance. However, much more is now being discovered about the vital role of other important nutrients for growth, development, immune system functioning and prevention of birth defects; zinc and folate are two of these.

Zinc. Global attention to zinc deficiency has accelerated rapidly over the past 15 years. However, there is still no information about the prevalence of this deficiency, although it is assumed to be widespread in areas lacking dietary diversity. Zinc is an essential component in over 300 enzymes needed by the body for metabolism (FAO/WHO, 2002). The best dietary sources of zinc are meat, particularly organ meats, and shellfish, while eggs and dairy products are also relatively good sources of zinc. The bioavailability of zinc is inhibited by phytate, which is present in large amounts in cereals and legumes. Thus people whose diet contains only minor amounts of animal-source foods (including dairy products), with large amounts of staple grains and pulses, will be at greater risk of zinc deficiency. Research is emerging on the role of zinc deficiency and the impact of zinc supplementation on pregnancy outcomes for both mother and foetus, and on the morbidity, growth and neuro-behavioural development of children. The clearest indicator of zinc deficiency is stunted child growth; there is evidence that zinc supplementation can improve the growth of stunted children (Brown and Wuehler, 2000). Some benefits in relation to incidence and prevalence of diarrhoea have also been noted with zinc supplementation. Evidence linking zinc to improvement in pregnancy outcomes and cognitive development of children is not strong, and more research is needed in these areas (Brown and Wuehler, 2000). Most importantly, there is a need to develop simple low-cost methods for assessing the zinc status of individuals so that a better assessment of the global prevalence of zinc deficiency can be conducted.

Folate. Folate is required for the synthesis of nucleic acids. Deficiency can arise from insufficient dietary intake as well as malabsorption resulting from gastrointestinal disorders and secondary deficiencies of B_6 and B_{12}, or iron (Stover and Garza, 2002). Liver is considered to be the richest source of this nutrient; folate is also present in a variety of vegetables. Folate has received considerable attention for its role in the prevention of foetal neural tube defect, a condition associated with inadequate folate stores in early pregnancy. Thus folate status before conception and during early pregnancy has become the focus of much of the discussion on this nutrient. There is increased risk of foetal neural tube defects if the folate status of pregnant women shifts from adequate to poor (FAO/WHO, 2002). It is for this reason that folate supplementation for women planning a pregnancy and during the first trimester has become a recommendation in many countries. An important distinction to note with folate is that recommendations during early conception are designed to prevent deficiency and are recommended even for people whose folate status is considered adequate. The supplementation strategy in this case focuses on prevention rather than correction of problems. Even though there has not been a large effort to determine the global prevalence of folate deficiency, the FAO/WHO Expert Consultation on Human Vitamin and Mineral Requirements has recommended that further investigation be conducted into the relationship between folate deficiency and incidence of neural tube defects in developing countries (FAO/WHO, 2002).

Progress in controlling micronutrient deficiencies

Micronutrient deficiencies remain a significant global public health concern. Although scientific knowledge is sufficient to solve the problems of micronutrient deficiencies, operational impediments prevent the implementation of solutions. Impediments include lack of political commitment and poor use of resources (Underwood, 1999). A recent report by the Micronutrient Initiative undertook a thorough analysis of trends in the prevalence of the three major deficiencies. This analysis revealed reductions in the prevalence of clinical VAD and significant improvements in goitre rate in countries with substantial iodization programmes, such as Bolivia, Cameroon, Peru and Thailand but virtually no progress in the control of IDA (Mason et al., 2001). However, it is equally important to note the difficulties encountered in estimating the global reduction of micronutrient deficiencies, owing to underestimation in past evaluations, lack of comparable information from one survey to another and improved detection skills in recent surveys (WHO, 2001b; Hunt and Quibria, 1999; Mason et al., 2001).

The importance of collecting data on subclinical and process indicators is becoming increasingly evident. Table 1 provides a list of clinical, subclinical and process (or programmatic) indicators for vitamin A, iron and iodine deficiencies. Process indicators are being increasingly utilized to detect programmatic improvements in control strategies, and are frequently included in nationally representative surveys such as multiple cluster indicator surveys or demographic and health surveys. When systematically collected, these indicators can also be used to demonstrate progress and are often easier to collect than clinical and subclinical indicators.

Innovative and multisectoral approaches to controlling micronutrient deficiencies have contributed to observed improvement in the global situation. One of the more successful recent strategies in the control of VAD has been to link the distribution of vitamin A capsules to national immunization days. The United Nations Children's Fund (UNICEF) estimates that 11 countries had vitamin A supplementation coverage rates of 70 percent or more for the targeted population of children under five years of age in 1996, and by 1999, 43 countries had reached this level of coverage (UNICEF, 2001). In the case of iodine deficiency, an estimated 72 percent of households in developing countries now use iodized salt, compared to 20 percent a decade ago (UNICEF, 2001).

Strategies to address micronutrient malnutrition

Three of the main strategies for addressing micronutrient malnutrition are dietary diversification, fortification (including biofortification) and supplementation. Most micronutrient deficiencies can be effectively addressed through dietary diversification. Fortification strategies are needed in areas where the traditional diet lacks a specific nutrient, such as iodine. Food-based approaches to

TABLE 1

Examples of indicators commonly used to detect vitamin A, iron and iodine deficiencies

TYPE OF INDICATOR	DEFICIENT MICRONUTRIENT		
	Vitamin A	Iron	Iodine
Clinical	Xerophthalmia and Bitot's spots	Haemoglobin, haematocrit	Goitre, visible or palpable
Subclinical	Serum retinol	Serum ferritin	Urinary iodine
Process/ Programmatic	Percentage of preschool children receiving vitamin A capsules	Percentage of households consuming adequately iodized salt	Percentage of pregnant women receiving iron supplementation

fulfilling micronutrient requirements have received strong support as a sustainable means of meeting the nutritional needs of population groups (WHO/FAO, 1996; FAO/WHO, 2002). These strategies are discussed in more detail below.

Supplementation

Supplementation is a technical approach in which nutrients are delivered directly by means of syrup or pills. Supplementation is most appropriate for targeted populations with a high risk of deficiency or under special circumstances, such as during pregnancy or in an acute food shortage. Under normal circumstances, supplementation programmes are used only as a short-term measure and are then replaced with long-term, sustainable food-based measures such as fortification and dietary modification, usually by increasing food diversity.

Fortification

Fortification strategies utilize widely accessible, commonly consumed foods to deliver one or more micronutrients. The most widespread effort to date has been fortification of salt with iodine. However, many other foods may be used as vehicles for a variety of micronutrients. Some of the more common combinations are wheat products (cereal, bread or pasta) with one or more nutrients including calcium, iron, niacin, riboflavin, thiamine and zinc. Milk can be fortified with vitamin D; fruit and fruit juices have been fortified with calcium and vitamin C. Fish sauce and soy sauce are also recognized as good fortification vehicles, and trials are under way to determine the efficacy of these foods as fortification tools (Mannar and Gallego, 2002; Chen, 2003).

Successful employment of fortification strategies requires centralized processing facilities, mechanisms for quality control, and social marketing and public education strategies (Nantel and Tontisirin, 2002; Uauy *et al.*, 2002). The required infrastructure is often weak or lacking in developing countries, which reduces the potential for the success of fortification measures. Adequate income and marketing channels are essential if these strategies are to succeed, but the poor and nutritionally vulnerable are frequently less able to purchase fortified food products. Moreover, infrastructure, including roads and transportation systems, is weak in many developing countries. In order for fortification programmes to be successful, these issues need to be addressed, particularly in rural and remote areas, where the majority of the populations at high risk live.

Biofortification

Consumption of a wide variety of foods, including those that contain an array of micronutrients, is still seen as the best long-term sustainable solution to eradicate hidden hunger. Along the path to achieving this goal, biofortification may help to improve the health and welfare of many populations. Biofortification, or plant breeding for the specific purpose of enhancing the nutritional properties of crop varieties, reflects the new application of an ancient technique. For centuries, farmers have bred crops to enhance specific traits such as improved yield, drought tolerance or insect resistance. Recently, breeding trials have been undertaken for the specific purpose of enhancing the nutritional value of crops with the specific objective of improving human nutrition. Gene-marking techniques make it possible for scientists to identify the specific plant genetic material that controls nutrient content so as to select the most beneficial ones for breeding purposes. Using genes that contain nutritionally superior traits has enabled scientists to produce crop varieties with higher nutrient content. There have been some reported successes, including high-protein maize, high-carotene sweet potato and cassava, and iron-enhanced rice (IFPRI, 2002).

Dietary diversification

Dietary diversity can be augmented by expanding the production, processing, marketing and consumption of a wide variety of foods. In treating the problem of micronutrient deficiencies, food-based approaches that focus on improving overall dietary quality, rather than merely delivering a single nutrient, are particularly useful. Several factors lend support to this approach. First, there are complex nutrient-nutrient interactions that increase bioavailability when nutrients are consumed simultaneously. For example, iron absorption is increased when it is combined with vitamin C (FAO, 1997). New evidence about the protective role of phytochemicals and antioxidants continues to emerge. These protective chemicals are easily obtained by consuming a wide variety of fruits and vegetables. Scientific knowledge linking nutrition and disease continues to evolve and expand, implicating an even wider range of nutrients with a variety of roles in health maintenance. Rickets, a disease associated with vitamin D deficiency, has now been connected to diets low in calcium. Demonstrating the existence of dependent relationships heightens the importance of promoting food-based approaches that focus on achieving sustained improvements in the overall diet.

There are several low-cost, food-based measures that can be promoted at the community level to improve micro nutrient status, some of which are presented in Box 1. Culturally appropriate dietary modifications should be developed to help people identify con crete actions that can improve both dietary supply and the absorption of micronutrients. This information needs to be disseminated to the public through traditional information channels.

BOX 1
Community-based strategies to improve micronutrient status

- Encouraging exclusive breastfeeding up to six months of age and continued breastfeeding for older infants
- Identifying and promoting use of culturally appropriate weaning foods rich in micronutrients
- Identifying and promoting use of traditional green leafy vegetables and fruits to add diversity to the diet
- Preserving micronutrients in fruits and vegetables by using solar drying or canning technologies
- Promoting small-scale community gardens
- Rearing small livestock
- Improving year-round supply of micronutrient rich foods

SOURCE: Adapted from FAO/ILSI (1997).

Factors for success: increased collaboration and political commitment

Developing communities face multiple problems. Therefore focusing on a single micronutrient deficiency or on a single strategy is not the most effective means to eliminate micronutrient deficiencies. The problems often result from a wider set of factors including health care, education, sanitation, water supply and housing (Nantel and Tontisirin, 2002). Complementary public health interventions that can help reduce micro nutrient mal nutrition include deworming, malaria prophylaxis, improved water and sanitation facilities and childhood immunization. Successful strategies are those that address all these issues in an integrated and coordinated fashion. Holistic strategies, using a mixture of direct and indirect interventions and public health measures, as well as education and awareness campaigns, have proved to be the most successful in reducing micronutrient malnutrition (Under wood, 1999). Communities themselves are best suited to determine which corrective actions to employ to address their problems. Collecting process indicators at this level can help direct community actions. The role of government and government counter parts is to support these actions through political commitment, training and the provision of basic services, including attention to micronutrients.

References

Brown, K. & Wuehler, S., eds. 2000. *Zinc and human health*. Ottawa, Micronutrient Initiative.

Chen, Chunming. 2003. Iron fortification of soy sauce in China. *Food, Nutrition and Agriculture*, 32, pp. 76–82.

FAO. 1997. *Human nutrition in the developing world*, by M. Latham. Rome.

FAO. 2002. *State of Food Insecurity in the World 2002*. Rome.

FAO/ILSI (International Life Sciences Institute). 1997. *Preventing micronutrient malnutrition: a guide to food-based approaches. A manual for policy makers and programme planners*. Rome/Washington, DC, FAO/ILSI.

FAO/WHO. 2002. *Human vitamin and mineral requirements*. Report of a joint FAO/WHO expert consultation. Rome.

Hunt, J. & Quibria, M., eds. 1999. *Investing in child nutrition in Asia*. Manila, Asian Development Bank.

ICCIDD (International Council for the Control of Iodine Deficiency Disorder). 2002. IDD fact card. New Orleans, ICCIDD Communications Focal Point, Tulane University School of Public Health and Tropical Medicine (available at www.tulane.edu/~icec/aboutidd.htm; accessed end May 2003).

International Food Policy Research Institute (IFPRI). 2002. *Biofortification: harnessing agricultural technology to improve the health of the poor* (available at www.ifpri.org/themes/grp06/papers/biofort.pdf; accessed end May 2003).

Mannar, V. & Gallego, E. 2002. Iron fortification: Country level experiences and lessons learned. *J. Nutr.*, 132: 856S–858S.

Mason, J.B., Lotfi, M., Dalmiya, N., Sethuraman, K., & Deitchler, M.; with Geibel, S., Gillenwater, K., Gilman, A., Mason, K. & Mock, N. 2001. *The micronutrient report: current progress in the control of vitamin A, iodine, and iron deficiencies*. Ottowa, Micronutrient Initiative/International Development Research Center (available at http://www.micronutrient.org/frame_HTML/resource_text/publications/mn_report.pdf; accessed end May 2003).

Nantel, G. & Tontisirin, K. 2002. Policy and sustainability issues. *J. Nutr.*, 132: 839S–844S.

Stover, P. & Garza, C. 2002. Bringing individuality to public health recommendations. *J. Nutr.*, 132: 2476S–2480S.

Uauy, R., Hertrampf, E. & Reddy, M. 2002. Iron fortification of foods: Overcoming technical and practical barriers. *J. Nutr.*, 132: 849S–852S.

Underwood, B. 1999. Perspectives from micronutrient malnutrition elimination/eradication programmes. *MMWR—Morbidity and Mortality Weekly Report*, 48: 37–42.

United Nations Children's Fund (UNICEF). 2001. *Review of the achievements in the implementation and results of the World Declaration on the Survival, Protection and Development of Children and Plan of Action for Implementing the World Declaration on the Survival, Protection and Development of Children in the 1990s*. Report of the Secretary General to the United Nations General Assembly, 27th Special Session. New York.

UNICEF. 2002. *Vitamin A global initiative* (available at www.unicef.org/vitamina; accessed end May 2003).

USAID (The United States Agency for International Development). 1992. *Economic rationale for investing in micronutrient programs: A policy brief based on new analyses*. Washington, DC, United States Agency for International Development, Bureau for Research and Development, Office of Nutrition, Vitamin A Field Support Project.

WHO (World Health Organization). 1996. *Indicators for assessing vitamin A deficiency and their application in monitoring and evaluating intervention programmes*. WHO/NUT/96.10. Geneva.

WHO. 2001a. *Iron deficiency anaemia: Assessment, prevention and control—a guide for programme managers*. Geneva.

WHO. 2001b. *Assessment of iodine deficiency disorders and monitoring their elimination—a guide for programme managers*. Second edition. Geneva.

WHO. 2002. Turning the tide of malnutrition, responding to the challenge of the 21st century (available at www.who.int/nut/documents/nhd_brochure.pdf; accessed end May 2003).

WHO/FAO. 1996. *Preparation and use of food-based dietary guidelines*. Geneva.

Note

[1]Vitamins A, B4, B12, C, D, E and K; thiamine, riboflavin, niacin, pantothenic acid and biotin, folate and folic acid, calcium, iodine, iron, magnesium and zinc.

Gina Kennedy is a Consultant in the Nutrition Planning, Assessment and Evaluation Service (ESNA) at FAO, Guy Nantel is a Senior Officer, ESNA and Prakash Shetty is Chief of ESNA.

From *Food Nutrition and Agriculture*, 2003.

Undernourishment around the world

Undernourishment, poverty and development

THE WORLD FOOD SUMMIT (WFS) in 1996 set the goal—to reduce the number of hungry people in the world by half before the year 2015. Four years later, that goal was echoed in the first of the Millennium Development Goals (MDGs), which set targets of reducing by half both the proportion of people who suffer from hunger and the proportion living on less than US$1 per day.

These targets are closely related; neither can be achieved without the other, and achieving both is essential to success in reaching the rest of the MDGs.

Poverty and hunger—mutual causes, devastating effects

Measures of food deprivation, nutrition and poverty are strongly correlated (see graphs). Countries with a high prevalence of undernourishment also have high prevalences of stunted and underweight children. In these countries, a high percentage of the population lives in conditions of extreme poverty. In countries where a high proportion of the population is undernourished, a comparably high proportion struggles to survive on less than US$1 per day.

Undernourishment, poverty and indicators for other Millennium Development Goals: 1995–2000

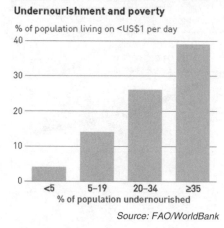

Undernourishment and poverty

% of population living on <US$1 per day

x-axis: % of population undernourished (<5, 5–19, 20–34, ≥35)

Source: FAO/WorldBank

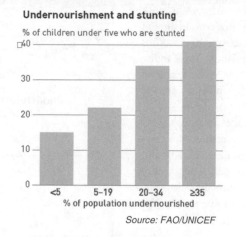

Undernourishment and stunting

% of children under five who are stunted

x-axis: % of population undernourished (<5, 5–19, 20–34, ≥35)

Source: FAO/UNICEF

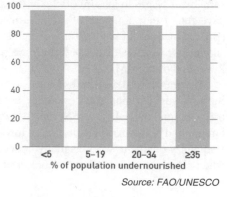

Undernourishment and female schooling

Ratio of girls attending primary school as % of ratio of boys

x-axis: % of population undernourished (<5, 5–19, 20–34, ≥35)

Source: FAO/UNESCO

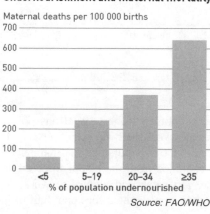

Undernourishment and maternal mortality

Maternal deaths per 100 000 births

x-axis: % of population undernourished (<5, 5–19, 20–34, ≥35)

Source: FAO/WHO

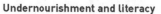

Undernourishment and literacy

Adult literacy rate (%)

x-axis: % of population undernourished (<5, 5–19, 20–34, ≥35)

Source: FAO/WHO

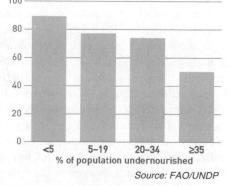

Undernourishment and improved water

% of population with access to improved water

x-axis: % of population undernourished (<5, 5–19, 20–34, ≥35)

Source: FAO/UNDP

Hunger impacts other Millennium Development Goals

Goal	Selected indicators	Impact of hunger
Achieve universal primary education	• net enrollment ratio • literacy rate	• reduces school attendance • impairs cognitive capacity
Promote gender equality	• ratio of girls to boys in primary education	• may reduce school attendance more for girls
Reduce child mortality	• under-five mortality rate	• associated with 60 percent of child deaths
Improve maternal health	• maternal mortality rate	• greatly increases risk of maternal death
Combat HIV/AIDS, malaria and other diseases	• HIV prevalence among pregnant women • death rates associated with malaria	• spurs migratory labour that increases spread of HIV • multiplies child death rates from two- to three-fold
Ensure environmental sustainability	• proportion of land area covered by forest	• leads to unsustainable use of forest lands and resources

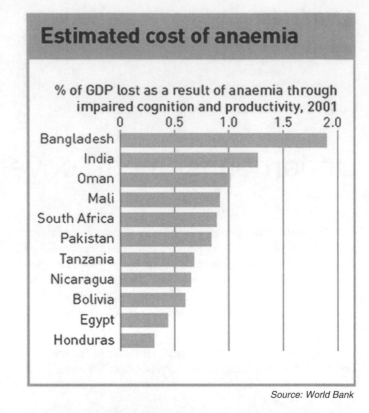

Source: World Bank

While poverty is undoubtedly a cause of hunger, hunger can also be a cause of poverty. Hunger often deprives impoverished people of the one valuable resource they can call their own: the strength and skill to work productively. Numerous studies have confirmed that hunger seriously impairs the ability of the poor to develop their skills and reduces the productivity of their labour.

Hunger in childhood impairs mental and physical growth, crippling the capacity to learn and earn. Evidence from household food surveys in developing countries shows that adults with smaller and slighter body frames caused by undernourishment earn lower wages in jobs involving physical labour. Other studies have found that a 1 percent increase in the Body Mass Index (BMI, a measure of weight for a given height) is associated with an increase of more than 2 percent in wages for those toward the lower end of the BMI range.

Micronutrient deficiencies can also reduce work capacity. Surveys suggest that iron deficiency anaemia reduces productivity of manual labourers by up to 17 percent. As a result, hungry and malnourished adults earn lower wages. And they are frequently unable to work as many hours or years as well-nourished people, as they fall sick more often and have shorter life spans.

Hunger and the poverty of nations

Widespread hunger and malnutrition impair economic performance not only of individuals and families, but of nations. Anaemia alone has been found to reduce GDP by 0.5–1.8 percent in several countries (see graph). Studies in India, Pakistan, Bangladesh and Viet Nam estimated conservatively that the combined effect of stunting, iodine deficiency and iron deficiency reduced GDP by 2 to 4 percent. Recent calculations by FAO suggest that achieving the WFS goal of reducing the number of undernourished people by half by the year 2015 would yield a value of more than US$120 billion. That figure reflects the economic impact of longer, healthier, more productive lives for several hundred million people freed from hunger.

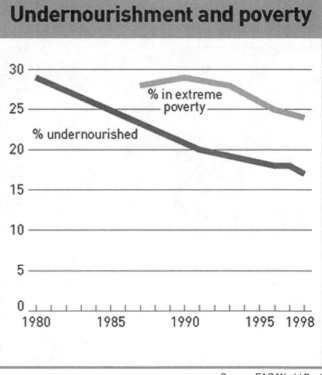

Source: FAO/World Bank

Nobel Prize-winning economist Robert Fogel has pointed out that hungry people cannot work their way out of poverty. He estimates that 20 percent of the population in England and France was effectively excluded from the labour force around 1790 because they were too weak and hungry to work. Improved nutrition, he calculates, accounted for about half of the economic growth in Britain and France between 1790 and 1880. Since many developing countries are as poor as Britain and France were in 1790, his analysis suggests reducing hunger could have a similar impact in developing countries today.

A key to Millennium Development Goals

Evidence clearly shows that failure to eliminate hunger will undermine efforts to reach the other MDGs as well (see box, "Hunger impacts other Millennium Development Goals").

Hopes for achieving universal primary education and literacy, for example, will be thwarted while millions of hungry children suffer from diminished learning capacity or are forced to work instead of attending school. Low birth weight, protein energy malnutrition, iron deficiency anaemia and iodine deficiency are all linked to cognitive deficiencies. Hunger also limits school attendance. In Pakistan, a relatively small improvement in height for age increased school enrolment rates substantially: 2 percent for boys, 10 percent for girls. This steep increase for girls suggests one way in which reducing hunger would also accelerate another of the MDGs—promoting gender equality.

Data and analysis confirm that reducing hunger and malnutrition could have a decisive impact on reducing child mortality, improving maternal health, and on combating HIV/AIDS, malaria and other diseases.

Towards the Summit commitments

Confronting the causes of malnutrition: the hidden challenge of micronutrient deficiencies

OVER 2 BILLION PEOPLE worldwide suffer from micronutrient malnutrition, often called "hidden hunger". Their diets supply inadequate amounts of vitamins and minerals such as vitamin A, iron, iodine, zinc, folate, selenium and vitamin C. Deficiencies usually occur when the habitual diet lacks diversity and does not include sufficient quantities of the fruits, vegetables, dairy products, meat and fish that are the best sources of many micronutrients.

Vitamin A and mortality, 1992

A World Health Organization study concluded that an improved vitamin A nutriture could prevent 1.3 to 2.5 million deaths each year among children aged six months to five years in the developing world.

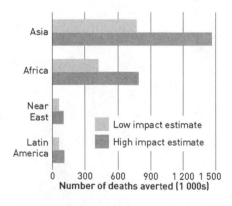

Source: WHO

Micronutrients are essential for human growth and development as well as normal functioning. The three most common forms of micronutrient malnutrition are deficiencies of vitamin A, iodine and iron. In developing countries, deficiencies of micronutrients often are not present in isolation but exist in combination (see map).

Children and women are the most vulnerable to micronutrient deficiencies—children because of the critical importance of micronutrients for normal growth and development, women because of their higher need for iron, especially during childbearing years and pregnancy.

> "We will implement policies aimed at . . . improving . . . access by all, at all times to sufficient, nutritionally adequate and safe food . . ."

Between 100 and 140 million children suffer from vitamin A deficiency. That figure includes more than 2 million children each year afflicted with severe visual problems, of whom an estimated 250 000 to 500 000 are permanently blinded.

Lack of vitamin A also impairs the immune system, greatly increasing the risk of illness and death from common childhood infections such as diarrhoea and measles (see graph).

162

Prevalence of micronutrient deficiencies in developing countries

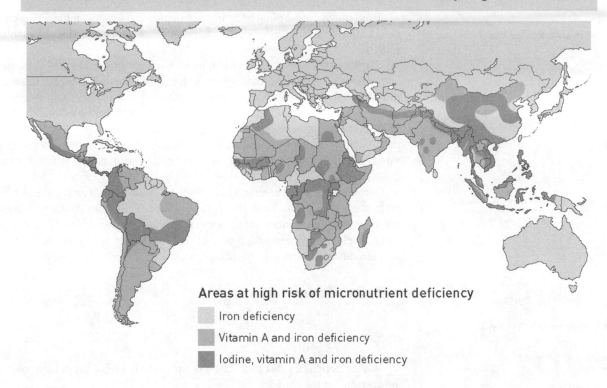

Areas at high risk of micronutrient deficiency

- Iron deficiency
- Vitamin A and iron deficiency
- Iodine, vitamin A and iron deficiency

Source: USAID

Dietary diversification reduces vitamin A deficiency

Home gardens boost consumption of micronutrient-rich food

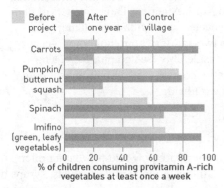

Before project | After one year | Control village

Carrots

Pumpkin/ butternut squash

Spinach

Imifino (green, leafy vegetables)

0 20 40 60 80 100
% of children consuming provitamin A-rich vegetables at least once a week

Source: Faber et al.

A home gardening programme focusing on production and consumption of vegetables rich in vitamin A and its precursor, beta carotene, has been successfully demonstrated by the Medical Research Council of South Africa in a mountainous, rural village in KwaZulu-Natal.

Prior to the programme, the diet of children in the village consisted mainly of maize porridge, bread and rice. The lack of variety and vitamin-rich foods resulted in high incidence of vitamin A deficiency. The programme changed that by promoting cultivation of vegetables, such as carrots, pumpkins and spinach, that are rich in beta carotene and by teaching villagers, especially women, the importance of including them regularly in their diet.

After only one year, the percentage of children consuming vitamin-A rich vegetables had increased significantly. And the increased diversity in their diets led to measurable improvements in vitamin A status.

The most devastating consequence of iodine deficiency is reduced mental capacity. Some 20 million people worldwide are mentally handicapped as a result of iodine deficiency, including 100 000 born each year with irreversible brain damage because their mothers lacked iodine prior to and during pregnancy.

Iron deficiency and the anaemia it causes are the most widespread of all forms of micronutrient malnutrition. Anaemia results in fatigue, dizziness and breathlessness following exertion.

Children with anaemia are less able to concentrate and have less energy for play and exploratory behaviours. In adults, anaemia diminishes work capacity and productivity by as much as 10–15 percent. And for pregnant women, anaemia substantially increases the risk of death in childbirth, accounting for up to 20 percent of maternal deaths in Asia and Africa.

The three main strategies for reducing micronutrient deficiencies are dietary diversity and food fortification along with supplements.

Most micronutrient deficiencies could be eliminated by modifying diets to include a greater diversity of nutrient-rich foods. Promoting home gardens, community fish ponds, and

Biofortification increases nutrient content of staple foods

Varietal differences suggest high biofortification potential for rice

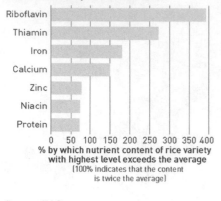

% by which nutrient content of rice variety with highest level exceeds the average
(100% indicates that the content is twice the average)

Source: FAO

Both conventional plant breeding techniques and genetic engineering can be used to develop varieties of staple food crops that are enriched with essential minerals.

"Golden rice" offered proof that biotechnology can produce both nutrients and controversy. Golden rice owes its colour and its name to beta carotene, introduced by transplanting genes from daffodils and bacteria. Critics have charged that the enriched rice will not provide enough beta carotene to satisfy vitamin A requirements. But supporters argue that it could provide 15 to 20 percent of daily requirements and significantly reduce the incidence and severity of vitamin A deficiency, particularly if consumed in conjunction with other nutrient-rich foods.

Conventional plant breeding also holds promise for enhancing the nutrient content of staple foods. Varieties of crops differ considerably in the quantities of nutrients that they contain (see graph). Advances in plant breeding techniques and biotechnology may make it possible to cross varieties that are relatively rich in micronutrients with high-yielding varieties preferred by farmers.

Iodine deficiency disorders

Access to iodized salt, 1995–98

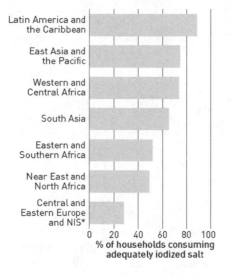

% of households consuming adequately iodized salt

NIS = newly independent states　　　*Source: FAO*

Iodine deficiency disorder (IDD) is particularly prevalent in the mountainous regions of the world.

The areas with the most severe deficiencies include the Himalayas, the Andes, the European Alps and the vast mountains of China. IDD is also common in frequently flooded lowlands. In both mountains and flooded areas, iodine that is naturally present in the soil is leached away, reducing the iodine content in locally grown crops.

Iodization of salt has virtually eliminated IDD in the mountainous regions of industrialized countries in Europe and North America. Three-quarters of the countries in the developing world have enacted legislation for iodizing salt, mostly over the past 15 years. More than two-thirds of households now get adequately iodized salt. But access varies considerably (see graph). Increasing access to iodized salt and improving quality control of its iodine content hold the key to eliminating iodine deficiency worldwide.

livestock and poultry production can contribute to increasing dietary diversity, while improving food supplies and incomes at the same time (see box on dietary diversification).

Another important food-based strategy is food fortification. The most successful of these initiatives is fortification of salt with iodine (see box). Other micronutrients can also be supplied to populations by enriching widely consumed foods such as milk and flour. In addition, recent advances in crop breeding and biotechnology have heightened the prospects for "biofortification"—developing crops with higher concentrations of micronutrients (see box).

Supplementation involves treating and preventing micronutrient deficiencies by administering capsules, tablets, syrups or other preparations. This medical approach is the method of choice when the deficiency is severe and life-threatening or when access to regular intake of the deficient micronutrient is limited. Use of high-dose vitamin A supplements can reduce mortality from acute measles by up to 50 percent.

Successful campaigns to eliminate micronutrient deficiencies often combine all of these strategies. Vitamin A intake, for example, can best be increased over the long term by adding nutrient-rich foods to the diet and fortifying staple foods, while providing supplements to high-risk groups in vulnerable areas.

Food Security, Overweight, and Agricultural Research—A View from 2003

ABSTRACT: Some of the poorest countries of the world are facing an apparent paradox. Food insecurity, undernutrition, and overweight exist side by side within the same country. Indeed, food-insecure households often contain an overweight member. Data from 11 mega-countries (countries with a population of more than 100 million) will be presented to illustrate the magnitude of the problem. These 11 countries represent more than 60% of the world's population. Agriculture is still a dominant industry. The links between food insecurity, nutritional status, and agriculture will be presented.

E. KENNEDY, D.SC.

Introduction

Enormous progress has been made since the 1974 World Food Summit. Dramatic increases in food supplies have occurred, in part due to effective investment in agricultural research. In addition over the past 30 years progress has been made in improving nutrition globally. For example, in developing countries, stunting in preschool-aged children decreased from 47.1% in 1980 to 32.5% in 2000

However, we now have a different dilemma. Increasingly, countries are finding that food insecurity and undernutrition exist side by side with problems of overnutrition and chronic disease.

The purpose of this paper is to examine the links between food security, overweight, and agriculture.

The double burden of disease

The phenomenon of hunger and malnutrition existing in the same countries and the same households with overweight and chronic disease has been labeled "the double burden of disease." World Health Organization (WHO) and the Food and Agriculture Organization of the United Nations (FAO) in 2003 released their report "Diet, Nutrition and the Prevention of Chronic Disease."

The old view of overweight and obesity was that these were problems for middle- and upper-income countries. The new view is that developing countries are increasingly suffering from high levels of overweight and obesity and other chronic diseases. This issue of dramatic rise in overweight and obesity is a message that has not gotten out to many policy makers and implementers in developing countries.

The WHO/FAO report highlights the fact that, in 2001, 60% of all deaths are due to chronic diseases; this represents 46% of the global burden of disease. By 2020, 75% of deaths worldwide are estimated to be due to noncommunicable diseases.

The challenge for international institutions, researchers, and national policy officials is, "How can food and agricultural policy meet the needs of the poor and undernourished while also tackling the problem of overweight and obesity?"

Mega Country Health Promotion Network

Indonesia is but one country that reflects the "double burden of disease"; in Indonesia, 1 out of 10 households has both underweight and overweight in the same family. Rates of overweight have been increasing worldwide. In Brazil, 49% and 45% of men and women, respectively, are overweight in urban areas. The rates in Brazil for overweight in rural areas are somewhat lower. In urban India, 19.9% of women are overweight and in Russia, 30.3% and 50.3% of men and women are overweight.

Thus, in December 2001, WHO created the Mega Country Health Promotion Network. The network includes 11 countries with populations of more than 100 million. These 11 countries represent more than 60% of the world's population. The 11 countries include: China, Japan, Bangladesh, India, Pakistan, Indonesia, Brazil, Mexico, Nigeria, Russia, and the USA. The purpose of this network is to identify public health strategies to decrease the burden of chronic disease including overweight and obesity.

Data from each of the 11 countries indicate that:

(1) There is a continuum in each country going from under-nutrition to over-nutrition. It is no longer an "either/or situation" for under- and over-nutrition. The point on this continuum where each country falls varies.

(2) The poor in each country, increasingly, have a greater risk of overweight and obesity.

(3) Urbanization of the population has brought about changes in diets and physical activity.

In this nutrition transition that is occurring worldwide, urban diets have shifted from basic staples to refined grains and more fats and sugars. There are now increased levels of total fat and saturated fat in the diet. The old view was that increases in fat in the diet were associated with middle and upper income countries and households. The new view is that fat consumption is not linked to national GNP. This pattern globally is similar to what occurred in the USA between the 1950s and 1970s. During this period in the US the dietary patterns of lower- and upper-income households became more similar.

The challenge for the Mega Country Health Promotion Network is to identify newer paradigms and approaches for promoting healthy lifestyles. The essential components of these approaches are:

- Comprehensive—many sectors need to be involved in the solution; no one approach by itself is likely to be successful.
- Each country must select the optimal mix of actions and policies to put in place.
- Public–private partnerships will be an important part of the strategies used.

The first core guiding principle in prevention of overweight and obesity is that Food Security is the foundation to good health and good nutrition. Even where overweight and obesity exists the poor are most at risk of food insecurity.

There has been a marked change globally in how we define and measure food insecurity. It's what some are calling the "newer faces of food security." Food security requires enough food—both quantity and quality—for an active and healthy life—but also that food be obtained in a socially acceptable manner. Therefore, households that need to rely on emergency food supplies—such as soup kitchens—are not food-secure, even where their energy intakes may be adequate.

In addition, international organizations such as the FAO are exploring newer methods for measuring food insecurity. The classic measure of food insecurity, kcals per individual, in the modern environment no longer sufficiently captures food insecurity. At the World Food Summit Plus Five meeting in Rome in June 2002, there was in-depth discussion of the use of qualitative or semi-quantitative measures of food insecurity that allow us to measure on a continuum from food-secure to food-insecure to food-insecure with hunger.

Role of agricultural research

In dealing both with problems of food insecurity/hunger and over-weight/obesity, agricultural research will continue to be essential. There are 4 key areas where the need for agricultural research is essential:

(1) Agricultural research will continue to be essential in increasing food supplies worldwide. All of the projections from FAO for meeting increasing demands for food supplies worldwide are premised on continued investment in agricultural research. Just a word of caution, we cannot be complacent about the support for agricultural research. Even when I was in USDA, we would regularly be asked if the support for agricultural research was still needed, given the overall sufficiency of world food supplies. My answer was an unequivocal, absolutely "yes".

(2) For small-farm households dependent on own farm production, agricultural research will continue to be needed to increase returns to land and returns to labor from agriculture.

(3) A general benefit to society is the low food prices that accrue from successful agricultural production.

(4) Finally, agricultural research through more effective agricultural technologies can help smooth out variations in food production, which can lead to seasonal variations in food prices.

There are other areas where agricultural research can make significant contributions. The potential for agricultural research to provide more nutritious foods at a low cost is enormous. This can be a particularly important role of agricultural research for the poor consumers. For example, lowering the price of fruits and vegetables to consumers would be an important way to improve the micronutrient content of the diet.

There are indirect effects of agricultural research that often are less apparent. Clearly, some farms in developing countries are so small as to be uneconomical. Agricultural research by promoting growth in the agricultural sector would also spur growth in the rural and urban nonfarm economy. The nonfarm economy increasingly will have to provide employment for the very small farmers who will need both farm and nonfarm income to have sufficient income. Of course, the rural poor rely on the nonfarm sector for employment as well as employment as hired labor on farms.

What else?

There are other factors influencing people's lifestyle choices that affect what we call "Healthy Lifestyles". Some of these factors include:

Access—this includes both physical access (are the foods available in the marketplace?) and economic access (can the consumer afford them?).

Culture—what people are used to eating, realizing that culture can change over time and people's preferences are obviously also subject to change over time.

Sedentary Lifestyles—which is a modern phenomenon.

Taste—which does not have to be explained. Changes in physical activity patterns have been changing rapidly throughout the world; this is true in both urban and rural areas, although the changes in relative energy expenditure are greater in the urban areas. Changes in level of energy output are:

Work-related levels of energy expenditure are declining—even in traditional occupations, such as agriculture. I chaired the FAO/WHO/IUNS expert consultation on Energy in Human Nutrition—

the report is soon to be released. Using more precise measures of energy expenditure, we find that for many activities, energy expenditures have been overestimated in the past.

Transportation-related energy expenditures have also changed. Again, this is a phenomenon worldwide. I like to use the personal example of Beijing. When I started going there in the last 1980s, walking was the common mode of transportation, then replaced by bicycles, now being replaced by cars.

Leisure-related activities are also changing to become less energy-intensive.

The combination of less intensive work, transportation, and leisure have meant that many people are consuming more kcals than is needed for energy expenditure. Hence overweight and obesity are increasing.

Policy and research challenges

The challenge for policy makers and research is to identify policies, programs, and approaches that deal with the new lifestyle realities. Consumers worldwide have gotten what they have asked for, cheaper food supplies, and a less energy-intensive lifestyle. How do we take this reality and think about ways to promote healthy lifestyles for healthy people?

A key part of this challenge is that there are fewer successful nutrition interventions for the urban poor. Even interventions that have been used in rural areas have focused on undernutrition, not overnutrition and chronic disease. Therefore, an essential first step is to identify models for healthy lifestyle promotion. Clearly, there is general agreement that this will involve a combination of a healthful diet and physical activity. But what is it we are asking policy makers and implementers to actually do?

It is likely that we will find common elements in interventions that "work". These include being comprehensive. It is unlikely that a single intervention or approach, by itself, will work. Agriculture is a key sector in the solution; but increasingly we see a need to link agriculture to other sectors.

Finally, policy makers, given resource constraints, including lack of money, are interested in exploring the potential of public–private partnerships for promoting healthy lifestyles—healthy people. The potential of public–private partnerships is enormous; we now need some success stories.

Edited by Manfred Kroger, Ph.D., Editor of the Proceedings of the 12th World Congress of Food Science and Technology

Author Kennedy is with the International Life Sciences Institute, One Thomas Circle, Washington, D.C. (E-mail: ekennedy@ilsi.org).

Global Food Companies in the Developing World

Benefactors, Malefactors, or Inevitable Change agents?

James E. Tillotson, PhD, MBA

Global food companies provide many advantages to developing countries, including foreign investment, employment, and both food technology and food safety. At the same time, they have been accused of being malefactors that encourage overconsumption. Our columnist provides his views.

As many American pundits are fussing and fuming over our domestic food industry's role—and their tasty products—in our ever-increasing weight and long-term health, two United Nations bodies, the World Health Organization (WHO) and the Food and Agriculture Organization (FAO), are also questioning the dietary role of these same companies in their global businesses in the developing world.

These international health organizations are questioning the role these food and beverage multinationals serve in the rapidly changing diets in the developing countries. Increasingly, these developing nations' diets are replicating our Western diets with their too ample calories, high-energy-dense/low-nutrient-content foods and beverages, high-fat, high-sugar, and high animal-content foods. WHO's and FAO's staff members are convinced that there exists a strong connection between the observed dietary changes and the business activities of these global food companies. These organizations are attempting to take what they consider to be appropriate remedial action. *What are all the issues?*

Currently, WHO and FAO are attempting to pursue aggressive policies that they believe will stem the duplication of obesity and diet-related chronic degenerative diseases that are becoming common in the industrial nations.[1] One of the underlying issues in this initiative is whether global food companies are acting as saviors, malefactors, or inevitable dietary change agents in the developing world.[2]

Compounding their concern is the fact that many developing nations do not have, and probably will not have

in the future, the necessary resources to deal with the large number of people whose health is compromised by nutrition-related chronic diseases associated with unwise consumption of our Western diet. *A daunting prospect, given the limited medical resources to treat chronic diseases.*

The explosive market growth of food and beverage products in the industrial countries is now occurring in the frontier nations.

These diet and health issues have been brought to center stage internationally by a recent joint report of the WHO/FAO last year—*Diet, Nutrition and The Prevention of Chronic diseases*—which calls for limiting the availability of foods that are high in sugars, fats, and salt; requiring daily physical education for students; and modifying nations' tax policies to promote healthier life styles.[3] As may be expected, this WHO/FAO initiative has become controversial with food and beverage multinationals and their governments, particularly with US interests.[4]

Anyone visiting those nations on the frontier of development can immediately understand their concerns regarding the influence that predominantly American-based global food and beverage companies already have on these nations' diets. *It appears to be significant.*

Our leading American brands of soft drinks, fun foods, and fast foods are successfully marketed in the developing world, using promotional methods similar to those used successfully in the industrial countries. Coca-Cola reports that today it sells more than 70% of its soft drinks in foreign countries, with high hopes for great future growth in the frontier nations.[5] KFC reportedly has more than 1,000 of its fast-food outlets already in China alone, and McDonald's has more than 580 outlets.[6] Unilever, an Anglo-Dutch multinational, currently is estimated to sell more than 25% of the entire world's packaged handheld ice-cream products annually in the world, much of it in the developing world.

As expected, because of the universal nature of people's *liking* for sweetness, fats, and oils, the companies marketing such products are highly successful in selling their tasty products to new hordes of willing developing world consumers. It is only human nature that they might like the same fun foods as much as Americans do.

What happened with the explosive market growth of consumer food and beverage products in the United States after World War II, particularly in the 1970s, 1980s, and 1990s, is now occurring in the rest of the world, including the developing countries. In the United States, this rapid industrialization of our diet has occurred predominantly during the last 50 years, but in the up-and-coming countries, this diet transformation is now often occurring in fast forward during only 1 to 2 decades. Such rapid dietary changes are difficult for any population to assimilate, even under the best of conditions. The WHO'S/FAO'S fear is that the rapidity of these dietary changes can be fatal for nutritionally uninformed people of the frontier nations.

No question about this food trend; food multinationals are currently touting their own great marketing successes in their annual reports, news releases, and management interviews. This is accompanied by disturbing silence on the diet and health implications of their marketing success to uninformed Third-World people.

However, in our laudable health zeal, snap judgments must be avoided. The issues involved are devilishly complex; they aren't solely about nutrition or science. What you see may be only part of what is really involved.

Food Globalization: Striking the Balance Between Benefits and Risks is Difficult

Food globalization involves other key issues, such as tariffs and farm subsidies, that also affect health, human welfare, and economics. These conflicting issues are often unclear and difficult to resolve individually. They require trade-offs between conflicting goals, usually with no win-win solutions. The issue of the multinational food companies in developing nations is far more complex than just good food or bad food dietary choices. It also involves serious social, economic, and political factors that are vitally important for these developing nations.

The Issues Surrounding Food Multinationals Are Gray, Not Black and White

In my opinion, the core dietary and health issue is straight-forward: will these developing nations go from widespread undernutrition or malnutrition to overnutrition that Western-type diets foster? There is strong evidence that this is already occurring in numerous developing countries. Obesity is now becoming a common problem in the developing world.[1] This is a sobering thought, given the potential health threat from nutrition-related noncommunicable diseases, such as hypertension, cardiovascular disease, diabetes, and various other diet-related and obesity-related diseases, which can commonly occur with unwise overconsumption of the aggressively marketed Western-type diet. *To what extent are the multinationals responsible?*

Despite any potentially negative health issues that may arise, we must also recognize that multinational food-oriented companies often can be, and are, *constructive* change agents for developing countries in their efforts to ensure an adequate and safe food supply for their people. Several food multinationals that have operated—in some cases for decades—in these countries are agribusinesses (Cargill), which import and distribute needed basic foodstuffs (grains and oils). Others either import or locally process basic foods of a beneficial nutritional nature (Nestle and Unilever).

Certainly, a strong case can be made on both economic and social grounds for allowing such companies to operate in the developing nations as their food supply industrializes, especially when local firms are, or will be, also producing the same sorts of foods. *The issues surrounding food multinationals are anything but black and white.*

Some multinational food companies are economically beneficial today because these countries attempt to bootstrap their food supplies into ones with greater food hygiene and food security. These companies are performing services, while also serving their own economic interests, which the developing nations' governments cannot or do not presently have the resources or know-how to provide for them. The economic development that results from the presence of multinationals also has the potential for alleviating other types of human suffering through raising incomes.

Global food companies provide needed resources and knowledge not readily available elsewhere for these countries. Thus, the role of multinational companies in these countries is complex, involving conflicting economic, social, and health issues. Their role cannot be simply dismissed as solely beneficial or detrimental but rather as offering a mixture of difficult trade-offs for the governments of these frontier countries that host the food multinationals.

One of the most pressing issues is balancing the important immediate economic benefits such companies offer to a nation's food supply against the potential long-term nutritional problems that the widespread introduction of some food and beverage consumer products might cause for developing countries.

Many of these global food and beverage companies desire to seek new commercial markets for their own economic ends because their domestic markets have become largely saturated.[7] Yet, as they enter these countries, these companies bring with them much needed foreign investments, commerce, employment, technology, business

- Foreign investment
- Increased commerce
- Increased employment
- Better food-processing technology
- Increased commercial knowledge
- Improved safety of food
- Increased food assurance

Figure 1. Advantages of multinational food companies for the developing countries.

- A great deal is known about the economic power of and the manner in which multinational food companies work, grow, and prosper.
- A great deal is also known about the nutritional sciences and what people should eat for good health.
- However, much less is known on how to combine the two fields of knowledge in public health programs for the benefit of the citizens both in the industrial countries and now in the developing countries! (A key research need.)

Figure 2. The public policy health paradox.

knowledge, and improvements in the safety and the quantity of the food supply to these developing countries—all economic and food inputs often desperately needed by those same countries. Ideally, both parties benefit.

The global companies can offer resources and knowledge to their populations that their own governments often cannot offer (Figure 1). All of these factors are significantly economically important and thus have great immediate appeal to their governments.

These attractive economic factors also must be balanced against potentially long-term negative health influences. Today, I believe we face a *public health policy paradox* in the developing nations (in the industrial countries also) in our understanding of how to accomplish this balancing feat between dietary health and economic goals (Figure 2).

Multinationals Are Not the Only Source of the Western-Type Diet

Local companies could produce, and in certain countries, *are* already producing similar products. In India, the locally developed soft drink Thumbs preferred by many is proving to be a strong market competitor to those of the multinational beverage companies (Thumbs was purchased by Coca-Cola), and in the Philippines, the domestically started fast-food chain Jolly Bee far outperforms the international fast-food chains and is now successfully entering business on the US West Coast. Some interpret the issue of the entry of multinationals in developing countries as more about globalization issues than diet and health.

Another needed question is: if it were possible to prevent the multinational food and beverage companies from entering developing nations, would the diets of such countries still become Westernized as incomes rose just because people like to eat that way? The answer is probably yes, based on our experience in the industrialized countries.

The Essential Food Policy Issue Is Rapid Diet Transformation: It Is Already Occurring, but When

The essential food policy issue for countries experiencing rapid diet transformation is no longer whether or when

this will occur but what are the appropriate public policies to pursue in the face of such *commercial food and beverage invasions.*

Acknowledging that multinationals can contribute overall benefits, both economically and nutritionally, developing countries, whose food markets are the target of multinationals, must undertake comprehensive benefit/risk analyses of this business trend. The frontier countries need to differentiate these companies from those marketing products of more questionable benefit to the health and diets of their countries. *Easily said, but how? We haven't been able to do this in the industrial countries yet.*

Bottom Line

International business interests and their respective governments often find that the involvement of these international health organizations can lead to controversy. The present initiative of WHO/FAO to help alleviate global obesity,[4] *Obesity: Preventing and Managing the Global Epidemic,* is being seriously questioned by our government.

A leading reason has been the scientific analysis of the dietary issues and the lack of research-based substantiation for the dietary recommendations of the report. The US government's challenge was put forward in a lengthy letter to the WHO from US Department of Health and Human Service (HHS) signed by William R. Steiger, Special Assistant to the Secretary for International Affairs.[8] Commercial business interests aggressively objected to the report's recommendations and conclusions. Andrew Briscoe, President of the of Sugar Association, noted in a letter to Gro Harlem Brundtland, then WHO director general, that his sugar trade association would, "exercise every avenue available to expose the dubious nature" (the report recommends limiting 10% of consumers' total caloric intake from "added sugars") including, "asking congressional appropriators to challenge funding of the US's $406 million contribution to the WHO."[9]

The HHS letter summarizes in detail numerous comments from various branches of HHS and the US Department of Agriculture concerning the report's science content.[8] The specific scientific issues of this WHO/FAO report are too extensive to treat here; however, I believe that there is no escaping the basic intent of the report that if continued, unwise dietary choices globally, particularly in the developing countries, will have dire health consequences.

Another particularly controversial aspect of the WHO report—and *potentially the most difficult to resolve between interested parties*—is its philosophic approach to future public policy and governmental action in attempting to curb the unwise overconsumption of Western-type diets—high caloric, sugars, animal fat, and salt content foods. The WHO report recommends a highly activist and interventionist government approach to the problem, calling for aggressive use of policy levers, such as taxation of high sugars, fats, and salt content foods; use of public tax incentives; and aggressive physical interventions and goals. *Aside from good intentions, one must ask whether these particular policy levers will work. Where is the proof?*

Beyond the specifics called for in remedies proposed in the WHO report is the basic philosophy concerning the role of government and its citizens in diet and health matters. Traditionally, the relationship in the United States has been that the basic responsibility for diet and health behavior *rests with the individual*, with the government's role being to keep the food supply safe, wholesome, and affordable and advising its citizens on a prudent diet.

The WHO report challenges this American laissez-faire approach. It calls for governments to become more active and more aggressive in attempting to shape the people's daily diets and food-related activities (physical activity), assuming that this overall strategy will be successful (although still largely untested). This could be the core issue in future public policies for diet and health efforts. The scientific issues that the report raises will probably be resolved, but this basic philosophic issue will be much harder to resolve, given the social, economic, and political factors beyond the science involved.

Notes

1. World Health Organization. *Diet, Nutrition and The Prevention of Chronic Diseases*. WHO Technical Report Series 916. Geneva: World Health Organization; 2003.

2. Tillotson JE. Multinational food companies and developing nations' diets. In: *Food Policy Options: Preventing and Controlling Nutrition Related Non-Communicable Diseases*. Washington, DC: World Health Organization and World Bank; 2002:29-47.

3. World Health Organization wants taxes to help alleviate obesity. *Nutr Today.* 2004; 39:4.

4. United States questions global obesity plan: the United States is challenging a strategy by the World Health Organization (WHO) to tackle obesity. BBC News. Available at: http://newsvote.bbc.co.uk. Accessed January 1, 2004

5. Coca-Cola still the world's most valuable brand. *Financial Times*, January 20, 2003, 16.

6. Liu L. KFC fast food to wing its way at last to Tibet & McDonald's plans to open 100 new outlets in China. Available at: http://www.1.chinadaily.com. Accessed January 15, 2004.

7. Tillotson JE. What does the future hold for American food companies? *Nutr Today.* 2002;37:192-194.

8. Letter to J.W. Lee, Director-General, World Health Organization from William R. Steiger, Special Assistant to the Secretary to the Secretary for International Affairs, US Department of Health and Human Services, January 5, 2004. Available at: http://cspinet.org/new/pdf/steigerltr.pdf. Accessed May 7, 2004.

9. Alden E. Buckley N. Sweet deals: 'Big Sugar' fights threats from free trade and a global drive to limit consumption. *Financial Times*, February 27, 2004, 8.

James E. Tillotson, PhD, MBA, is currently Professor of Ford Policy and International Business at Tufts University. Before returning to the academic world, Dr Tillotson worked in industry, holding various research and development positions in the food and chemical sectors. Correspondence: James E. Tillotson, PhD, MBA, PO Box Ten, Cohasset, MA 02025-0100 (e-mail: james.tillotson@tufts.edu).

Contribution of Indigenous Knowledge and Practices in Food Technology to the Attainment of Food Security in Africa

RUTH ONIANG'O, JOSEPH ALLOTEY, SERAH J. MALABA

ABSTRACT: Indigenous knowledge and practices are important aspects of a society's culture and its technology. They include accumulated knowledge, as well as skills and technology of the local people, usually derived from their direct interaction with their local environment. These aspects need due recognition and full understanding and utilization because of the valuable contributions to food security, especially in African communities. Africa's people have traditionally utilized indigenous knowledge, skills and structures, most often locally developed and handed down in the course of centuries. Insufficient attention has been given to this local knowledge within the mainstream food security development and management interventions. However, there is now increasing awareness of the fact that technology includes not only energy sources and tools, but also knowledge and skills, as well as social organizations. It is, therefore, imperative to approach indigenous communities as partners and collaborators in all food security endeavors in order to realize the objective of sustainability. African communities offer a vast array of indigenous knowledge and practices in food technology that are favorable to the food supply, as well as to food quality and food safety and thus directly contribute to food security. As such, indigenous knowledge and practices in food technology that have proved capable of ensuring food security need to be implemented before considering the introduction of external ones if food security is to be realized in Africa. Emphasis of the same should be especially made for foods that are adapted to local conditions thus improving food access, safe food availability, and utilization to meet local and regional needs. This paper seeks to outline the numerous contributions and enormous potentials that indigenous knowledge and practices in food technology have in ensuring food security in Africa.

Introduction

Africa experiences the stark reality of hunger in the midst of plenty. Since the early 1970s, Africa has periodically experienced episodes of drought with famine, civil unrest with food deficits, and structural adjustment programs with food distribution dislocations. Indeed, during these last 3 decades, Africa has prominently featured as a basket case; and food aid has almost become a fixture of the social condition of several African countries [1].

Specifically, between 1990–1992 and 1997–1999, food deprivation has increased in practically all African countries with the exception of a few, such as, Sudan, Chad, Nigeria, and Ghana [2]. Almost one-half of the sub-Saharan African population is food-insecure, and about one-third of the pre-school children are malnourished. More than 4 million preschool children die every year, mostly from nutrition-related illnesses [3].

This state of human condition was never the case in Africa. In 1938 Africa exported cereals; in 1950 Africa was self-sufficient; in 1976 Africa was importing 10 million tons of cereals a year; in 1978, 13 million tons of cereals imported; in 1983, 31 million tons of cereals imported; from 1983–1985 disastrous drought and food shortages were experienced in Africa [4]

The food quantity, food quality, and nutritional insecurity that Africa faces today can be mitigated and sustainably reversed. As food is uniquely part of a people's integral culture, as well as a key socio-cultural survival mechanism, a manifest change can be realized through the appreciation of Africa's indigenous knowledge.

Indigenous knowledge (IK)

Indigenous knowledge is knowledge that is unique to a given culture or society [5]. Communities use IK at the local level as the basis of decision making pertaining to vital activities in which food security is included. As such, IK is the most important and often only asset for many poor, rural societies and its significance increases as other resources disappear or dwindle.

Building on this IK to ensure food security in Africa can be particularly effective as this is an asset that the people of Africa control and certainly one with which they are very familiar. Utilizing IK will help increase the sustainability of food security efforts because the IK integration process provides for mutual learning and adaptation, which in turn contributes to the empowerment of local communities. Building on IK systems will empower local communities in Africa, enabling them to shape their own food security agenda by actively participating in it.

IK in agriculture

Traditional agricultural practices provide valuable lessons to be learned from local farmers who, through their own innovations and experimentation on farms, have perfected tools such as the hoe and the plough, developed seeds and plants through preservation and selection, and designed crop mixtures and rotations leading to improved productivity.

Practices like fallow, mixed farming, and intercropping were contained in the IK systems long before the introduction of the Green Revolution. These practices provide advantages that are now recognized for ensured fertility of soils, control of pests as well as variety of food sources, among others [6].

Classically, in subsistence agriculture, farmers grew and used traditional food crops because the practice was familiar. They understood traditional food plants, selected varieties to meet the needs and constraints of their environment, and trusted seed from their own land races to produce a reliable crop [6].

Many of these traditional plants make an important contribution to crop productivity. Grown as rotation crops between successive main crops, they may have the advantage of reducing the build-up of pests and diseases. When interplanted they may act as an ecological barrier to diseases. By acting as ground cover, traditional food plants help to prevent soil erosion, reduce evaporation and suppress weed growth. Grown as green manure and ploughed in, traditional plants can increase soil organic matter and improve soil structure. In addition, legumes fix atmospheric nitrogen, enriching the soil for the following crop or for nearby plants [7].

It is necessary to understand the knowledge of traditional agriculture. This knowledge should be harnessed to ensure food security. Besides, the farmers who have been involved in the selection and conservation of food plants need to be recognized for their role in the conservation of germplasm used in breeding programmes while being encouraged to continue conservation of such germplasm.

Africa's indigenous knowledge has thrived over the years. So far over 90% of the food production in sub-Saharan Africa is attributed to traditional peasant or low-resource farmers. These farmers rely on age-tried methods that depend on expansion of area under cultivation to achieve about 80% of the annual increases in food and agricultural production. Knowledge of things around us can be put to effective use in satisfying our everyday needs [8]

Africa's indigenous food crops

Africa's traditional food crops are underexploited, yet they have been accepted by communities through habit and tradition and are appropriate as well as desirable food sources. In terms of technology input, subsistence agriculture in African tropics has totally depended on traditional farming methods and low inputs of labor-saving technologies [9].

People are accustomed to traditional food crops, know how to cultivate them and prepare them, and enjoy eating dishes made from them. For example, to see them through the hungry season, rural people grow traditional food plants near their homes. Many of these crops are drought-resistant, can be grown without expensive inputs, and have good storage qualities [7].

Traditional food crops fall into 2 broad categories: those consumed as traditional dietary staples, such as cassava, yam, plantain, sweet potato, millets, and sorghum, and those that serve as ingredients in accompanying relishes and sauces, which include a wide variety of legumes, oilseeds, seeds, and vegetables [7].

Traditional staples

Roots, tubers, bananas, and plantains account for some 40% of total food supplies (in terms of food energy) for about one-half of the population of sub-Saharan Africa, where overall food supplies are at very low levels [7]. The major root and tuber crops grown in Africa include cassava, yam, sweet potatoes, and cocoyams. Cassava and yams are among the principal staple crops in many countries on the west coast of Africa, including Nigeria, Cameroon, Ghana, Benin, Togo, and Cote d' Ivoire [10]. Cassava is grown and consumed extensively in Zaire also. On the other hand, in East Africa and Madagascar, cassava and sweet potatoes are important crops and constitute major staples [11].

Traditional staples are known to be more resilient to domestic climate. Roots and tubers are the major contributors to food security, particularly in years of cereal crop failures. Most countries have grown more roots and tubers to combat famine, hunger, and mitigate drought impact [12]. These crops have low input requirements, which is desirable among poor farmers.

Oil crops

Oil crops are essential components of food security, because of their high energy value and the high protein value of the meals, especially the leguminous crops such as soybeans, groundnuts, beans, and peas. Countries on the coastal fringes of West Africa grow palm oil, coconut palms, cotton crops, and sunflower, which can also provide both oil and meals [12]. The processing of nuts and oil seeds that include groundnuts, sunflower seed, sesame seed, olive oil, and palm oil enables Africa to meet part of its vegetable oil requirements. These should be effectively exploited, as there is great potential.

Fruits and vegetables

Africa is endowed with a large variety of fruits and vegetables. Indigenous vegetables are plants whose fruit, leaves, pods, or roots are consumed as relish and they have originated in Africa or have been cultivated in Africa over a long period of time [13]. They include crops that are wild, semi-wild, or domesticated.

Indigenous fruits and vegetables are noted for meeting the energy and protein requirements of populations. These plants also have the vitamins that provide the necessary nutrients the populace need, especially in the region's harsh environment [14]. Traditional green leafy vegetables are rich sources of vitamin A, C, folic acid, thiamine, vitamin B2, niacin, calcium, phosphorus, iron, and zinc. They contribute significantly as sources of protein. The protein is high in lysine, an amino acid insufficient in diets based on most cereals and root crops [15].

Traditional vegetables are familiar in terms of taste, methods of cultivation, and preparation. They are cheaper to grow, as they require minimal labor and management and very little cultivation. Most, especially *Solanum nigrum* and *Amaranthus*, may be harvested severally as need arises. In addition to the afore-mentioned, traditional vegetables are much more resistant to diseases, nutrient deficiency, and water stress than the exotic vegetables [12].

The post-harvest technology and processing methods employed with these fruits and vegetables are diverse, varying from simple mechanical equipment and sun-drying techniques to highlevel technology. Fruits and vegetables are processed into products such as jams, jelly, fruit preserves sauces, juices, nectars, squashes, wines, vinegar, dried and pickled vegetables, sauces, and flour.

Milk

Traditionally, milk is churned to make butter and sour milk, which are especially popular in southern Sudan and among pastoralists all over Africa [7]. The Somali community adds the aromatic hoary basil (*Ocium americanum*) to milk as a flavoring agent. To most pastoralists, fresh blood obtained by darting the jugular vein of an animal (usually a cow) is an important food, especially in times of food shortage. Blood is normally mixed with milk and stirred vigorously into a uniform brown mixture [7].

The nomadic tribes of Sudan make a type of cheese called *kush*, which is eaten with sorghum porridge. The camel herders put milk into a bag that is fastened to the saddle of a camel, and the milk (*gariss*) is allowed to ferment.

In undocumented instances, a cheese-like product, *wagashi*, is prepared from cow milk. Preheated fresh cow milk is coagulated with juice from the leaves of *Calotropis pro-* cera and put in a basket to drain before it is formed into round balls. *Wagashi* is then fried and is consumed in the place of meat with gravy. In addition, among some communities in Kenya, fresh or sour milk is added to African leafy vegetables to enhance taste and vitamin C bioavailability, boost protein intake, and allow long shelf-life as is the case when sour milk is added.

Meat

Traditionally, in Africa meat from cattle, sheep, goats, and pigs is used unprocessed. However, generally, meat is preserved by drying, smoking, or salting [7].

In Ethiopia and northern Kenya, among the pastoralists, meat that is cut into long pieces (*quanta*) is smeared with powdered pepper, salted, and dried by hanging it above the fireplace for 5-7 days [14]. Among the Somali, dried meat (*otkac* or *nyirnyir*) is prepared from camel meat (*hilib* gel). Strips of sun-dried meat are cut into small pieces that are fried (usually in oil with garlic and *iliki*) and immersed in camel ghee (*subag*). *Nyirnyir* can last for several months and is usually eaten with tea, honey, chapatti, and *enjera* [7]. Quails, which are wild birds that resemble small chickens, are also considered a delicacy in East Africa [7].

Insects

Despite their vast numbers, insects represent an underexploited resource in many parts of Africa. About 500 insect species are known to be consumed worldwide [16]. Insects eaten include green bugs (*Hemiptera*), termites (*Isoptera*), various caterpillars, crickets, and grasshoppers. These insects are widely used in the rural areas of the north-eastern part of southern Africa and may make an important contribution to the protein and fat of the local diet [18].

During the rainy season, the flying reproductive forms of termites emerge from termite mounds. These are trapped, dried or roasted, and eaten or preserved in honey, or used as a snack and occasionally in sauces. A variety of caterpillars are also harvested and eaten [7].

Fish

Fresh water and sea fish constitute an important source of protein in the diets of many African populations, although consumption of fish by low-income groups has not progressed significantly [10]. However, the poor in Kenya's Nyanza Province mostly eat minnows/whitebait (*omena*) because they are cheap and plentiful.

Processing methods used to prevent fish spoilage include salting, drying, smoking, pickling, fermentation, canning, and freezing. Fish is salted by rubbing dry salt into the flesh, or by immersing the fish in brine while natural air-drying of fish uses the combined action of the sun and wind, whereby fish to be dried are put on a raised platform or racks. Fish-smoking in traditional smoking kilns is a widely employed practice in Africa. In most tropical developing fisheries, however, smoking is used not only to impart desirable flavors, but also, and more more importantly, to accelerate the drying process. Smoked products in tropical countries have storage properties, which enable them to be marketed without the use of sophisticated refrigeration systems. Smoking is often combined with a period of sun-drying and/or preliminary brining. The temperature of smoking varies from place to place depending on consumer preference and the type of smoking kiln or oven available for use. Most products, however, are hot-smoked, with the smoking temperature cooking the product.

Documented practices of IK

The traditional technologies for processing perishable foods or for the pre-treatment of originally unpalatable foods such as cassava have created stable foodstuffs that are not only edible but also nutritious and enjoyable. A few of these have been documented as successes of IK:

Sun-drying of fruits, vegetables, and edible insects

In Zimbabwe, older women sun-dry food in 2 main ways. One method is to immerse fresh vegetables in salted boiling water for a few minutes and then to dry them in the sun for about 3 days. These are then stored in a safe, dry place. This method is also used to dry edible insects such as white ants, termites, and caterpillars [18].

Another method is to directly spread the food in the sun. The food is first salted if there is danger of decaying during the drying process, as is the case with mushrooms and tomatoes. Food drying is an important activity for women as they bear responsibility for food preparation, even during the dry seasons [11].

Palm wine making technique

Kongo-lori farmers from the South of Congo-Brazzaville in the Democratic Republic of Congo have maintained palm wine making techniques from the 16th century [18]. These techniques have enabled them to produce much appreciated wines. The palm wine is produced locally and sold in cities and rural areas in cans containing 10 liters. The wines are appreciated and in demand by local populations, and constitute an important market in the capital city of Brazzaville [18].

Palm produce

Extraction of kernels from the palm fruit involves crude processing, which in the case of oil extraction implies boiling or fermenting the fruit, depulping by pounding or mashing with the feet in a container, and squeezing the depulped fiber by hand to obtain the oil. The palm nuts obtained during the process are dried, usually for a month and later cracked between stones or with the aid of stones to extract the palm kernel. The fruit of the oil palm is useful not only for its oil which is used in the production of edible oil, fats, and soups, but also for its press cake which is used to supplement animal feeds [19]. Palm kernel press cake is cheaper than other feeds and contains a favorable calcium-to-phosphorus ratio and for this reason it makes a valuable contribution to protein build-up of a compound animal feed.

Salt production

The Moundang and Toupouri people, who live in the Mayo-Kebbi district in the nothern province of Cameroon, have developed a technology to make salt from dry stalks of sorghum plants [18]. The stalks are gathered and burned, and the remaining ash is sieved and boiled in water until it becomes whitish. After cooling, the liquid is left to coagulate. At that stage, it is ready for consumption as a substitute for salt. This salt, called *garlaka*, is produced by women who are said to earn up to 250.000 cfa francs per year in selling it [18].

Small-scale community vegetable and fruit gardens

Community and family vegetable and fruit gardens play a significant role in increasing small-scale production of micronutrient-rich foods. The home garden is the most direct means of supplying families with most of the nonstaple foods they need year-round [11]. Growing of vegetables as intercrops, that is, mixing vegetables among trees or staple crops, eases land constraints [11].

Solar drying techniques

In many African countries, women use solar drying techniques for fruits, vegetables, mushrooms, and tubers. Drying is also often used to preserve meat, fish, and roots. Cassava and bananas are also preserved by fermentation followed by drying, as is the case with *gari* and the preservation of *ensete*, a banana-type plant [11]. Reducing the moisture in food prevents growth of the microorganisms that cause foods to decay. At the same time, enzymatic and biochemical activities are practically stopped or reduced at very low levels. Foods preserved by drying can be kept at ambient temperatures for long periods and provide nutrients when fresh produce is not available [7].

Storage of roots, tubers, bananas, and plantains

Fresh roots and tubers are highly perishable and cannot be stored for long periods. Cassava, for example, has to be processed within 48 hours of harvesting to avoid deterioration of quality [10]. Fresh cassava, therefore, is best left unharvested until needed. As they exhibit a period of dormancy, curing extends the storage life of sweet potatoes and yams. As an alternative, yams, cocoyams, and cassava may be stored in underground pits after harvesting [7]. In some instances, root crops such as cassava can be grown as a food reserve, left in the ground for up to 2 y and used as the main source of energy during lean times [7].

In West Africa, yams are stored for 6 to 9 mo but if they begin to run low, fruits, seeds, and nuts that grow in abundance at different times of the year usually supplement them [7].

Processing of these crops is generally conducted on a small scale in the rural areas. The unit operations in regard to the processing of roots and tubers include peeling, cleaning, grating, fermentation, de-watering, heating or roasting, milling, and sieving.

Cereal and legume grains

For these crops, the drying stage is all-important to reduce attack and damage by insects and fungi. Threshing or shelling follows after which the grains are then stored in traditional grain cribs [11]. These operations reduce the fiber content and may extend the storage life of the foodstuff. In humid areas, the cribs are ventilated to facilitate both the drying and storing of grain. Some cribs are raised on a platform and a fire is lit under the structure for insect control by natural fumigation. Smoke enters through holes into the platform and escapes through the roof. Thus, the wall must have few openings, so the structure will function as a chimney. Before consumption, many grains are ground, pounded or milled, and sieved to provide various grades of flour.

Cowpeas and other grain legumes may be treated as follows: soaked in water and boiled; roasted; milled into flour; fried in oil; steamed. These processing techniques are employed to eliminate anti-nutritive factors and improve the overall value of the food. Cowpeas are eaten in the form of oily seeds, green pods, green seeds, and tender green leaves. Dry cowpeas are processed into a wide variety of dishes, ranging from soups to snacks. The utilization of cowpeas is limited to perishable traditional food products that are processed as and when needed by traditional methods. The utilization of cereals such as maize follows a variety of processing procedures including soaking, dehulling, grinding, roasting, boiling, fermentation, and germination. Cereals and legumes can be utilized in making various combinations of food mixtures and such mixtures can be used as a basis for infant and children foods, which are equally good as imported foods.

Hunting and foraging

Hunting and gathering are food procuring methods which do not involve production in the sense of investing in the environment and waiting to harvest whatever has withstood the constraints of drought and pests. Hunting communities had hunting guilds and closely monitored traditional practices of group hunting ensured that the environmental resources were well maintained. Great care was taken not to kill unnecessarily. Very young or pregnant animals were not killed and this ensured constant renewal of edible wild animals. Hunting was not performed carelessly or too frequently [11].

Fermentation

Fermentation is widely employed in Africa to preserve vegetables, meat, fish, roots, and tubers, and also to manufacture alcoholic beverages [10].

Fermentation is a traditional way of preserving vegetable surpluses which, when used, enhances the overall flavor of the meal. The technique provides a suitable environment for lactic acid bacteria to grow, thus imparting an acid flavor to the vegetable.

On the other hand, roots and tubers are mainly fermented to add variety to the diet. Cassava and sweet potatoes are the most commonly fermented ones. Two well known types of fermented cassava are *gari* and *fufu*, products of natural fermentation.

Fermentation also provides a low-cost way of preserving meat and fish, as well as adding variety to the diet. There is a wide range of fermented meat products from Sudan that include fermented strips of fatty meat, and similar products made from intestines and offal [10]. Fermented meat products, by comparison with fermented products of other food commodities, are less widely reported.

Alcoholic beverages constitute the largest category of fermented products in Africa [10]. Most of these beverages are processed from fruits. Banana beer, a popular drink in Uganda, Rwanda, Burundi, Gabon, and Cameroon, is made by allowing banana juice to ferment. Palm wine and coconut wine are made through the same process. The examples cited are few of many hundreds of foods produced by fermentation processes that are consumed all over Africa.

Qorasum

Qorasum is a woman's indigenous food preservation technology that is used for storage and preservation of food, particularly milk. It can extend the life of fresh milk in the desert for up to 24 h. Yogurt and sour milk can be preserved for up to 2 mo. *Qorasum* is also used to impart flavor and aroma to foods and it also ensures the proper maintenance of vessels of food storage. It plays a critical role in the preservation of milk, fat, and meat products, all of which are vital in pastoralist nutrition.

A dried taproot of the maderra tree (*Cordia sinensis*) is split into several pieces, 6 inches long and 1 inch thick. The ends of these faggots are placed in the fire until they ignite. They are then pulled out of the flame, and the flame blown out and are popped one by one into the open container. The lid is closed and the vessel shaken for several minutes, taking the lid off intermittently to release pressure before repeating the process again. After several rounds of shaking and releasing pressure, the pieces are poured out and placed carefully back into the fire to begin the process from fire to shaking to fire again, 3 to 5 times. When the last piece has come out of the container, a sort of rag pounded from bark and soaked in fat is used to clean the inside of the container after which it is ready to store milk. Variations of this process are repeated all day long by pastoral women all over Kenya. The Gabra call this technology *qorasum* [20].

In most parts of Africa, the bulk of the agricultural produce is processed using simple indigenous knowledge and practices. Women use these techniques predominantly and they provide income and employment. For example, cereals and legumes play an important role in the diet of the majority of the population and in issues related to their production, storage, marketing, and processing are very important. The outcome expected is to provide Africans with adequate and nutritionally balanced diets at affordable prices, both now and in the future. The cereals grown in Ghana can be used in many various foods using indigenous knowledge and technology. Some of the foods from maize include fried cakes (*akpiti*), steamed or baked dumplings (*abolo*), boiled maize porridge, cornwine (*nmeda*), or just corn on the cob. Legumes are used in various forms in Ghana, such as boiled beans, cakes (*akara*), bean stews, bambara porridge (*aboboe*), roasted or boiled groundnuts, groundnut paste, groundnut soup, and groundnut cakes. Certainly in Africa indigenous knowledge and practices cannot be overlooked.

Conclusion

The indigenous knowledge and practices outlined by this paper present an opportune basis on which food security interventions in Africa may be built as they have the potential, if exploited, to ensure food security in Africa. The challenge, however, is that systematic documentation of IK has not been done. This is largely attributed to its oral and rural nature that makes it largely invisible. Moreover, the introduction of "western food" constitutes a threat to indigenous food crops that have survived the test of time. This, therefore, calls for research and adequate citation of IK before its appreciation and incorporation in the existing interventions. As IK is dynamic and based on innovation, adaptation, and experimentation, it presents an existent possibility for improving food and livelihood security in Africa. In addition, greater recognition must be accorded IK if its potential is to be exploited.

Notes

1. http://www.ift.org/iftsa/featurearchive/africa.html

2. COASAD/UN-HABITAT. 2002. Food Security in English-Speaking African Countries. Report of the Proceedings of a Joint COASAD/UN-HABITAT Workshop on Food Security for Parliamentarians from English-Speaking African Countries, Gigiri, Nairobi, Kenya, 30 April–2 May, 2002.

3. Toward Eradicating Hunger and Poverty. Life and Work of Per Pinstrup-Andersen and Anwar Dil. 2003.

4. African Farmer Nr1 p. 5–12. 1988.

5. Grenier L. 1998. Working with indigenous knowledge: A Guide for Researchers. IDRC, Ottawa.

6. Kabuye CHS. 2002. Indigenous knowledge for biodiversity and development. Proceedings of the national workshop on indigenous knowledge, National Museums of Kenya.

7. Katz HS, Weaver WW. 2003. Encyclopedia of food culture Volume 1.

8. Okigbo BN. 1987. Overview of technical crisis in subsistence Agriculture. In: Amoako-Atta B, editor. Subsistence Agriculture in Africa: Problems and Prospects. UNESCO/ABN. p 57–92.

9. Nyiira ZM. 1987. The status of subsistence Agriculture in Africa. In: Amoako- Atta B, editor. Subsistence Agriculture in Africa: Problems and Prospects. UNESCO/ABN. p 28–56.

10. RANDFORUM/UNDP. 1995. Sourcebook on African Food Technology. Production and Processing Technologies for Commercialization.

11. FAO. 1997. Agriculture, food and nutrition for Africa. A Resource Book for Teachers of Agriculture.

12. Scott GJ, Rosegrant MW, Ringler C. Roots and Tubers for 21st Century: Trends, Projections and Policy Options. 2020 Vision for Food, Agriculture and the Environment. Discussion Paper 31.

13. Schippers RR. 2000. African Indigenous Vegetables. An Overview of the Cultivated Species Natural Resources Institute, Univ. of Greenwich.

14. UNDRO. 1988. Peasant Survival Strategies in Ethiopia. *UNDRO News* No.8 (July/August).

15. JICA-Dept. of Social Services (K). Traditional vegetables in Kenya. User's Manual.

16. Groombridge B. 1992. Global biodiversity. Status of the Earth's living resources.

17. Crafford JE. 1991. Insects as a source of food, folklore and folk taxonomy in Venda. Proceedings of the Eighth Entomological Congress.

18. http://www.worldbank.org/afr/ikdb/ik_results.cfm

19. Kuku FO, Umeh EO. 1979. The effect of five lipolytic mold species on the protein content of palm kernels. Tech Rep Nr 7. Rep Nig Stored Prod Res Inst 1976–77. p. 75–7.

20. Ramos Elorduy de Conconi J. 1996. Insect consumption as a means of national identity. In: Jain SK. Ethnobiology in Human Welfare. p 9–12.

Edited by Manfred Kroger, Ph.D., Editor of the Proceedings of the 12th World Congress of Food Science and Technology

Author **Oniang'o** is Professor of Food Science and Nutrition, Editor-in-Chief, African Journal of Food, Agriculture, Nutrition and Development (AJFAND) and Chair, Kenya Union of Food Science and Technology (KUFoST). Author **Allotey** is Associate Professor, Post Harvest Food Systems, Univ. of Botswana, Private Bag 0022, Gaborone, Botswana. Author **Malaba** is Student Intern, African Institute of Knowledge Management. Authors **Oniang'o and Malaba** are with the Rural Outreach Program: Josem Trust Place, Ground Floor, Bunyala Road, Upper Hill, P.O. Box 29 Nairobi, KENYA. Direct inquiries to author Oniang'o (E-mail: oniango@iconnect.co.ke).

Helping Solve Hunger in America

ROBERT FORNEY

June 5, 2003, is National Hunger Awareness Day, designed to help raise awareness that hunger exists in America.

Americans know that there is hunger in underdeveloped and war-torn countries around the globe, but they may not realize that there is hunger in the United States as well. In a focus group conducted in 2001 by the Advertising Council, the nation's leading producer of public-service advertisements, one participant said, "If there were hungry children in America, we'd know about it. The press would report on it, and we would feed those children and solve the problem."

> **Besides arranging for food donations, food industry professionals can help solve hunger in a number of ways.**

The fact is that there is hunger in America. Last year, the U.S. Dept. of Agriculture reported that 33 million Americans were food insecure—they didn't know if they would be able to buy the food they needed to feed their families. The Census Bureau announced last fall that, for the first time in a decade, the number of people living in poverty had grown and real earnings had dropped for the average American worker. America's Second Harvest, the nation's largest hunger-relief charity, reported in its landmark study, *Hunger in America: 2001,* that it feeds 23 million hungry Americans, 9 million of whom are children.

Amid the stress of the war and terrorism, American families are facing a more personal sort of stress. More than two million jobs have been lost in the past two years. Discouraged workers have exhausted their savings and emptied their retirement accounts. They have been forced to ask family and friends for aid. And when all other resources are gone, they turn to hunger-relief charities to feed their families. These new demands at food pantries, soup kitchens, and shelters have strained the hunger-relief system.

America's Second Harvest, a national umbrella organization dedicated to creating a hunger-free America, sup-

ports a network of more than 200 regional food banks and food-rescue organizations that collect, sort, warehouse, and then distribute the food and personal-care products that are donated by companies across the country. More than 50,000 hunger relief charities in the U.S. depend on organizations affiliated with America's Second Harvest for the food they give directly to hungry Americans. These include national organizations such as Catholic Charities, the Red Cross, Meals on Wheels, and the Salvation Army, as well as community and faith based organizations created to help people on a local level.

America's Second Harvest makes it easy for food manufacturers, producers, retailers, and restaurants to donate food they cannot sell. Sometimes, food ends up in packages that are mislabeled, dented, or underfilled; or products are the wrong shape, size, or color; or there may just be more on hand than can be sold before its shelf life expires; or excess product may be left over from events. Companies willing to donate such products can call 800-771-2303, and America's Second Harvest will make arrangements to accept delivery of the donation, make arrangements for shipping to a regional affiliate that can distribute the food, and provide receipts acknowledging the donation.

Last year, America's Second Harvest network distributed 1.8 billion lb of food—including 17,820 lb of product donated by the exhibitors at the close of the Institute of Food Technologists' 2002 Annual Meeting & Food Expo® last June. Every day, America's Second Harvest works with industry professionals to capture potential waste and distribute it through its network of hunger-relief agencies that serve every county in America.

Besides arranging for food donations, food industry professionals can help solve hunger in a number of ways. They can make sure that meetings are held at facilities that participate in "food rescue" programs so that leftovers are distributed to hunger-relief organizations; volunteer at a soup kitchen; teach parents how to prepare healthy meals; add a panel about how food industry people can help end hunger at professional conferences; or invite a local, regional, or national hunger-relief professional to be a guest speaker at meetings.

Food industry professionals can also share their expertise with America's Second Harvest by volunteering to serve on Corporate Inspection Teams that visit regional food banks and share their knowledge of logistics, marketing, storage, and other food-specific business matters. They can also volunteer to participate in two national programs that particularly depend on the support of foodservice professionals. The first program, Community Kitchen, is a technical training course that provides unemployed people with foodservice skills. These programs rely to a great extent on professionals who are willing to volunteer to share their knowledge with students. The second program is called Kids Cafe. There are more than 600 of these after-school feeding programs at America's Second Harvest affiliates across the country. They, too, seek professional volunteers to help plan new kitchens at local Kids Cafes, provide menu or foodservice assistance, and teach participating children about nutrition and food preparation.

More information about these and other ways to help solve hunger in America can be obtained by contacting America's Second Harvest at 312-263-2303 or visiting www.secondharvest.org.

Robert Forney is President and CEO, America's Second Harvest, 35 E. Wacker Dr., Suite 2000, Chicago, IL 60601.

Assessment of Allergenic Potential of Genetically Modified Foods: An Agenda for Future Research

Speakers and participants in the workshop "Assessment of the Allergenic Potential of Genetically Modified Foods" met in breakout groups to discuss a number of issues including needs for future research. These groups agreed that research should progress quickly in the area of hazard identification and that a need exists for more basic research to understand the mechanisms underlying food allergy. A list of research needs was developed. *Key words:* biotechnology, food allergy, genetically modified food, hazard identification, research needs. *Environ Health Perspect* 111: 1140–1141 (2003). doi:10.1289/ehp.5815 available via *http:/dx.doi.org/*[Online 19 December 2002].

MaryJane K. Selgrade,[1] Ian Kimber,[2] Lynn Goldman,[3] and Dori R. Germolec[4]

Potential benefits that may be derived from biotechnologies involving genetically modified organisms could be enormous. Potential risks of allergenicity possibly associated with their use will likely be manageable, provided appropriate information is available to decision makers. At the end of the workshop "Assessment of the Allergenic Potential of Genetically Modified Foods," speakers and participants met in small groups to discuss information needs. Five groups considered the following key issues: *a*) use of human clinical data, *b*) animal models to assess food allergy, *c*) biomarkers of exposure and effect, *d*) sensitive populations, *e*) dose-response assessment, and *f*) postmarket surveillance. The groups were asked to consider two general questions: On the basis of current information, what can we do to assess the potential allergenicity of genetically modified food, and what do we need to know to improve this process, i.e., what are the most critical research needs? The first question is the topic discussed in another article in this mini-monograph (Germolec et al. 2003). The research needs are the topic of this article. Just as research provided the tools to generate genetically modified food, it can also provide the tools needed for effective safety evaluation and risk assessment/management.

Regulatory problems are rarely stated in scientific terms. The problem in this case is we wish to avoid inadvertently introducing an allergenic protein into the food supply. One task for this workshop was to translate this problem into research needs. Because there is a sense of urgency to develop tools for hazard identification, much of the conversation revolved around the short-term research required to develop test methods for this purpose. This discussion focused largely on the potential allergens and how to distinguish these from other proteins. However, it was recognized also that more long-term (basic) research is needed on the characteristics of food allergens, allergic disease, and the mechanisms underlying susceptibility to food allergy. This discussion considered more broadly the factors leading to allergic sensitization, including the nature of the allergen, and how genetics, life stage, and other environmental influences might affect susceptibility.

Hazard Identification: Immediate Needs

Research needed to improve hazard identification fell into three categories:

development of animal models, identification and characterization of food allergens, and establishment of well-defined clinical serum banks. All were deemed important to improve the Food and Agriculture Organization of the United Nations/World Health Organization (FAO/WHO) decision tree (FAO/WHO 2001) or to replace it with a better approach. Also discussed was the need to improve human skin test technology for incorporation in a decision tree. Animal models are needed that could be used not only for hazard identification purposes but also to determine relative potency, to derive sensitization and elicitation thresholds, and to define the conditions under which tolerance (failure to develop an allergic response to potential food allergens) is induced. Identification, characterization, purification, and banking of food allergens (and nonallergens) are needed for two reasons: to provide positive (and negative) controls for animal and serum bank tests and for use in defining the characteristics that confer on food proteins the ability to induce allergic sensitization, that is, to establish structure-activity relationships. Serum from clinically well-defined allergic individuals needs to be banked for use in

Table 1. Summary of research needs.

Hazard identification
  Development, evaluation, and validation of animal models
  Establishment of clinically well-defined banks of human serum containing antibodies to allergens
  Improved human skin test technology
  Identification, purification, and banking of both known protein allergens and proteins believed not to be allergenic
  A systemic approach to recording adverse events (case studies)
  Definition of relative potency and thresholds for sensitization and the elicitation of allergic reactions
  Development, refinement, standardization, and validation of test protocols
Basic mechanistic
  Development of animal models of allergic disease
  Studies of the qualitative and quantitative relationships between antigen-specific IgE and overt disease
  Investigation of the influence of route, duration, timing, and nature of exposure on the development of sensitization
  Studies of the factors that contribute to susceptibility to food allergy
  Investigation of the mechanisms underlying food allergy
  Investigation of potential windows of vulnerability during development
  Identification of unique situations that cause children or other individuals to be at greater risk
  Epidemiology to establish the incidence of food allergy and whether it is changing
  Studies of the potential role of non–IgE-mediated reactions in food allergy

screening proteins of unknown allergenicity. Development of proteomic approaches to screen potential allergens (specific IgE on a chip) was also suggested as a research need. Characterization of allergens and development of serum banks require a systematic process for recording adverse events and obtaining informed consent for use of serum obtained in epidemiologic and experimental studies. Once developed, all tests for hazard identification will require standardization and validation—no small task. These research needs are summarized in Table 1.

Basic Mechanistic Research

Appropriate animal models (not necessarily the same as those used for hazard identification) and human clinical and epidemiologic studies are needed to assess the correlation between antigen-specific IgE and clinical disease and to investigate the influence of the route, duration, and nature of exposure on the development of sensitization. An important research need is to investigate the mechanisms underlying food allergy, including the development of and failure to develop oral tolerance, and identification of possible windows of vulnerability during immune development (including in utero and during lactation) or unique exposure conditions that might place children at greater risk. The mechanisms underly-

ing the development of tolerance to ingested antigens, whether by passive (anergy) or active (suppressor cells) processes, are poorly understood and may be crucial to understanding what makes a protein allergenic and what makes an individual susceptible. The contributions of in utero exposure, gut immaturity, and exposure via breast milk to children's risk of sensitization also need to be determined. Studies (possibly using tansgenic mice) are needed to assess the heritable factors that contribute to susceptibility to food allergy. Epidemiology is needed to determine whether the incidence of food allergy in the industrialized world, like the incidence of other types of allergic disease, is increasing.

The natural history of non–IgE-mediated food allergies (although somewhat beyond the scope of this current workshop) was also considered an important long-term research need. Questions were raised as to whether certain foods were associated with this type of allergy and whether IgE is a reasonable surrogate marker in this instance or if other biomarkers would be more appropriate. The context in which food is presented, including the matrix, concomitant infections, and other sources of gut inflammation, also deserves further attention with respect to both IgE- and non–IgE-mediated food allergies. Basic mechanistic research needs are summarized in Table 1.

Recommendations

In summary, there was consensus that research should progress quickly in the area of hazard identification to improve or replace the FAO/WHO decision tree. Support was particularly strong for the development, standardization, and validation of appropriate animal model(s) for this purpose. It was also generally agreed that there is much we do not know about the development of food allergies, and that more basic research in this area would help us to control the risks more effectively and efficiently. More work is needed than any one funding organization is likely to be able to support. Therefore, it is recommended that there be significant coordination between these organizations and an integrated approach to tackling this problem. Open and free exchange of information as it becomes available is needed to facilitate these research endeavors

[1]National Health and Environmental Effects Research Laboratory, Office of Research and Development, U.S. Environmental Protection Agency, Research Triangle Park, North Carolina, USA; [2]Syngenta Central Toxicology Laboratory, Alderley Park, Macclesfield, Cheshire, United Kingdom; [3]Johns Hopkins University Bloomberg School of Public Health, Baltimore, Maryland, USA; [4]Laboratory of Molecular Toxicology, National Institute of Environmental Health Sciences, Research Triangle Park, North Carolina, USA

References

FAO/WHO. 2001. Evaluation of Allergenicity of Genetically Modified Foods. Report of a Joint FAO/WHO Expert Consultation of Allergenicity of Foods Derived from Biotechnology, 22–25 January 2001, Rome, Italy. Available: http://www.fao.org/es/esn/gm/allergygm.pdf [accessed 11 September 2002)

Germolec DR, Kimber J, Goldman L, Selgrade MJK. 2003. Key issues for the assessment of the allergenic potential of genetically modified foods: breakout group reports. Environ Health Perspect 111: 1131–1139.

From *Environmental Health Perspectives*, June 2003. Printed by the National Institute of Environmental Health Sciences.

Glossary

Absorption   The process by which digestive products pass from the gastrointestinal tract into the blood.

Acid/base balance   The relationship between acidity and alkalinity in the body fluids.

Amino acids   The structural units that make up proteins.

Amylase   An enzyme that breaks down starches; a component of saliva.

Amylopectin   A component of starch, consisting of many glucose units joined in branching patterns.

Amylose   A component of starch, consisting of many glucose units joined in a straight chain, without branching.

Anabolism   The synthesis of new materials for cellular growth, maintenance, or repair in the body.

Anemia   A deficiency of oxygen-carrying material in the blood.

Anorexia nervosa   A disorder in which a person refuses food and loses weight to the point of emaciation and even death.

Antioxidant   A substance that prevents or delays the breakdown of other substances by oxygen; often added to food to retard deterioration and rancidity.

Arachidonic acid   An essential polyunsaturated fatty acid.

Arteriosclerosis   Condition characterized by a thickening and hardening of the walls of the arteries and a resultant loss of elasticity.

Ascorbic acid   Vitamin C.

Atherosclerosis   A type of arteriosclerosis in which lipids, especially cholesterol, accumulate in the arteries and obstruct blood flow.

Avidin   A substance in raw egg white that acts as an antagonist of biotin, one of the B vitamins.

Basal metabolic rate (BMR)   The rate at which the body uses energy for maintaining involuntary functions such as cellular activity, respiration, and heartbeat when at rest.

Basic four   The food plan outlining the milk, meat, fruits and vegetables, and breads and cereals needed in the daily diet to provide the necessary nutrients.

Beriberi   A disease resulting from inadequate thiamin in the diet.

Beta-carotene   Yellow pigment that is converted to vitamin A in the body.

Biotin   One of the B vitamins.

Bomb calorimeter   An instrument that oxidizes food samples to measure their energy content.

Buffer   A substance that can neutralize both acids and bases to minimize change in the pH of a solution.

Calorie   The energy required to raise the temperature of one gram of water one degree Celsius.

Carbohydrate   An organic compound composed of carbon, hydrogen, and oxygen in a ratio of 1:2:1.

Carcinogen   A cancer-causing substance.

Catabolism   The breakdown of complex substances into simpler ones.

Celiac disease   A syndrome resulting from intestinal sensitivity to gluten, a protein substance of wheat flour especially and of other grains.

Cellulose   An indigestible polysaccharide made of many glucose molecules.

Cheilosis   Cracks at the corners of the mouth, due primarily to a deficiency of riboflavin in the diet.

Cholesterol   A fat-like substance found only in animal products; important in many body functions but also implicated in heart disease.

Choline   A substance that prevents the development of a fatty liver; frequently considered one of the B-complex vitamins.

Chylomicron   A very small emulsified lipoprotein that transports fat in the blood.

Cobalamin   One of the B vitamins (B_{12}).

Coenzyme   A component of an enzyme system that facilitates the working of the enzyme.

Collagen   Principal protein of connective tissue.

Colostrum   The yellowish fluid that precedes breast milk, produced in the first few days of lactation.

Cretinism   The physical and mental retardation of a child resulting from severe iodine or thyroid deficiency in the mother during pregnancy.

Dehydration   Excessive loss of water from the body.

Dextrin   Any of various small soluble polysaccharides found in the leaves of starch-forming plants and in the human alimentary canal as a product of starch digestion.

Diabetes (diabetes mellitus)   A metabolic disorder characterized by excess blood sugar and urine sugar.

Digestion   The breakdown of ingested foods into particles of a size and chemical composition that can be absorbed by the body.

Diglyceride   A lipid containing glycerol and two fatty acids.

Disaccharide   A sugar made up of two chemically combined monosaccharides, or simple sugars.

Diuretics   Substances that stimulate urination.

Diverticulosis   A condition in which the wall of the large intestine weakens and balloons out, forming pouches where fecal matter can be entrapped.

Edema   The presence of an abnormally high amount of fluid in the tissues.

Emulsifier   A substance that promotes the mixing of foods, such as oil and water in a salad dressing.

Enrichment   The addition of nutrients to foods, often to restore what has been lost in processing.

Enzyme   A protein that speeds up chemical reactions in the cell.

Epidemiology   The study of the factors that contribute to the occurrence of a disease in a population.

Essential amino acid   Any of the nine amino acids that the human body cannot manufacture and that must be supplied by the diet, as they are necessary for growth and maintenance.

Essential fatty acid   A fatty acid that the human body cannot manufacture and that must be supplied by the diet, as it is necessary for growth and maintenance.

Fat   An organic compound whose molecules contain glycerol and fatty acids; fat insulates the body, protects organs, carries fat-soluble vitamins, is a constituent of cell membranes, and makes food taste good.

Fatty acid   A simple lipid—containing only carbon, hydrogen, and oxygen—that is a constituent of fat.

Ferritin   A substance in which iron, in combination with protein, is stored in the liver, spleen, and bone marrow.

Fiber   Indigestible carbohydrate found primarily in plant foods; high fiber intake is useful in regulating bowel movements, and may lower the incidence of certain types of cancer and other diseases.

Glossary

Flavoprotein   Protein containing riboflavin.

Folic acid (folacin)   One of the B vitamins.

Fortification   The addition of nutrients to foods to enhance their nutritional values.

Fructose   A six-carbon monosaccharide found in many fruits as well as honey and plant saps; one of two monosaccharides forming sucrose, or table sugar.

Galactose   A six-carbon monosaccharide, one of the two that make up lactose, or milk sugar.

Gallstones   An abnormal formation of gravel or stones, composed of cholesterol and bile salts and sometimes bile pigments, in the gallbladder; they result when substances that normally dissolve in bile precipitate out.

Gastritis   Inflammation of the stomach.

Glucagon   A hormone produced by the pancreas that works to increase blood glucose concentration.

Glucose   A six-carbon monosaccharide found in sucrose, honey, and many fruits and vegetables; the major carbohydrate found in the body.

Glucose tolerance factor (GTF)   A hormone-like substance containing chromium, niacin, and protein that helps the body to use glucose.

Glyceride   A simple lipid composed of fatty acids and glycerol.

Glycogen   The storage form of carbohydrates in the body; composed of glucose molecules.

Goiter   Enlargement of the thyroid gland as a result of iodine deficiency.

Goitrogens   Substances that induce goiter, often by interfering with the body's utilization of iodine.

Heme   A complex iron–containing compound that is a component of hemoglobin.

Hemicellulose   Any of various indigestible plant polysaccharides.

Hemochromatosis   A disorder of iron metabolism.

Hemoglobin   The iron-containing protein in red blood cells that carries oxygen to the tissues.

High-density lipoprotein (HDL)   A lipoprotein that acts as a cholesterol carrier in the blood; referred to as "good" cholesterol because relatively high levels of it appear to protect against atherosclerosis.

Hormones   Compounds secreted by the endocrine glands that influence the functioning of various organs.

Humectants   Substances added to foods to help them maintain moistness.

Hydrogenation   The chemical process by which hydrogen is added to unsaturated fatty acids, which saturates them and converts them from a liquid to a solid form.

Hydrolyze   To split a chemical compound into smaller molecules by adding water.

Hydroxyapatite   The hard mineral portion (the major constituent) of bone, composed of calcium and phosphate.

Hypercalcemia   A high level of calcium in the blood.

Hyperglycemia   A high level of "sugar" (glucose) in the blood.

Hypocalcemia   A low level of calcium in the blood.

Hypoglycemia   A low level of "sugar" (glucose) in the blood.

Incomplete protein   A protein lacking or deficient in one or more of the essential amino acids.

Inorganic   Describes a substance not containing carbon.

Insensible loss   Fluid loss, through the skin and from the lungs, that an individual is unaware of.

Insulin   A hormone produced by the pancreas that regulates the body's use of glucose.

Intrinsic factor   A protein produced by the stomach that makes absorption of B_{12} possible; lack of this protein results in pernicious anemia.

Joule   A unit of energy preferred by some professionals instead of the heat energy measurements of the calorie system for calculating food energy; sometimes referred to as "kilojoule."

Keratinization   Formation of a protein called keratin, which, in vitamin A deficiency, occurs instead of mucus formation; leads to a drying and hardening of epithelial tissue.

Ketogenic   Describes substances that can be converted to ketone bodies during metabolism, such as fatty acids and some amino acids.

Ketone bodies   The three chemicals—acetone, acetoacetic acid, and betahydroxybutyrie—that are normally involved in lipid metabolism and accumulate in blood and urine in abnormal amounts in conditions of impaired metabolism (such as diabetes).

Ketosis   A condition resulting when fats are the major source of energy and are incompletely oxidized, causing ketone bodies to build up in the bloodstream.

Kilocalorie   One thousand calories, or the energy required to raise the temperature of one kilogram of water one degree Celsius; the preferred unit of measurement for food energy.

Kilojoule   *See* Joule.

Kwashiorkor   A form of malnutrition resulting from a diet severely deficient in protein but high in carbohydrates.

Lactase   A digestive enzyme produced by the small intestine that breaks down lactose.

Lactation   Milk production/secretion.

Lacto-ovo-vegetarian   A person who does not eat meat, poultry, or fish but does eat milk products and eggs.

Lactose   A disaccharide composed of glucose and galactose and found in milk.

Lactose intolerance   The inability to digest lactose due to a lack of the enzyme lactase in the intestine.

Lacto-vegetarian   A person who does not eat meat, poultry, fish, or eggs but does drink milk and eat milk products.

Laxatives   Food or drugs that stimulate bowel movements.

Lignins   Certain forms of indigestible carbohydrate in plant foods.

Linoleic acid   An essential polyunsaturated fatty acid.

Lipase   An enzyme that digests fats.

Lipid   Any of various substances in the body or in food that are insoluble in water; a fat or fat-like substance.

Lipoprotein   Compound composed of a lipid (fat) and a protein that transports both in the bloodstream.

Low-density lipoprotein (LDL)   A lipoprotein that acts as a cholesterol carrier in the blood; referred to as "bad" cholesterol because relatively high levels of it appear to enhance atherosclerosis.

Macrocytic anemia   A form of anemia characterized by the presence of abnormally large blood cells.

Macroelements (also macronutrient elements)   Those elements present in the body in amounts exceeding 0.005 percent of body weight and required in the diet in amounts exceeding 100 mg/day; include sodium, potassium, calcium, and phosphorus.

Malnutrition   A poor state of health resulting from a lack, excess, or imbalance of the nutrients needed by the body.

Maltose   A disaccharide whose units are each composed of two glucose molecules, produced by the digestion of starch.

Marasmus   Condition resulting from a deficiency of calories and nearly all essential nutrients.

Melanin   A dark pigment in the skin, hair, and eyes.

Metabolism   The sum of all chemical reactions that take place within the body.

Microelements (also micronutrient elements; trace elements)   Those elements present in the body in amounts under 0.005 percent of body weight and required in the diet in amounts under 100 mg/day.

Monoglyceride   A lipid containing glycerol and only one fatty acid.

Monosaccharide   A single sugar molecule, the simplest form of carbohydrate; examples are glucose, fructose, and galactose.

Monosodium glutamate (MSG)   An amino acid used in flavoring foods, which causes allergic reactions in some people.

Monounsaturated fatty acid   A fatty acid containing one double bond.

Mutagen   A mutation-causing agent.

Negative nitrogen balance   Nitrogen output exceeds nitrogen intake.

Niacin (nicotinic acid)   One of the B vitamins.

Nitrogen equilibrium (zero nitrogen balance)   Nitrogen output equals nitrogen intake.

Nonessential amino acid   Any of the 13 amino acids that the body can manufacture in adequate amounts, but which are nonetheless required in the diet in an amount relative to the amount of essential amino acids.

Nutrients   Nourishing substances in food that can be digested, absorbed, and metabolized by the body; needed for growth, maintenance, and reproduction.

Nutrition   (1) The sum of the processes by which an organism obtains, assimilates, and utilizes food. (2) The scientific study of these processes.

Obesity   Condition of being 30 percent above one's ideal body weight.

Oleic acid   A monounsaturated fatty acid.

Organic foods   Those foods, especially fruits and vegetables, grown without the use of pesticides, synthetic fertilizers, etc.

Osmosis   Passage of a solvent through a semipermeable membrane from an area of higher concentration to an area of lower concentration until the concentration is equal on both sides of the membrane.

Osteomalacia   Condition in which a loss of bone mineral leads to a softening of the bones; adult counterpart of rickets.

Osteoporosis   Disorder in which the bones degenerate due to a loss of bone mineral, producing porosity and fragility; normally found in older women.

Overweight   Body weight exceeding an accepted norm by 10 or 15 percent.

Ovo-vegetarian   A person who does not eat meat, poultry, fish, milk, or milk products but does eat eggs.

Oxidation   The process by which a substrate takes up oxygen or loses hydrogen; the loss of electrons.

Palmitic acid   A saturated fatty acid.

Pantothenic acid   One of the B vitamins.

Pellagra   Niacin deficiency syndrome, characterized by dementia, diarrhea, and dermatitis.

Pepsin   A protein-digesting enzyme produced by the stomach.

Peptic ulcer   An open sore or erosion in the lining of the digestive tract, especially in the stomach and duodenum.

Peptide   A compound composed of amino acids that are joined together.

Peristalsis   Motions of the digestive tract that propel food through the tract.

Pernicious anemia   One form of anemia caused by an inability to absorb vitamin B_{12}, owing to the absence of intrinsic factor.

pH   A measure of the acidity of a solution, based on a scale from 0 to 14: a pH of 7 is neutral; greater than 7 is alkaline; less than 7 is acidic.

Phenylketonuria (PKU)   A genetic disease in which phenylalanine, an essential amino acid, is not properly metabolized, thus accumulating in the blood and causing early brain damage.

Phospholipid   A fat containing phosphorus, glycerol, two fatty acids, and any of several other chemical substances.

Polypeptide   A molecular chain of amino acids.

Polysaccharide   A carbohydrate containing many monosaccharide subunits.

Polyunsaturated fatty acids   A fatty acid in which two or more carbon atoms have formed double bonds, with each holding only one hydrogen atom.

Positive nitrogen balance   Condition in which nitrogen intake exceeds nitrogen output in the body.

Protein   Any of the organic compounds composed of amino acids and containing nitrogen; found in the cells of all living organisms.

Provitamins   Precursors of vitamins that can be converted to vitamins in the body (e.g., beta-carotene, from which the body can make vitamin A).

Pyridoxine   One of the B vitamins (B_6).

Pull date   Date after which food should no longer be sold but still may be edible for several days.

Recommended Daily Allowances (RDAs)   Standards for daily intake of specific nutrients established by the Food and Nutrition Board of the National Academy of Sciences; they are the levels thought to be adequate to maintain the good health of most people.

Rhodopsin   The visual pigment in the retinal rods of the eyes which allows one to see at night; its formation requires vitamin A.

Riboflavin   One of the B vitamins (B_2).

Ribosome   The cellular structure in which protein synthesis occurs.

Rickets   The vitamin D deficiency disease in children characterized by bone softening and deformities.

Saliva   Fluid produced in the mouth that helps food digestion.

Salmonella   A bacterium that can cause food poisoning.

Saturated fatty acid   A fatty acid in which carbon is joined with four other atoms; i.e., all carbon atoms are bound to the maximum possible number of hydrogen atoms.

Scurvy   A disease characterized by bleeding gums, pain in joints, lethargy, and other problems; caused by a deficiency of vitamin C (ascorbic acid).

Standard of identity   A list of specifications for the manufacture of certain foods that stipulates their required contents.

Starch   A polysaccharide composed of glucose molecules; the major form in which energy is stored in plants.

Stearic acid   A saturated fatty acid.

Sucrose   A disaccharide composed of glucose and fructose, often called "table sugar."

Sulfites   Agents used as preservatives in foods to eliminate bacteria, preserve freshness, prevent browning, and increase storage life; can cause acute asthma attacks, and even death, in people who are sensitive to them.

Teratogen   An agent with the potential of causing birth defects.

Thiamin   One of the B vitamins (B_1).

Thyroxine   Hormone containing iodine that is secreted by the thyroid gland.

Toxemia   A complication of pregnancy characterized by high blood pressure, edema, vomiting, presence of protein in the urine, and other symptoms.

Glossary

Transferrin A protein compound, the form in which iron is transported in the blood.

Triglyceride A lipid containing glycerol and three fatty acids.

Trypsin A digestive enzyme, produced in the pancreas, that breaks down protein.

Underweight Body weight below an accepted norm by more than 10 percent.

United States Recommended Daily Allowance (USRDA) The highest level of recommended intakes for population groups (except pregnant and lactating women); derived from the RDAs and used in food labeling.

Urea The main nitrogenous component of urine, resulting from the breakdown of amino acids.

Uremia A disease in which urea accumulates in the blood.

Vegan A person who eats nothing derived from an animal; the strictest type of vegetarian.

Vitamin Organic substance required by the body in small amounts to perform numerous functions.

Vitamin B complex All known water-soluble vitamins except C; includes thiamin (B_1), riboflavin (B_2), pyridoxine (B_6), niacin, folic acid, cobalamin (B_{12}), pantothenic acid, and biotin.

Xerophthalmia A disease of the eye resulting from vitamin A deficiency.

Index

Index

Gussow, Joan, 29–30

H

HDL (high-density-lipoprotein) cholesterol, 8, 9–11, 37, 40
health claims, 107–108
Health Eating Index (HEI), 13
heart disease, 54; fat and, 8, 9, 10–11, 12, 13; fiber and, 55; omega-3 fatty acids and, 34–35; vitamins and, 120–121
HIV, 149
hormone replacement therapy (HRT), soy and, 112, 113
hunger, in U.S., 178–179
hydrogenation, 37

I

immune system, vitamins and, 121–122
indigenous knowledge (IK), contributions of, in food security in Africa, 172–177
Indonesia, 165
inflammatory conditions, omega-3 fatty acids and, 35
inflammatory proteins, 101
insects, food security in Africa and, 174
insulin resistance, 44
inulin, 55–56
iodine, 121; deficiency, 154, 156
iron, 5, 75–76, 121, 152–153, 156
Islam, food choices and, 22
isoflavones, soy and, 112–115. *See also* phytoestrogens

J

Jenny Craig, low-carbohydrate diets and, 18
Judaism, dietary laws of, 22
Jungle, The (Sinclair), 133

K

kava, 145
kidnetic.com, 74, 94
Kids Cafe, 179
Kraft Foods, 73; low-carbohydrate diets and, 16, 17

L

LDL (low-density-lipoprotein) cholesterol, 9–10, 40
leptin, 100, 101
life expectancy, caloric restriction and, 116–118
lignins, 58
liposuction, 102
low-carbohydrate diets, 40–42; influence of, on marketplace, 14–18
low-fat diets, prostate cancer and, 67–68
lutein: age-related macular degeneration and, 51–52, 53-54; cataracts and, 49, 50
lycopene, 110; prostate cancer and, 68–69

M

magnesium, 121

malaria, among malnourished children, 151
malnutrition, 149, 150–151
manganese, 121
marketing, by global food companies, 27, 88–91, 168–169
measles, among malnourished children, 151
meat, 3, 12, 86; food security in Africa and, 174; organic, 137; prostate cancer and, 67
Mega Country Health Promotional Network, of WHO, 165–167
menopausal symptoms, soy and, 113–114
mercury, fish and, 35–36, 134, 142, 143
metabolic syndrome, 44
micronutrient deficiencies, 152–158
milk, 3; food security in Africa and, 174
monoculture, food sustainability and, 30
monounsaturated fats, 8–9, 10, 37, 38

N

nutrigenomics, 19–21, 63–65
nuts, 12, 41, 52

O

oatmeal, 74, 76
oats, 56
obesity, 11; human ancestral history and, 85–87; marketing by food companies and, 88–91; social change and, 95–99
oil crops, food security in Africa and, 173–174
oils, 3; vegetable, 38
omega-3 fatty acids, 12, 34–36
orange-juice manufacturers, low-carbohydrate diets and, 16
organic farming, 136–137
organic foods, food safety and, 133–134
osteoporosis, 12; vitamins and, 122
overweight: age-related macular degeneration and, 52; cataracts and, 50; human ancestral history and, 85–87; Mega Country Health Promotional Network and, 165–167

P

Paleolithic Prescription, The (Eaton), 44
palm fruit, 175
personalized nutrition, 19–21, 63–65
pesticides, 133, 134, 137
phosphorous, 121
physical activity, 6; obesity and, 95–99
phytoestrogens, 58
polydextrose, 58
polyunsaturated fat, 8–9, 10, 37, 38, 54
potassium, 7, 12, 121
potato industry, low-carbohydrate diets and, 16
potatoes, monoculture and, 30
poultry, 3, 12
probiotics, 75
prostate cancer, 66–69; fat and, 11, 66–67; soy and, 69, 112–113
publishing industry, low-carbohydrate diets and, 17–18
Pure Foods, 14
pyrrolizidine alkaloids, 145

Q

qorasum, 176–177
Quaker Oats, 74

R

red wine, 63
religion, mindful eating and, 22–24
renal disease, omega-3 fatty acid and, 35
resistant starch, 57–58
rice, 56
Russet potatoes, monoculture and, 30

S

salmon, 141, 142
Saltzman, Brad, 14
Sara Lee, 16–17
saturated fat, 8, 13, 37
school nutritional programs, adolescents and, 77–81
seafood, 3
secoisolariciresinol diglucoside (SDG), 58
selenium, 121, 122; prostate cancer and, 68
sight: age-related macular degeneration and, 50–52, 53–54; cataracts and, 48–50
Sinclair, Upton, 133
skin aging, vitamins and, 120
social change, obesity prevention and, 95–99
sodium, 7
soft drink consumption, 2
soy, 64, 112–115; prostate cancer and, 68, 112–113
spirituality, mindful eating and, 22–24
St. John's wort, 110
starch, resistant, 57–58
structure/function claims, 112
sugar, 3, 86, 87
sun-drying, food security in Africa and, 175
supplementation, micronutrient deficiency and, 157
supplements. *See* dietary supplements
sweeteners, 3
Syndrome X, 44

T

tea, diabetes and, 71. *See also* green tea
This Organic Life: Confessions of a Suburban Homesteader (Gussow), 29
tomatoes: lycopene-enhanced, prostate cancer and, 68–69
trans fat, 11, 13, 37–39
turmeric, 64, 65
type 2 diabetes, 11–12; omega-3 fatty acids and, 35. *See also* diabetes

U

ulcerative colitis, omega-3 fatty acid and, 35
Unilever, 16
United States Department of Agriculture (USDA), 107; food guide pyramid and, 4, 5, 7, 8–13
U.S. Pharmacopoeia (USP), 111
usnic acid, 145

Test Your Knowledge Form

We encourage you to photocopy and use this page as a tool to assess how the articles in *Annual Editions* expand on the information in your textbook. By reflecting on the articles you will gain enhanced text information. You can also access this useful form on a product's book support Web site at *http://www.dushkin.com/online/*.

NAME: DATE:

TITLE AND NUMBER OF ARTICLE:

BRIEFLY STATE THE MAIN IDEA OF THIS ARTICLE:

LIST THREE IMPORTANT FACTS THAT THE AUTHOR USES TO SUPPORT THE MAIN IDEA:

WHAT INFORMATION OR IDEAS DISCUSSED IN THIS ARTICLE ARE ALSO DISCUSSED IN YOUR TEXTBOOK OR OTHER READINGS THAT YOU HAVE DONE? LIST THE TEXTBOOK CHAPTERS AND PAGE NUMBERS:

LIST ANY EXAMPLES OF BIAS OR FAULTY REASONING THAT YOU FOUND IN THE ARTICLE:

LIST ANY NEW TERMS/CONCEPTS THAT WERE DISCUSSED IN THE ARTICLE, AND WRITE A SHORT DEFINITION:

We Want Your Advice

ANNUAL EDITIONS revisions depend on two major opinion sources: one is our Advisory Board, listed in the front of this volume, which works with us in scanning the thousands of articles published in the public press each year; the other is you—the person actually using the book. Please help us and the users of the next edition by completing the prepaid article rating form on this page and returning it to us. Thank you for your help!

ANNUAL EDITIONS: Nutrition 05/06

ARTICLE RATING FORM

Here is an opportunity for you to have direct input into the next revision of this volume.
We would like you to rate each of the articles listed below, using the following scale:

1. **Excellent: should definitely be retained**
2. **Above average: should probably be retained**
3. **Below average: should probably be deleted**
4. **Poor: should definitely be deleted**

Your ratings will play a vital part in the next revision.
Please mail this prepaid form to us as soon as possible.
Thanks for your help!

RATING	ARTICLE	RATING	ARTICLE
	1. The Changing American Diet: A Report Card		32. Are Your Supplements Safe?
	2. Dietary Guidelines for Americans 2005: Executive Summary		33. Tainted Food
			34. Certified Organic
	3. Rebuilding the Food Pyramid		35. Send in the Clones
	4. The Low-Carb Frenzy: The Force That is Reshaping the Food Industry and Our Bodies		36. Hooked on Fish? There Might Be Some Catches
			37. Ensuring the Safety of Dietary Supplements
	5. Getting Personal with Nutrition		38. Hunger and Mortality
	6. Food, Spirituality, Mindful Eating		39. The Scourge of "Hidden Hunger": Global Dimensions of Micronutrient Deficiencies
	7. Who's Filling Your Grocery Bag?		
	8. Moving Towards Healthful Sustainable Diets		40. Undernurishment, Poverty and Development
	9. Omega-3 Choices: Fish or Flax?		41. Confronting the Causes of Malnutrition: The Hidden Challenge of Micronutrient Deficiencies
	10. Revealing Trans Fats		
	11. Going Beyond Atkins		42. Food Security, Overweight, and Agricultural Research—A View From 2003
	12. Good Carbs, Bad Carbs		
	13. Eye Wise: Seeing Into the Future		43. Global Food Companies in the Developing World—Benefactors, Malefactors or Inevitable Change Agent?
	14. Feast For Your Eyes: Nutrients That May Help Save Your Sight		
	15. Fortifying with Fiber		44. Contribution of Indigenous Knowledge and Practices in Food Technology to the Attainment of Food Security in Africa
	16. Diet and Genes		
	17. Prostate Cancer: More Questions than Answers		
	18. Coffee, Spices, Wine: New Dietary Ammo Against Diabetes?		45. Helping Solve Hunger in America
			46. Assessment of Allergenic Potential of Genetically Modified Foods: An Agenda for Future Research
	19. Meeting Children's Nutritional Needs		
	20. The Role of the School Nutrition Environment for Promoting the Health of Young Adolescents		
	21. How We Grew So Big		
	22. Pandemic Obesity: What is the Solution?		
	23. A Call to Action: Seeking Answers to Childhood Weight Issues		
	24. Social Change and Obesity Prevention: Where Do We Begin?		
	25. Fat: More Than Just a Lump of Lard		
	26. Q & A on Functional Foods		
	27. Herbal Lottery		
	28. The Latest Scoop on Soy		
	29. How Low Can You Go?: Cutting Calories to Extend Life?		
	30. Multiple Choices: The Right Vitamins For You		
	31. Food-Friendly Bugs Do The Body Good		

(Continued on next page)

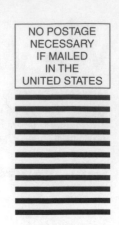

BUSINESS REPLY MAIL
FIRST CLASS MAIL PERMIT NO. 551 DUBUQUE IA

POSTAGE WILL BE PAID BY ADDRESEE

McGraw-Hill/Dushkin
2460 KERPER BLVD
DUBUQUE, IA 52001-9902

NO POSTAGE
NECESSARY
IF MAILED
IN THE
UNITED STATES

ABOUT YOU

Name   Date

Are you a teacher? ☐   A student? ☐
Your school's name

Department

Address   City   State   Zip

School telephone #

YOUR COMMENTS ARE IMPORTANT TO US!

Please fill in the following information:
For which course did you use this book?

Did you use a text with this ANNUAL EDITION? ☐ yes ☐ no
What was the title of the text?

What are your general reactions to the *Annual Editions* concept?

Have you read any pertinent articles recently that you think should be included in the next edition? Explain.

Are there any articles that you feel should be replaced in the next edition? Why?

Are there any World Wide Web sites that you feel should be included in the next edition? Please annotate.

May we contact you for editorial input? ☐ yes ☐ no
May we quote your comments? ☐ yes ☐ no